MULTIDRUG RESISTANCE-
ASSOCIATED PROTEINS

Vehicle   **Genipin**

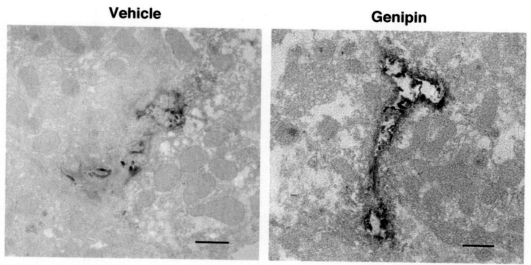

Figure 15. Immunohistochemical localizations of Mrp2 in the SDR livers (electron-microscopic view). Liver sections were prepared from rat livers 30 minutes after intravenous administration of vehicle or genipin. The Mrp2 protein was localized mostly in canalicular microvilli in vehicle-treated livers, whereas the localization was predominant in both microvilli and canalicular membrane in genipin-treated livers. Bars, 1.0 μm.

Vehicle   **Genipin**

Mrp2

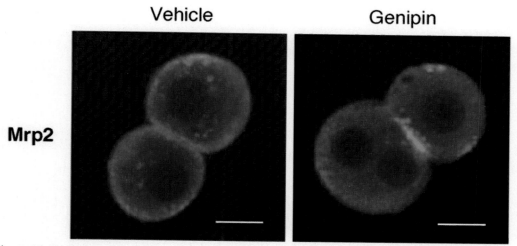

Figure 16. Redistribution of Mrp2 to apical domain in hepatocyte couplets. Hepatocyte couplets were cultured for 1 hour in the presence or absence of 100 μM genipin. The cells were fixed and labeled with a pAb raised against rat Mrp2 followed by a secondary fluorescently labeled Ab. Images were taken from representative couplets by confocal laser microscopy. Optical sections taken from the middle part are shown. Bars, 10 μm.

The redistribution of Mrp2 in genipin-treated livers is most likely due to an increased reinsertion of Mrp2 into the canalicular membrane or to a decreased retrieval into the subapical compartment, assuming that the endocytosis/exocytosis equilibrium is shifted toward the canalicular membrane. The increased Mrp2 density in the canalicular membrane of genipin-treated livers is strongly supported by the results of immunohistochemical Mrp2 localizations in genipin-treated livers. Since only the short-term effects of genipin treatment on livers were investigated in this study, it seems reasonable to assume that changes in the membrane density of Mrp2 protein during this short period of time would mainly be observed at the site of first contact of carrier protein-transporting vesicles with their target membrane, as discussed previously [62]. Fusion of vesicles with the apical membrane of hepatocytes is assumed to occur mainly along the circumference, and early alterations in the membrane density of Mrp2 should occur at this site.

Although the mechanism by which genipin enhances the redistribution of Mrp2 protein into bile canaliculi remains to be clarified, we may exclude several possibilities of mechanistic factors as follows: First, genipin 1-O-□-D-glucuronide, the main metabolite of genipin [59], was detected in the bile of SDRs but not in that of EHBRs, the observation suggesting that genipin is secreted into the bile via Mrp2 in glucuronide forms. Unconjugated genipin and GSH-conjugated genipin are detected only in small amounts, if any, in SDRs. However, the rapid redistribution of Mrp2 protein into the bile canaliculi induced by genipin could not be explained by the idea that genipin 1-O-□-D-glucuronide is a mere Mrp2 substrate, because it has been reported that the intravenous administration of Mrp2 substrates does not enhance Mrp2 function in perfused rat liver [63-65]. Second, cAMP regulates transport activity at the canalicular membrane by stimulating exocytosis and/or fusion of vesicles containing Mrp2 [66]. However, we did not find any significant increase in the hepatic cAMP concentrations after genipin treatment in rats. Third, UDC was suggested to stimulate biliary secretion, due in part to stimulation of the insertion of Mrp2 protein into the canalicular membrane via Ca^{2+}- and □-protein kinase C (PKC)-dependent mechanisms [62]. However, the immunoblot analysis of the PKC isozymes did not reveal any significant induction of the translocation of the PKC isozymes to a particulate membrane fraction, a key step for the activation of PKC.

Effects of oral administration of ICKT, geniposide and genipin on Mrp2-mediated choleretic activity in SDRs were investigated. ICKT (2 g/kg/day), geniposide (150 mg/kg/day) or genipin (100 mg/kg/day) was orally administered for 7 days, and the choleretic activity was assessed by measuring basal bile flow, rate of biliary secretion of GSH and hepatic GSH concentration. ICKT, geniposide or genipin treatment all resulted in significant increases in the basal bile flow and rate of biliary secretion of GSH to similar degrees (Table 1). Moreover, significant increases in hepatic GSH concentrations were observed in ICKT-, geniposide- and genipin-treated groups. The potent enhancement of bilirubin secretion and bile formation of genipin and geniposide as well as ICKT may explain the well-known beneficial effect of ICKT on jaundice and cholestasis, at least partly. The confirmation of the effect of ICKT and its ingredients on human MRP2 in the experimental study using chimeric mice having humanized liver and in the clinical study in patients with biliary drainage for obstructive jaundice is now in progress .

**Table 1. Comparison of the Choleretic Activities of ICKT, Geniposide,
and Genipin *in Vivo***

Group	Bile						Liver		
	Bile flow (μL/min/100g•B.W.)			GSH secretion rate (nmol/min/100g•B.W.)			GSH concentration (μmol/g•liver)		
H_2O	5.4	±	0.2	12.6	±	0.9	5.5	±	0.1
ICKT (2 g/kg)	7.4	±	$0.3^{\ddagger}$	25.1	±	$1.4^{\ddagger}$	7.1	±	$0.1^{\ddagger}$
Geniposide (150 mg/kg)	6.8	±	$0.3^{\dagger}$	23.3	±	$1.4^{\ddagger}$	6.8	±	$0.2^{\ddagger}$
Genipin (100 mg/kg)	7.6	±	$0.4^{\ddagger}$	27.5	±	$2.9^{\ddagger}$	6.9	±	$0.3^{\ddagger}$

Rats were orally administered with ICKT, geniposide or genipin for 1 week. Bile was collected over a 30 minute period to estimate the choleretic activity and GSH secretion rate. Blood was collected from an abdominal artery and then livers were removed. The GSH levels of bile and liver were determined using a GSH assay kit.

Each value represents the mean ± SEM (n = 10).

$^{\dagger}P<0.05$, $^{\ddagger}P<0.01$: significantly different from the vehicle-treated group.

6,7-DIMETHYLESCURETIN
(SCOPARONE OR 6,7-DIMETHOXYCOUMARIN)

The mechanism of action of 6,7-dimethylescuretin, a major ingredient of *Artamisia Capirallis* Spica, has been elucidated in the recent studies by Huang et al concerning Yin Zhi Huang [5], a Chinese herbal drug closely related to ICKT. Yin Zhi Huang contains extracts from four different plants: *Artemisia capillaris*, *Gardenia jasminoides* Ellis, *Rheum officinale* Baillon, and *Scutellaria baicalensis* Georgi. Three of four constituent herbs are common to those of ICKT. Yin Zhi Huang, the decoction of *Artemisia Capillaris*, and 6,7-dimethylescuretin accelerated the clearance of exogenously injected bilirubin. The effect of the agents has been suggested to be mediated by the constitutive androstane receptor (CAR, NR1I3), a key regulator of bilirubin clearance in the liver, because the effect was completely abrogated in CAR KO mice (Figure 10). In primary hepatocytes from both wild type mice and mice expressing only human CAR, 6,7-dimethylescuretin activated CAR and accelerated bilirubin clearance in vivo accompanied with the increase in transcription of various components involved in bilirubin metabolic pathways; a sinusoidal organic anion transporter (OATP2), carrier protein Ligandin (Glutathione S transferase A1 and/or A2), conjugation enzyme UDP-glucuronosyltransferase 1A1 (UGT1A1), and MRP2. While the possible stimulatory effect on CAR by ICKT has not been investigated directly, the well-known contribution of 6,7-dimethylescuretin to the beneficial effect of ICKT suggests the drug has a similar action.

CAPILLARISIN AND OTHER CHORELETIC COMPOUNDS

Capillarisin has been isolated from *Artemisia Capillaris* as a choleretic agent more potent than 6,7-dimethylesculetin [67]. However, the content of capillarisin in Inchin-ko-to is rather small [68-71] therefore whether capillarisin contributes to the choleretic effect of Inchin-ko-to is still undetermined [72]. The detailed mechanism by which capillarisin exerts choleretic effect is also to be clarified in the future. However, in an *in vitro* experiment, capillarisin has been observed to markedly induce Mrp1, a basolateral membrane efflux transporter for GSH-conjugates. Effects of this ingredient on expression levels of other Mrp family members are being investigated in our laboratories. Other choleretic compounds such as p-hydrocyacetophenone, capillartemisin A, B and B1, artepillin A and C, scopoletin, isoscopoletin and capillene from *Artemisia capillaris* [73,74] has been preliminarily reported but further investigation has not been performed.

CLINICAL STUDIES

Unfortunately, although no well-controlled, clinical human studies have been conducted, some case studies has been reported. Many of the literature reporting the beneficial effects of ICKT for various types of hepatobiliary diseases has been written in Japanese. It is likely that some of the beneficial effects of ICKT may be related to the stimulation of MRP2 expression and function (choleresis) and cytoprotection in the liver of patients. Onji et al [75] has reported that combined use of ursodeoxycholate and ICKT in patients with primary biliary cirrhosis resulted in clinical and biochemical improvement including a decrease of bilirubin in all patients. Kobayashi et al [76] has reported the beneficial effect of ICKT in postoperative biliary artesia patients. Postoperative biliary artesia patients with elevated ALT and gamma-glutamyl transpeptidase ((γ-GTP) but normal serum total bilirubin levels (T-Bil) has been treated with ICKT for 2 years. All patients had been receiving ursodeoxycholate for at least 1 year without improvement before ICKT treatment. All subjects tolerated the drugs well and completed the study without difficulty. The liver function parameters of AST, ALT, γ-GTP, total bile acid (TBA), and T-Bil as markers of liver failure, and those of hyaluronic acid (HA), prolylhydroxylase, procollagen type III, type IV collagen as markers of liver fibrosis were measured before and after treatment. The percentage of subjects who improved (as defined by > 25% decrease in the parameter for each patient) after the treatment was 72% for ALT, γ-GTP, TBA and 67% for HA, respectively. The mean values of all serum markers significantly decreased after ICKT treatment. Another paper [77] evaluated the efficacy of ICKT on the treatment of liver fibrosis in patients with biliary artesia without jaundice reported that most patients showed significant decrease in AST, ALT and γ-GTP after 1 to 3 year ICKT treatment. Arai et al [78] reports a case of severe acute hepatitis with unknown etiology treated with ICKT. The patients having grade I hepatic encephalopathy, liver atrophy and massive ascites was treated with transfusion of fresh frozen plasma (FFP) and glucagon-insulin therapy to improve liver failure and lacturose and kanamycin to prevent encephalopathy. The values of AST and ALT decreased after these treatment, however, that of prothrombin time remained unimproved and that of T-Bil continued to increase. Additional treatment with glyccyrrhizin, ursodeoxycholate and ICKT showed no apparent beneficial effect. However, after stopping kanamycin treatment, the values of T-Bil and prothrombin time began to improve. An abdominal CT study at 3 months showed that the liver had increased in size. These studies of course have not established the efficacy and safety of ICKT in the treatment of hepatobiliary diseases. However, they encourage further extensive research which may open the road to the development of new pharmacotherapeutic strategies aimed at a wide variety of the diseases.

CONCLUSIONS

A series of our studies and other reports on the expression of plasma membrane transporters in patients with cholestatic liver diseases have provided valuable information on the crucial role of specific transporters such as MRP2 and BSEP in the pathogenesis of cholestasis. They conclude that the transcription and immunohistochemical expression levels of MRP2 may be altered in the livers of cholestatic patients, and that both the decreased mRNA levels and the diminished canalicular membrane localization may be associated with the impairment of bile formation and secretion.

ICKT, one of Kampo medicines, has been approved as an ethical drug and is used for the treatment of liver diseases in Japan by physicians who have been educated in Western medicine. Recent experimental studies concerning the effects and the mechanism of action of the drug and its ingredients have addressed the possibility of development of new pharmacotherapeutic strategies aimed at a wide variety of liver diseases. A choleretic effect of the administration of ICKT and its ingredients may be due to a "bile acid-independent" mechanism through a selective stimulation of exocytosis and insertion of Mrp2 in the bile canaliculi (redistribution), thus resulting in potent Mrp2-mediated bile formation and secretion in rats. The confirmation of the effect of ICKT on human MRP2 in the experimental study using chimeric mice having humanized liver and in the clinical study in patients with biliary drainage for obstructive cholestasis is now in progress. Moreover, it becomes evident that ICKT potentiates the expression of Mrp3 and Mrp4, inducible transporters for organic anion transporters, in livers of experimental animals. The mechanism induced by the drug for the stimulatory effect on Mrp2-mediated transport appears to be different from that induced by ursodeoxycholate, the established therapeutic drug for cholestasis, thus indicating the possibility of development of new pharmacotherapeutic strategies aimed at stimulation and restoration of defective Mrp2 expression and function in various types of cholestatic liver diseases, many of which are currently untreatable.

REFERENCES

[1]   Yamamura, Y. *Preface*. In: Recent Advances in the Pharmacology of Kampo (Japanese Herbal) Medicines, International Congress Series 854. E. Hosoya and Y. Yamamura (Eds). *Excerpta Medica 1988*, 3.

[2]   Aburada M, Sasaki H, Harada M. Pharmacological studies of gardeniae fructus. II. Contribution of the constituent crude drugs to choleretic activity of Inchin-ko-to in rats. *Yakugaku Zasshi* 1976;96:147-153 [English abstract].

[3]   Yamamoto M, Ogawa K, Morita M, Fukuda K, Komatsu Y. The herbal medicine Inchin-ko-to inhibits liver cell apoptosis induced by transforming growth factor beta 1. *Hepatology* 1996;23:52-59.

[4]   Yamamoto M, Miura N, Ohtake N, Amagaya S, Ishige A, Sasaki H, Komatsu Y, Fukuda K, Ito T, Terasawa K. Genipin, a metabolite derived from the herbal medicine Inchin-ko-to, and suppression of fas-induced lethal liver apoptosis in mice. *Gastroenterology* 2000;118:380-389.

[5]   Huang, W., J. Zhang, and D.D. Moore. A traditional herbal medicine enhances bilirubin clearance by activating the nuclear receptor CAR. *J Clin Invest* 2004, 113: 137-43.

[6]   Yamasaki M, Masae A, Arai I, Huang XX, Nobori T, Nishijima A, Sakaguchi S, et al. Effects of the Japanese herbal medicine "Inchin-ko-to" (TJ-135) on concanavalin A-induced hepatitis in mice. *Clin Sci* 2000;99:421-431.

[7]   Takeda S, Iizuka A, Funo S, Sudo K, Kikuchi N, Yoshida C, Aburada M, et al. Effect of Chinese prescription "Inchin-ko-to" on experimental hepatobiliary injury induced by a-naphthylisocyanate [English abstract]. *Wakan-Yaku* 1984;1:230-234.

[8]   Trauner M, Meier PJ, Boyer JL. Molecular pathogenesis of cholestasis. *N Eng J Med* 1998;339:1217-1227.

[9]   Müller M, Jansen PLM. The secretory function of the liver: new aspects of hepatobiliary transport. *J Hepatol* 1998;28:344-354.

[10] Trauner M, Boyer JL. Bile salt transporters: Molecular characterization, function, and regulation. Physiol Rev 2003;83:633-671.

[11] Buchler M, Konig J, Brom M, Kartenbeck J, Spring H, Horie T, Keppler D. cDNA cloning of the hepatocyte canalicular isoform of the multidrug resistance protein, cMrp, reveals a novel conjugate export pump deficient in hyperbilirubinemic rats. *J Biol Chem* 1996;271:15091- 15098.

[12] Paulusma CC, Bosma PJ, Zaman GJ, Bakker CT, Otter M, Scheffer GL, Scheper RJ, et al. Congenital jaundice in rats with a mutation in a multidrug resistance-associated protein gene. *Science* 1996;271:1126-1128.

[13] Madon J, Eckhardt U, Gerloff T, Stieger B, Meier PJ. Functional expression of the rat liver canalicular isoform of the multidrug resistance-associated protein. *FEBS Lett* 1997;406:75-78.

[14] Ito K, Suzuki H, Hirohashi T, Kume K, Shimizu T, Sugiyama Y. Functional analysis of a canalicular multispecific organic anion transporter cloned from rat liver. *J Biol Chem* 1998;273:1684-1688.

[15] Konig J, Nies AT, Cui Y, Leier I, Keppler D. Conjugate export pumps of the multidrug resistance protein (MRP) family: localization, substrate specificity, and MRP2-mediated drug resistance. *Biochem Biophys Acta* 1999;1461:377-394.

[16] Kullak-Ublick GA, Beuers U, Paumgartner G. Hepatobiliary transport. *J Hepatology* 2000;32:3-18.

[17] Keppler D, König J. Expression and localization of the conjugate export pump encoded by the MRP2 (cMRP/cMOAT) gene in liver. *FASEB J* 1997;11:5-9-516.

[18] Trauner M, Arrese M, Soroka CJ, Ananthanarayanan M, Koeppel TA, Schlosser SF, Suchy FJ, et al. The rat canalicular conjugate export pump (Mrp2) is down-regulated in intrahepatic and obstructive cholestasis. *Gastroenterology* 1997;113:255-264.

[19] Erlinger S: Bile flow. In: Arias M, Boyer JL, Fausto N, Jakoby WB, Schachter DA, eds. The liver: Biology and Pathobiology. 3rd Ed. New York: Raven Press, Ltd. 1994:769-786.

[20] Oude-Elferink RP, Meijer DK, Kuipers F, Jansen PL, Gröen AK, Groothuis GM. Hepatobiliary secretion of organic compounds: molecular mechanisms of membrane transport. *Biochem Biophys Acta* 1995;1241:215-268.

[21] Bossard R, Strieger B, O'Neill B, Fricker G, Meier PJ. Ethinylestradiol treatment induces multiple canalicular membrane transport alterations in rat liver. *J Clin Invest* 1993;91:2714-2720.

[22] Bolder U, Ton-Nu HT, Schteingart CD, Frick E, Hofmann AF. Hepatocyte transport of bile acids and organic anions in endotoxemic rats: impaired uptake and secretion. *Gastroenterology* 1997;112:214-225.

[23] Ballatori N, Truong AT. Glutathione as a primary osmotic driving force in hepatic bile formation. *Am J Physiol* 1992;263:G617-624.

[24] Koyama K, Takagi Y, Ito K, et al. Experimental and clinical studies on the effect of biliary drainage in obstructive jaundice. *Am J Surg* 1981;142:293-299.

[25] Pitt HA, Cameron JL, Postier RG, et al. Factors affecting mortality in biliary tract surgery. *Am J Surg* 1981;141:66-72.

[26] Dixon JM, Armstrong CP, Duffy SW, et al. Factors affecting morbidity and mortality after surgery for obstructive jaundice: A review of 373 patients. *Gut* 1983;24:845-852.

[27] Aronsen KF. Liver function studies during and after complete extrahepatic biliary obstruction in the dog. *Acta Chir Scand* 1961;275:Suppl 1-114.

[28] Hansson JA, Hoevel J, Simert G, et al. Clinical aspects of nonsurgical percutaneous transhepatic bile drainage in obstructive lesions of the extrahepatic bile ducts. *Ann Surg* 1979;189:58-61.

[29] Norlander A, Kalin B, Sundblad R. Effect of percutaneous transhepatic drainage upon liver function and postoperative mortality. *Surg Gynecol Obstet* 1982;155:161-166.

[30] Shoda J, Kano M, Oda K, Kamiya J, Nimura Y, Suzuki H, Sugiyama Y, Miyazaki H, Todoroki T, Stengelin S, Kramer W, Matsuzaki Y, Tanaka N. The Expression Levels of Plasma Membrane Transporters in Cholestatic Liver of Patients Undergoing Biliary Drainage and Its Association With the Impairment of Biliary Secretory Function. *Am J Gastroenterol* 2001;96:3368-3378.

[31] Hirohashi T, Suzuki H, Ito K, et al. Hepatic expression of multidrug resistance-associated protein-like proteins maintained in Eisai Hyperbilirubinemic rats. *Mol Pharmacol* 1998;53:1068-1075.

[32] Kool M, van der Linden M, de Hass M, et al. MRP3, an organic anion transporter able to transport anti-cancer drugs. *Proc Natl Acad Sci USA* 1999;96:6914-6919.

[33] Hirohashi T, Suzuki H, Sugiyama Y. Characterization of the transport properties of cloned rat multidrug resistance-associated protein 3 (MRP3). *J Biol Chem* 1999;274:15181-15185.

[34] König J, Rost D, CuiY, Keppler D. Characterization of the human multidrug resistance protein isoform MRP3 localized to the basolateral hepatocyte membrane. *Hepatology* 1999;29:1156-1163.

[35] Robert SK, Ludwig J, Larusso NF. The pathology of biliary epithelia. *Gastroenterology* 1997;112:269-279.

[36] Hirohashi T, Suzuki H, Takikawa H, et al. ATP-dependent transport of bile salts by rat multidrug resistance-associated protein 3 (MRP3). *J Biol Chem* 2000;275:2905- 2910.

[37] Kubitz R, Wettstein M , Warskulat U, et al. Regulation of the multidrug resistance protein 2 in the rat liver by lipopolysaccharide and dexamethasone. *Gastroenterology* 1996;116:401-410.

[38] Vos TA, Hooiveld GJEJ, Koning H, et al. Up-regulation of the multidrug resistance genes, mrp1 and mdr1b, and down-regulation of the organic anion transporter, mrp2, and the bile salt transporter, spgp, in endotoxic rat liver. *Hepatology* 1998;28:1637-1644.

[39] Chojkier M. Regulation of liver-specific gene expression. In: Boyer JL, Ockner RK, eds. *Progress in liver diseases.* Vol. 13. Philadelphia: W.B. Saunders, 1995:37-61.

[40] Yamada T, Arai T, Nagino M, Oda K, Shoda J, Suzuki H, Sugiyama Y, Nimura Y. Impaired expression of hepatic multidrug resistanc3e protein 2 is associated with posthepatectomy hyperbilirubinemia in patients with biliary cancer. *Langenbecks Arch Surg* 2005;390:421-429.

[41] Nimura Y, Hayakawa N, Kamiya J, et al. Hepatic segmentectomy with caudate lobe resection for bile duct carcinoma of the hepatic hilus. World J Surg 1990; 14:535-544.

[42] Nagino M, Nimura Y, Hayakawa N, et al. Logistic regression and discriminant analyses of hepatic failure after liver resection for carcinoma of the biliary tract. *World J Surg* 1993; 17:250-255.

[43] Pichlmayr R, Weimann A, Klempnauer J, et al. Surgical treatment in proximal bile duct cancer. A single-center experience. *Ann Surg* 1996; 224:628-638.

[44] Miyazaki M, Ito H, Nakagawa K, et al. Aggressive surgical approaches to hilar cholangiocarcinoma: hepatic or local resection? *Surgery* 1998; 123:131-136.

[45] Neuhaus P, Jonas S, Bechstein W, et al. Extended resections for hilar cholangiocarcinoma. *Ann Surg* 1999; 230:808-818.

[46] Kosuge T, Yamamoto J, Shimada K, et al. Improved surgical results for hilar cholangiocarcinoma with procedures including major hepatic reaction. *Ann Surg* 1999; 230:663- 671.

[47] Tsao JI, Nimura Y, Kamiya J, et al. Management of hilar cholangiocarcinoma. Comparison of an American and a Japanese experience. Ann Surg 2000; 232:166-174.

[48] Nagino M, Kamiya J, Uesaka K, et al. Complications of hepatectomy for hilar cholangiocarcinoma. *World J Surg* 2001; 25:1277-1283.

[49] Arai T, Yoshikai Y, Kamiya J, Nagino M, Uesaka K, Yuasa N, Oda K, Sano T, Nimura Y. Bilirubin impairs bactericidal activity of neutrophils through an antioxidant mechanism *in vitro*. *J Surg Res* 2001;96:107-113.

[50] Welsh FKS, Ramsden CW, MacLennan K, Sheridan MB, Barclay GR, Guillou PJ, Reynolds JV. Increased intestinal oerniability and altered mucosal immunity in cholestatic jaundice. *Ann Surg* 1998;227:205-212.

[51] Paulusma CC, Kothe MJC, Bakker CTM, et al. Zonal down-regulation and redistribution of the multidrug resistance protein 2 during bile duct ligation in rat liver. *Hepatology* 2000; 31:684- 693.

[52] Lee JM, Trauner M, Soroka CJ, Stieger B. Expression of the bile salt export pump is maintained after chronic cholestasis in the rat. *Gastroenterology* 2000;118:163-172.

[53] Soroka CJ, Lee JM, Azzaroli F, Boyer JL. Cellular localization and up-regulation of multidrug resistance-associated protein 3 in hepatocytes and cholangiocytes during obstructive cholestasis in rat liver. *Hepatology* 2001; 33:783-791.

[54] Kawaguchi T, Sakisaka S, Mitsuyama K, et al. Cholestasis with altered structure and function of hepatocyte tight junction and decreased expression of canalicular multispecific organ anion transporter in a rat model of colitis. *Hepatology* 2000;31:1285-1295.

[55] Kanai M, Nimura Y, Kamiya J, et al. Preoperative intrahepatic segmental cholangitis in patients with advanced carcinoma involving the hepatic hilus. *Surgery* 1996;119:498-504.

[56] Zollner G, Fickert P, Zenz R, Fuchsbichler A, Stumptner C, Kenner L, Ferenci P, et al. Hepatobiliary transporter expression in percutaneous liver biopsies of patients with cholestatic liver diseases. *Hepatology* 2001;33:633-646.

[57] Fickert P, Zollner G, Fuchsbichler A, Stumtner C, Pojer C, Zwnz R, Lammert F, et al. Effects of ursodeoxycholic and cholic acid feeding on hepatocellular transporter expression in mouse liver. *Gastroenterology* 2001;121:170-183.

[58] Taguchi H, Endo T, Nakajima K, Aburada M. Studies on the constituents and evaluation of Gardenia Fructus. [abstract in English]. *Proc Symp Wakan-Yaku* 1975;9:85-91.

[59] Takeda S, Endo T, Aburada M. Pharmacological studies on iridoid compounds. III. The choleretic mechanism of iridoid compounds. *J Pharmacobiodyn* 1981;4:612-23.

[60] Takeda S, Yuasa K, Endo T, Aburada M. Pharmacological studies on iridoid compounds. II. Relationship between structures and choleretic actions of iridoid compound. *J Pharmacobiodyn* 1980;3:485-92.

[61] Shoda J, Miura T, Utsunomiya H, et al. Genipin enhances Mrp2 (Abcc2)-mediated bile formation and organic anion transport in rat liver. *Hepatology* 2004;39:167-78.

[62] Beuers U, Bilzer M, Chittattu A, Kullak-Ublick GA, Keppler D, Paumgartner G, Dombrowski F. Tauroursodeoxycholic acid inserts the apical conjugate export pump, Mrp2, into canalicular membranes and stimulates organic anion secretion by protein kinase C-dependent mechanisms in cholestatic liver. *Hepatology* 2001;33:1206-1216.

[63] Fukumura S, Takikawa H, Yamanaka K. Effect of organic anions and bile acid conjugates on biliary excretion of pravastatin in the rat. *Pharm Res* 1998;15:72-76.

[64] Blizer M, Lauterburg BH. Peptidoleukotrienes increase the efflux of glutathione from perfused rat liver. *Prostaglandins Leukot Essent Fatty Acids* 1993;49:715-721.

[65] Huang L, Smit JW, Meijer DKF, Vore M. Mrp2 is essential for estradiol-17b (b-D-glucuronide)-induced cholestasis in rats. *Hepatology* 2000;3:266-272.

[66] Roelofsen H, Soroka CJ, Keppler D, Boyer JL. Cyclic AMP stimulates sorting of the canalicular organic anion transporter (Mrp2/cMOAT) to the apical domain in hepatocyte couplets. *J Cell Sci* 1998;111:1137-1145.

[67] Komiya T, Tsukui M, Oshio H. Studies on "Inchin-ko-to". I. Capillarisin, a new choleretic substance. [abstract in English]. *Yakugaku Zasshi* 1976;96:841-54.

[68] Kagawa K, Okuno I, Noro Y. Colorimetric determination of capillarisin. *Shoyakugaku Zasshi* 1984;38:133-137.

[69] Okuno I, Kagawa K, Noro Y, Namba T. Pharmacological studies on the crude drug "Inchinko" in Japan (VI). Seasonal variation in chemical constituents of Artemisia capillaris THUNB. Shoyakugaku Zasshi 1983;37:199-203.

[70] Akahori A, Kagawa K, Okuno I. Determination of scoparone, capillarin and capllin in the crude drug "Inchinko" [abstract in English]. *Shoyakugaku Zasshi* 1978;32:177-184.

[71] Wang X, Saito K, Kano Y. On the evaluation of the preparation of Chinese medicinal prescriptions (VII) HPLC analysis of the components in "Inchin-ko-to" and "Inchin-gorei-san". *Shoyakugaku Zasshi* 1993;47:243-248.

[72] Yamahara J, Matsuda H, Sawada T, Mibu H, Fujimura H. Biologically active principles of crude drugs. Pharmacological evaluation of Artemisiae capillaris FLOS. [abstract in English]. *Yakugaku Zasshi* 1982;102:285-291.

[73] Okuno I, Uchida K, Nakamura M, Sakurai K. Studies on choleretic constituents in Artemisia capillaris THUNB. *Chem Pharm Bull (Tokyo)* 1988;36:769-775.

[74] Kitagawa I, Fukuda Y, Yoshihara M, Yamahara J, Yoshikawa M. Capillartemisin A and B, two new choleretic principles from Artemisiae capillaris herba. *Chem Pharm Bull (Tokyo)* 1983;31: 352-355.

[75] Onji M, Kikuchi T, Michikata K, Yamashita Y, Ohta Y. Combined use of ursodeoxycholic acid and Inchin-ko-to in jaundiced patients with primary biliary cirrhosis. *J Med Pharm Soc WAKAN-YAKU* 1990;7:161-167.

[76] Kobayashi H, Horikoshi K, Yamataka A, Lane GJ, Yamamoto M, Miyano T. Beneficial effect of a traditional herbal medicine (inchin-ko-to) in postoperative biliary atresia patients. *Pediatr Surg Int* 2001;17:386-9.

[77] Iinuma Y, Kubota M, Yagi M, Kanada S, Yamazaki S, Kinoshita Y. Effects of the herbal medicine Inchinko-to on liver function in postoperative patients with biliary atresia — a pilot study. *J Pediatr Surg* 2003;38:1607-11.

[78] Arai M, Yokosuka O, Fukai K, et al. A case of severe acute hepatitis of unknown etiology treated with the Chinese herbal medicine Inchin-ko-to. *Hepatol Res* 2004;28:161-165.

INDEX

C

D

E

H

K

Kampo medicine, 212, 231
karyotype, 93, 103
kidney, 21, 44, 83, 84, 161, 162, 163, 165, 172, 174, 177, 199, 200, 202, 203
kidneys, xi, 9, 11, 84, 179, 187, 199
kinetic, 169
kinetic studies, 169
kinetics, viii, 49, 52, 53, 54, 59, 74, 177
knowledge, ix, 82, 107, 149, 170

L

labeling, 6, 7, 79, 97, 220
lactate dehydrogenase, 93
Langerhans cells (LC), 172
large intestine, 163
lateral sclerosis, 155
LDL, 134
lead, viii, ix, x, 32, 51, 59, 82, 107, 123, 138, 203, 213, 218
lesions, viii, x, 49, 50, 54, 65, 70, 72, 100, 122, 132, 138, 139, 140, 142, 144, 145, 146, 147, 148, 149, 151, 152, 153, 155, 156, 157, 180, 181, 183, 185, 197, 198, 199, 202, 204, 233
leucine, 14
leukemia, ix, 22, 47, 51, 52, 69, 74, 75, 82, 83, 85, 87, 88, 89, 90, 95, 96, 102, 103, 104, 106, 107, 108, 109, 110, 111, 112, 113, 115, 117
leukotrienes, 2, 3, 6, 22
lifespan, 166
lifestyle, 197
ligands, 74, 77, 225
likelihood, 126, 197
limitation, 54
linkage, 12, 186
links, 9
lipid peroxidation, 127, 134
lipids, 127
lipoproteins, 127
liver, ix, xi, 4, 5, 7, 9, 10, 11, 12, 14, 19, 20, 22, 23, 28, 82, 83, 101, 107, 115, 130, 159, 161, 162, 163, 174, 179, 187, 198, 199, 200, 202, 208, 211, 212, 213, 214, 215, 216, 217, 218, 219, 220, 221, 222, 223, 225, 226, 228, 229, 230, 231, 232, 233, 234, 235, 236
liver damage, 213
liver disease, xii, 161, 212, 221, 231, 234, 235
liver failure, 218, 219, 220, 221, 230

localization, x, xi, 63, 84, 107, 127, 129, 133, 135, 136, 138, 141, 172, 174, 178, 208, 209, 211, 213, 216, 217, 218, 220, 221, 222, 227, 231, 232, 235
location, 162, 169
locus, xi, 12, 180, 185, 186, 205, 210
lovastatin, 123
LTC, 4
lumen, 163
lung cancer, 5, 20, 44, 50, 52, 54, 71, 72, 73, 75, 78, 83, 84, 85, 103, 105, 107, 108, 117, 171
lying, 182
lymph, 72, 96, 175
lymph node, 72, 96, 175
lymph nodes, 175
lymphocytes, 89, 96
lymphoid, 164
lymphoma, 54, 88, 96

M

macrophage inflammatory protein (MIP), 175
macrophages, 127, 141, 161
magnetic resonance, 35, 156
magnetic resonance imaging, 35, 156
major histocompatibility complex, 155
males, 84, 184
malignancy, viii, 49, 84, 88, 98
malignant melanoma, 98
malignant tumors, 33, 36, 42, 44, 50, 54, 71, 84
mammalian brain, 169
management, 45, 117
manganese, 15
mannitol, 168
mapping, 205
Marfan syndrome, 187
marrow, 161, 163
mass, xi, 211
mast cells, 161
maturation, x, 94, 112, 113, 137, 142, 150
MBP, x, 137, 138, 141, 142, 144, 148, 150, 151
measurement, 17, 36, 37, 42, 54
measures, 76
median, 40, 42, 86, 101
Mediterranean, 199
medulloblastoma, 34
melanoma, 83, 103, 114, 117
membrane permeability, 74
membranes, x, xii, 11, 63, 67, 137, 139, 151, 154, 160, 199, 201, 212, 213, 214, 235
men, 140
messenger ribonucleic acid, 46, 75
messenger RNA, xi, 75, 79, 109, 211, 221
messenger RNA (mRNA), 166

N

Q

R

T

MULTIDRUG RESISTANCE-ASSOCIATED PROTEINS

CHRISTOPHER V. AIELLO
EDITOR

Nova Science Publishers, Inc.
New York

Library of Congress Cataloging-in-Publication Data

Multidrug resistance-associated proteins / Christopher V. Aiello (editor).
    p. ; cm.
Includes bibliographical references and index.
ISBN 13 978-1-60021-298-7
ISBN 10 1-60021-298-0
1. Multidrug resistance. 2. Proteins--Pathophysiolgy. 3. Tumor proteins. 4. Molecular neurobiology. I. Aiello, Christopher V.
[DNLM: 1. Multidrug Resistance-Associated Proteins--genetics. 2. Drug Resistance, Multiple. 3. Multidrug Resistance-Associated Proteins--pharmacokinetics. 4. Nervous System Diseases--drug therapy. QU 55 M96085 2006]
QR177.M85   2006
615'.7--dc22   2006018903

Published by Nova Science Publishers, Inc. ✦New York

CONTENTS

070119707

PREFACE

Organisms are said to be drug-resistant when drugs meant to neutralize them have reduced effect. When an organism is resistant to more than one drug, it is said to be multi-drug resistant. The most prominent example of this is antibiotic resistance. Drug resistance is also found in some tumor cells, which makes it more difficult to use chemotherapy to attack tumors made of those cells. When a drug such as an antibiotic is administered, those which have a genetic resistance to the drug will survive and reproduce, and the new population will be drug-resistant. This book provides in depth research on multi-drug resistance and its impact on neurology. This includes studies on GS-X Pump/Multidrug Resistance Proteins, Quantitation of O6 - Methylguanine, Therapeutic Responses to Chemotherapy, Profiles in Cancer, Neurodegenerative Diseases and Multiple Sclerosis.

Chapter 1 - The ATP binding cassette (ABC) proteins form one of the largest protein families encoded in human genome. Hitherto more than 48 genes ecoding human ABC proteins have been identified and sequenced. It has been reported that mutations of ABC protein genes are causative in several genetic disorders in humans. Many human ABC proteins are involved in membrane transport of drugs, xenobiotics, endogenous substances or ions, thereby exhibiting a wide spectrum of biological functions. The "ABCC" gene family (according to the new nomenclature or human ABC transporter genes) encomprises the multidrug resistance-associated proteins, sulfonylurea receptors, and cystic fibrosis transmembrane conductance regulator. Molecular cloning studies have identified ten members of the human MRP sub-family including ABCC11, ABCC12, and ABCC13 (pseudo gene) that have recently been cloned in our laboratory. This review addresses the historical background and discovery of the ATP-driven xenobiotic export pumps (GS-X pumps) encoded by the *ABCC(MRP1)* and *ABCC2(MRP2/cMOAT)* genes, the biological functions of ABC transporters in the MRP class, and the regulation of gene expression of GS-X pumps by oxidative stress.

Chapter 2 - O^6-methylguanine-DNA methyltransferase (MGMT) is a drug-resistance gene for nitrosoureas. The level of MGMT varies widely according to the type of tumor, and even varies among tumors of the same histological classification. MGMT mRNA was measured in 65 neuroepithelial tumor specimens from 54 patients almost that had received 1-(4-amino-2-methyl-5-pyrimidynyl) methyl – 3 - (2-chloroethyl) – 3 - nitrosourea hydrochloride (ACNU) after the resection of the tumor by real-time reverse transcription-polymerase chain reaction (RT-PCR) using TaqMan probe and normalized to the level of the internal control.

The absolute value of MGMTmRNA normalized to the level of GAPDH in 65 neuroepithelial tumor specimens was $1.20 \times 10^4 \pm 1.19 \times 10^4$ copy/µg RNA(mean ± standard deviation). The mean value of 35 glioblastomas ($1.20 \times 10^4 \pm 1.00 \times 10^4$ copy/µg RNA) was not significantly different from that of 7 low grade gliomas ($1.13 \times 10^4 \pm 0.60 \times 10^4$ copy/µg RNA) ($P= 0.4241$ by Student's t-test). The mean value of 36 primary tumors ($1.01 \times 10^4 \pm 0.92 \times 10^4$ copy/µg RNA) was not significantly different from that of the recurrent 21 tumors after ACNU therapy ($1.46 \times 10^4 \pm 1.53 \times 10^4$) ($P= 0.0920$ by Student's t-test). Similarly, in 8 patients who had been measured of MGMTmRNA more than twice, no significant elevations of MGMTmRNA after ACNU treatment were observed.

The response rate, more than 50% tumor regression rate, to ACNU of 28 patients who had MGMTmRNA less than 6×10^3 copy/µg RNA was 58.3% and that of 37 patients who had it more than 6×10^3 copy/µg RNA was 23.1%. Significant difference was observed in the response rates of these two groups ($P = 0.0421$ by Fisher's exact probability test). The value normalized MGMTmRNA < 6000 copy/µg RNA was the only significant factor predicted the initial effect of therapy with ACNU among some prognostic factors such as age, Kernofsky's performance status, histological grading, surgical reduction rate, and combination therapy.

A hundred and twenty-four adjuvant therapy individualized by the results of RT-PCR has been used to treat 100 patients with neuroepithelial tumors since 1997. Immediate after the operation, the mRNA expression for drug-resistance genes was investigated in 124 frozen samples of tumors (10 astrocytomas, 2 oligodendrogliomas, 9 anaplastic oligodendrogliomas, 40 anaplastic astrocytomas, 56 glioblastoma multiformes, and 7 medulloblastomas) by conventional RT-PCR in 51 samples, semi-quantitative RT-PCR in 12 samples, real-time RT-PCR using SYBR Green I in 55 samples, and real-time RT-PCR using TaqMan probe in 6 samples, all with the specific primers for MGMT. Eighty-five tumors were treated with ACNU because relative low expression value of MGMTmRNA and residual 39 tumors who had had relatively high MGMTmRNA were treated with platinum-compounds. The response rate of the individual adjuvant therapy (IAT) was 40.0% for glioblastoma multiformes, 51.4% for anaplastic astrocytomas, and 50.0% for all evaluable therapies. Two years survival rate of 45 glioblastoma patients was 55.6% at present.

These results suggest that quantitation of MGMTmRNA is the excellent method for predicting for the effect of ACNU in glioma therapy. Our IAT based on the results of real-time RT-PCR may lead to a simple and beneficial glioma therapy. A prospective randomized multi-center study should be performed to confirm the efficacy of this new method for glioma therapy

Chapter 3 - Lipophilic cationic nuclear tracers, technetium-99m-sestamibi (^{99m}Tc-MIBI) and technetium-99m-tetrofosmin (^{99m}Tc-TF), have been investigated as tumor imaging agents in various kinds of malignancy. They may not only delineate lesions but also provide information pertaining to tumor characteristics. There is sufficient evidence that these tracers are substrates of cell surface molecules, P-glycoprotein (P-gp) and multi-drug resistance associated proteins (MRP); therefore, they may enable scintigraphic pre-therapeutic prediction of tumor responses to chemotherapy. That is, tumors that do not take up these tracers are likely to fail to respond to chemotherapy. Furthermore, effectiveness of modulators to reverse the resistance attributable to these molecules may be monitored by changes in the tracer accumulation. In this paper, tracer kinetics of ^{99m}Tc-MIBI and ^{99m}Tc-TF in MRP-expressing tumor cell lines and their limitations to assess reversal effects of classical modulators on the function of MRP are demonstrated based on our experimental results. In addition, recent findings regarding the feasibility of scintigraphic monitoring on translational inhibition of mRNA coding MRP with antisense oligodeoxynucleotide are discussed.

Chapter 4 - Age has an important prognostic impact in therapy of cancer. Adults usually have a worse prognosis compared to children with the same type of cancer. This may be due to: (1) different, unfavourable cancer biology, (2) poor treatment tolerance, (3) cellular drug resistance, (4) higher expression of drug resistance related proteins, (5) development of other mechanisms of resistance. Regarding possible mechanisms of resistance, an almost endless number can be envisaged along the signal transduction pathways triggered by anticancer drugs. The difference in current cure rate between adult and childhood cancer may be caused by differences in regulation of drug resistance, both primary and acquired. The aim of this study was the systematic review of the literature on the role and impact of Multidrug Resistance-Associated Protein's (MRP's) expression in various types of childhood and adult cancer. This paper describes an update in differences of research on the biology of MRP's of various types of childhood and adult cancer with stress on differences in protein expression and clinical outcome. A panel of proliferative disorders is reviewed, including hematological malignancies, with emphasis on acute leukemias, both at diagnosis and at relapse; as well as brain tumors, bone tumors, soft tissue sarcomas, rhabdomyosarcomas, neuroblastomas and liver tumors. A large variety and discrepancy of results is presented in performed studies. MRP's are physiologically present in various tissues. MRP's are also markers of immature cells, thus are shown to be more often present in acute myeloid leukemia in adults, however recent data suggest the possible relevance of MRP's family in childhood acute lymphoblastic leukemia. In general, their overexpression is more often observed in solid tumors, which occur more frequently in adults. MRP seems to be disease specific, so overall distribution of cancer determine the occurrence and clinical prognostic impact in malignancies in adults. It may correlate and contribute to worse clinical outcome of cancer in adults. The impact of MRP's and association with resistant disease in childhood and adult cancer is analysed in this review, with emphasis on results of multivariate analyses, variety of diseases and possible geographical influence. Possible strategies of modulation or circumvention of resistance caused by MRP's are reviewed. In summary, it seems that the greater the age, the higher the drug resistance. Age itself, more than drug resistance profile, reflects factors with more direct effect on chemotherapy response in adult cancer. This might contribute to the difference in outcome between children and adults with malignancies. Induction of drug resistance proteins during chemotherapy and co-existence of various mechanisms are common phenomena in adult cancer. Differences in resistance to different drugs might contribute to the impact of age on cancer outcome. The underlying mechanisms for these differences are still largely unknown; however, knowledge about drug resistance mechanisms can lead to the development of new therapeutic options.

Chapter 5 - The blood-brain barrier (BBB) efficiently protects the brain against xenobiotics and plays an important part in the development of drug resistance in a wide range of neurological disorders such as brain cancer, epilepsy and infectious diseases. In this regard, the function of the members of the ABC transporter family, such as P-glycoprotein (P-gp) and multidrug resistance-associated proteins (MRP), in the integrity of the BBB recently has been the subject of intensive research. In particular, the importance of brain-to-blood transport across the BBB has garnered increasing attention as a potential mechanism in the pathogenesis of neurodegenerative disorders. According to the concept of "proteopathies", many neurodegenerative disorders such as Alzheimer's disease (AD), Creutzfeldt-Jakob-Disease (CJD), Parkinson's Disease (PD) and Huntington's Disease (HD) are the result of the aberrant polymerization and accumulation of misfolded proteins within the brain. In addition to their role in protecting the brain from exogenous toxins, there is now evidence that cellular transport proteins help to regulate the levels of some pathogenic proteins in the brain. In this review, we discuss the possible role of drug efflux transporters, especially P-gp, in neurodegeneration, and consider how a fuller understanding of this process might promote the development of more efficacious treatment strategies.

Chapter 6 - Little is known about the proteins involved in axonal damage (AD) which associates with demyelination during multiple sclerosis (MS). Axon transections, amyloid precursor protein accumulation and abnormal expression of the non-phosphorylated form of neurofilaments (NF) have been described. Characterization of AD is a main concern for at least two purposes. First, AD is probably involved in central nervous system (CNS) atrophy, and in patients permanent disability. Second, its impact on remyelination is unknown. Indeed, although neurons are dispensable for oligodendrocytes (OL), the myelinating cells in the CNS, to synthesize myelin-like membranes, neurons enhance this process *in vitro*. Thus, it may be that AD inhibits, in turn, remyelination.

To get insight into these axonal cytoskeleton alterations, we have analyzed by immunohistochemistry 18 chronic plaques from autopsy samples, originating from 6 MS patients (1 progressive, 5 remitting-progressive forms; mean disease duration : 18.5 years). In comparison to the normal appearing white matter decreased number of axons immunostained for the 3 NF subunits, βtubulin, and GAP-43 were - with demyelination and loss of oligodendrocytes (OL) - the hallmarks of plaques, and were extremely severe in 2/3. AD intensity did not correlate with demyelination : although severe demyelination always associated with a 90% decrease in NF+ axons, such severe NF loss also occurred in some plaques despite a moderate demyelination, suggesting it depends too upon other factors. CNP+ and MBP+ OL decreased by the same extent within one plaque, indicating that most OL have reached their final maturation. Nevertheless, residual cells show a lower capability to remyelinate axons, since the ratio of MBP+ fibers per OL decreased also.

These results enlarge previous descriptions of cytoskeleton and NF abnormalities in MS, since the expression of the 3 subunits of NF are decreased, providing evidence that their intimate constituents are impaired. As previously described in animal models, this decrease could lead to axonal atrophy (and slowness of axon potential conduction). Moreover severe impairment of NF associates with decreased tubulin expression which could result in altered axoplasmic transport. Finally one can hypothesized that the expression or localization of NF associated proteins (which copurify with NF) could be altered too.

Thus, the body of these results suggests that NF abnormalities are the core of more severe AD than previously hypothesized in MS. Detailing these lesions will help our understanding of permanent disability in MS patients, as well as cues to prevent them. Whether AD might be involved in MS remyelination impairment - which is one of the actual major target of therapeutic hopes such as cell grafts – is under current investigation at the laboratory.

Chapter 7 - Multidrug Resistance-associated Proteins (MRPs) are membrane proteins transporting organic anions. MRP1, MRP2, MRP4, and MRP5 (ABCC1, ABCC2, ABCC4, and ABCC5) and orphan organic anion efflux pump activities are detected in the brain. MRP1 is known to be a major basolateral transporter in epithelial cells, also expressed in the choroid plexus. MRP2 is a major apical canalicular multispecific organic anion transporter in the liver, also detected at brain blood capillaries. MRP4 and MRP5 are expressed in the choroid plexus and brain capillary endothelial cells. We discuss the putative roles of MRPs and orphan organic anion efflux pumps in the brain.

Chapter 8 - The 6th member of the sub-family C known as ABCC6 (*alias* MRP6), was first characterized by Kool and co-workers in 1999. ABCC6 is closely related to ABCC1 (*alias* MRP1), the defining member of the sub-family C, which is involved in multidrug-resistance. Predictive analysis indicated that ABCC6 displays a transmembrane structure similar to ABCC1 with three groups of 5, 6 and 6 membrane-spanning domains. In human and rodent, *ABCC6* appears to be constitutively expressed in the liver and kidneys and the encoded 1503 amino acids protein was localized on the basolateral membrane of hepatocytes and renal polarized cells. The substrate specificity of ABCC6 is unknown and only a few molecules were found to be actively transported in vesicular studies. Despite its similarity with ABCC1, there is no indication that ABCC6 is associated with chemotherapy resistance as no correlation between expression and drug resistance was ever observed.

Pseudoxanthoma elasticum (PXE) is an autosomal recessive disorder characterized by a generalized accumulation of calcified elastic fibers that results in dermal abnormalities. The skin manifestations are the prevailing characteristics of PXE and are associated with ocular and vascular symptoms. The PXE phenotype is highly heterogeneous and no correlation between the multiple gene alterations and the variable symptoms could be established. The genetic linkage analysis that permitted the identification of the first few mutations failed to reveal any locus heterogeneity suggesting that ABCC6 is solely responsible for PXE. Up to now, more than 140 mutations have been identified. The vast majority of these disease-causing changes are single nucleotide substitutions resulting in missense, nonsense and splice variants while a few others are large and small deletions or insertions. Most of the nucleotide variants seemed to cluster in specific domains of the protein such as the ATP-binding folds or a large cytoplasmic loop suggesting that PXE arises from the lack of transport activity. In prototypic elastic fiber diseases or in disorders caused by mutations in other ABCC genes, the development of the phenotype is usually consistent with the apparent function of the encoded protein. In contrast, there is no obvious connection between ABCC6 and elastic fiber synthesis or deposition. Therefore, it was suggested that PXE is a metabolic disease with ABCC6 involved in a detoxification process. At the present time, a handful of divergent approaches based on mouse models and *in vitro* studies aim specifically at gathering clues about these obscure and most likely indirect processes resulting from the absence of ABCC6 function in unspecified tissues and ultimately affecting elastic fibers.

Chapter 9 - Plants contain abundant bioactive materials. A Kampo (Chinese/Japanese herbal) medicine, Inchinkoto (ICKT), and its ingredients exert potent choleretic effects by a "bile acid-independent" mechanism. However, details underlying the choleresis have not been fully clarified. The ATP-dependent, apical conjugate export pump, termed multidrug resistance-associated protein 2 (Mrp2; Abcc2), is the major driving force for bile acid-independent bile flow. Therefore, the experiments were designed to determine whether ICKT or its ingredients potentiate Mrp2-mediated choleresis *in vivo*. Biliary secretion of Mrp2 substrates and protein mass, subcellular localization, and the steady-state messenger RNA (mRNA) level of Mrp2 were assessed in rat liver after an infusion of genipin, an intestinal bacterial metabolite of geniposide that is a major ingredient of ICKT. The function of Mrp2 was also assessed by the ATP-dependent uptake of Mrp2-specific substrates using canalicular membrane vesicles (CMVs) from the liver. Infusion of genipin rapidly increased bile flow and biliary secretion of bilirubin conjugates and reduced glutathione, but did not increase bile acid secretion. The ATP-dependent uptake of Mrp2 substrates was significantly stimulated in the CMVs from the liver. These effects were not observed in Eisai hyperbilirubinemic rats (Mrp2-deficient rats). Under these conditions, genipin treatment increased the protein mass of Mrp2 in the CMVs but not the mRNA level. In immunoelectron-microscopic studies, a significant increase in Mrp2 density in the canalicular membrane was observed in the genipin-treated liver when compared to the vehicle-treated liver. Genipin, a major active ingredient in ICKT, may enhance the bile acid-independent secretory capacity of hepatocytes, mainly by an Mrp2-mediated mechanism through stimulation of exocytosis and insertion of the transporter protein into canalicular membranes. Therefore, ICKT may be a potent therapeutic agent for a number of cholestatic liver diseases.

In: Multidrug Resistance-Associated Proteins
Editor: Christopher V. Aiello, pp. 1-29

ISBN 1-60021-298-0
© 2007 Nova Science Publishers, Inc.

Chapter 1

THE GS-X PUMP/MULTIDRUG RESISTANCE PROTEINS (MRP): ROLE OF GLUTATHIONE IN THEIR FUNCTION AND GENE REGULATION[*]

Toshihisa Ishikawa[1†], Hiroshi Nakagawa[1] and Macus Tien Kuo[2]

[1] Department of Biomolecular Engineering, Graduate School of Bioscience and Biotechnology, Tokyo Institute of Technology, Yokohama, Japan
[2] Department of Molecular Pathology, The University of Texas M. D. Anderson Cancer Center, Houston, Texas, USA

ABSTRACT

The ATP binding cassette (ABC) proteins form one of the largest protein families encoded in human genome. Hitherto more than 48 genes ecoding human ABC proteins have been identified and sequenced. It has been reported that mutations of ABC protein genes are causative in several genetic disorders in humans. Many human ABC proteins are involved in membrane transport of drugs, xenobiotics, endogenous substances or ions, thereby exhibiting a wide spectrum of biological functions. The "ABCC" gene family (according to the new nomenclature or human ABC transporter genes) encomprises the multidrug resistance-associated proteins, sulfonylurea receptors, and cystic fibrosis transmembrane conductance regulator. Molecular cloning studies have identified ten members of the human MRP sub-family including ABCC11, ABCC12, and ABCC13 (pseudo gene) that have recently been cloned in our laboratory. This review addresses the historical background and discovery of the ATP-driven xenobiotic export pumps (GS-X pumps) encoded by the *ABCC(MRP1)* and *ABCC2(MRP2/cMOAT)* genes, the biological

[*] The authors dedicate this review article to Drs. Naoyuki Taniguchi and Helmut Sies for their great contribution to glutathione and oxidative stress research.

[†] Address for Correspondence : Toshihisa Ishikawa, Ph.D. Professor, Department of Biomolecular Engineering, Graduate School of Bioscience and Biotechnology, Tokyo Institute of Technology, Nagatsuta 4259-B-60, Yokohama 226-8501, Japan. Tel: 045-924-5800. Fax: 045-924-5838 ; E-mail: tishikaw@bio.titech.ac.jp

functions of ABC transporters in the MRP class, and the regulation of gene expression of GS-X pumps by oxidative stress.

I. INTRODUCTION

Plant and animal cells eliminate a broad range of lipophilic toxins from the cytosol after their conjugation with glutathione (GSH) (Isikawa, 1992; Martinoia et al., 1993; Li et al., 1995; Ishikawa et al., 1997; Rea et al., 2003). This transport process is mediated by *GS-X* pumps, organic anion transporters with Mg^{2+}-ATPase activity. The term "*GS-X* pump" was originally proposed based on its transport activity and high affinity for glutathione S-conjugates (GS-conjugates), glutathione disulfide (GSSG), and cysteinyl leukotrienes (Ishikawa, 1992). Accumulating evidence suggests that *GS-X* pumps have broad substrate specificities toward different types of organic anions and thereby play a physiologically important role in inflammation, oxidative stress, xenobiotics metabolism, and antitumor drug resistance.

Glutathione (GSH) is a ubiquitous tripeptide thiol (L-Y-glutamyl-L-cysteinyl-glycine) that is present in virtually all eukaryotes (Meister and Anderson, 1983). It is a vital intra- and extra-cellular cytoprotectant (Droge, 2002; Reed, 1990) and an effective reactive oxygen species (ROS) scavenger. It is estimated that GSH biosynthesis originated about 3.5 billion years ago. GSH is found in the vast majority of eukaryotes, whereas in eubacteria, GSH biosynthesis is limited to only two groups, *i.e.*, cyanobacteria and purple bacteria (Fahey and Sundquist, 1991). The former appeared on earth about 35 billion years ago and was capable of oxygenic photosynthesis. The cyanobacteria are considered to have given rise to plant chloroplasts, whereas the purple bacteria is considered to have introduced the ancestor responsible for eukaryotic mitochondria. GSH production appears to be closely associated with those prokaryotes responsible for the oxygen-producing and oxygen-utilizing pathways of eukaryotes, suggesting that the ability of GSH biosynthesis may have been acquired by eukaryotes during the endosymbiotic process that give rise to chloroplasts and mitochondria (Fahey and Sundquist, 1991). In fact, GSH plays a pivotal role in protection of living cells under oxidative stress (Chance et al., 1979; Sies, 1985).

In aerobic cells, ROS which consist of oxygen radicals including superoxide anions [O_2^-], hydroxy radical [˙OH] and hydrogen peroxides [H_2O_2], play important roles in many important cellular physiological functions, including growth, differentiation, apoptosis, and aging (reviewed in Finkel, 2003). Under normal physiological conditions, there is a balance between oxidants and antioxidants, or reduction-oxidation (redox) homeostasis. Cytotoxic agents, including antitumor agents, xenobiotics, and carcinogens, induce oxidative stress. One of the important strategies in counteracting these stresses is the GSH system (reviewed in Winvard et al., 2005). Under oxidative stress, GSH is oxidized by GSH peroxidase to GSSG which is eliminated by the GS-X pump, commonly known as multidrug resistance protein (MRP) efflux proteins. Excess GSSG can be catalytically reduced back to GSH by the NADPH-dependent GSSG reductase (Figure 1). GSH also regulates the activities and biosynthesis of other redox-regulating enzymes, such as superoxide dismutase, DT-diphorases (NQO1 and NQO2). Because of its abundance (1 to10 mM inside the cells) (Smith et al., 1996; Hwang et al., 1992), the GSH/GSSG represents a major redox regulation system in the cells.

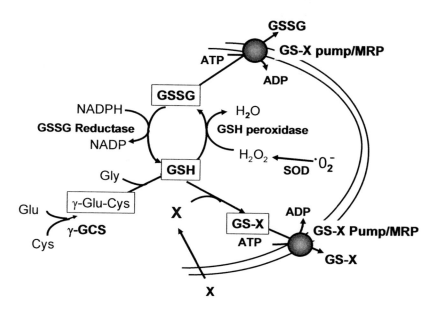

Figure 1. Role of GS-X pump/MRP1 transporter in regulation of intracellular redox conditions and elimination of xenobiotics. Xenobiotic compound (X) entering the cell is conjugated by GSH. The resulting GS-X conjugate is eliminated by GS-X pump/MRP1 using ATP as energy source. Biosynthesis of GSH is carried out by the rate-limiting enzyme, □-GCS, and glutathione synthetase. Under oxidative conditions, GSH is oxidized to GSSG by GSH peroxidase. GSSG is either eliminated by the GS-X pump or reduced by GSSG reductase. See Ishikawa et al. (1986a) for the original illustration.

GSH also serves as a cofactor for conjugation reactions involved in the elimination of various xenobiotics such as chemical carcinogens, environmetal pollutants, and antitumor agents (Sies and Ketterer, 1988). The formation of hydrophilic glutathionyl conjugates is catalyzed by glutathione S-transferases (GSTs), a family of so-called phase II enzymes that mediate the conjugation reaction in a substrate-dependent fashion (Townsend and Tew, 2003; Hayes et al., 2005). These GST isoenzymes are also involved in the endogenous biosynthesis of leukotrienes, prostaglandins, testosterone, and progesterone. Among their substrates, GSTs conjugate 4-hydroxynonenal, leukotriene A_4, and the signaling molecules 15-deoxy-□^{12,14}-prostaglandin J_2 (15□-PGJ$_2$) and □^{7}-prostaglandin A_1 (Suzuki et al. 1997; Isikawa et al., 1998). The GS-X pump is used to shuffle these glutathionyl metabolites into the appropriate cellular compartments (Ishikawa, 1992; Ishikawa et al., 1997).

II. HISTORICAL BCKGROUND OF GS-X PUMP RESEARCH

In 1969, the pioneering work was made by Srivastava and Beutler (1969) who reported that elimination of GSSG from human erythrocytes to the incubation medium is a unidirectional and energy-dependent process (see Table 1 for historical studies). GSSG transport occurred even against a concentration gradient of GSSG, and the transport was halted almost entirely when endogenous ATP was depleted by preliminary incubation of erythrocytes in a glucose-free medium for 8 hours or by the presence of fluoride in the incubation medium. Their report provided the first evidence that GSSG efflux is mediated not by simple diffusion but rather by active membrane transport. Although they suggested energy-dependence of GSSG transport, it was not elucidated whether ATP is directly required. In 1980, the transport of GSSG across the plasma membrane was proven to be an ATP-dependent "primary" active process in inside-out membrane vesicles from human erythrocytes (Kondo et al., 1980). Subsequently, ATP-dependent GSH conjugate transport was demonstrated by Board (1981), Kondo *et al.* (1982) and Labelle *et al.* (1986).

In 1984, Ishikawa and Sies reported that GSSG and GS-conjugates are released from the isolated perfused heart (Ishikawa and Sies, 1984). Because the heart is continuously exposed to highly oxygenated blood from the lungs, cardiomyopathy may result from oxidative damage inflicted by hyperoxia or administration of certain anticancer drugs, *e.g.*, doxorubicin, has been described. GSSG efflux was suggested to be an important defense mechanism against oxidative stress (Ishikawa et al., 1986a). The relationship of GSSG efflux rate *vs.* cytosolic free ATP/ADP ratio shows that GSSG efflux rate is half-maximal at (ATP/ADP)free=10 (Ishikawa et al., 1986b), suggesting an ATP-dependent transport process. GSSG efflux from the heart is not affected by epinephrine, nor-epinephrine or dibutyryl cyclic AMP, suggesting that GSSG transport is independent of $\Box$- or β-adrenergic hormonal regulations (Ishikawa et al., 1986b). Using plasma membrane vesicles prepared from rat hearts, Ishikawa et al. demonstrated ATP-dependent primary active transport of GSSG and GS-conjugates (Ishikawa, 1989). The cardiac *GS-X* pump was shown to have high affinities for GS-conjugates with long aliphatic carbon chain (Ishikawa et al., 1986b). Ishikawa et al. was the first to provide evidence that leukotriene C4 (LTC4), a pro-inflammatory mediator, is an endogenous substrate for the GS-X pump (Ishikawa, 1989; Ishikawa et al., 1989).

In the liver, GSSG and GS-conjugates are predominantly excreted into bile. Akerboom *et al.* reported that hepatobiliary transport of GSSG is inhibited by GS-conjugates, suggesting the existence of a common transport system for hepatobiliary transport of both GSSG and GS-conjugates (Akerboom et al., 1982). Membrane potential was speculated to be a potential driving force for the transport of GSSG and GSH conjugates, but Kobayashi and coworkers provided evidence for ATP-dependent primary active transport of S-(2,4-dinitrophenyl)-glutathione (GS-DNP) using rat hepatocyte canalicular membrane vesicles (Kobayashi et al., 1990). Moreover, Kobayashi *et al.* (1991) reported that transport of *p*-nitrophenyl-glucuronide across rat liver canalicular membrane is an ATP-dependent process. Inhibition of the transport of the glucuronide conjugate by GS-DNP suggested that the hepatobiliary elimination of glucuronide conjugates is mediated by the hepatic GS-X pump.

Table 1. Historical studies leading to the identification of *MRP* genes encoding the GS-X pump

1969	The first report on energy-dependent GSSG elimination from human erythrocytes	Srivastava and Beutler
1980	ATP-dependent GSSG transport in inside-out membrane vesicles of erythrocytes	Kondo et al.
1981	ATP-dependent GSSG transport in inside-out membrane vesicles of erythrocytes	Board
1982	ATP-dependent transport of GS-conjugate in erythrocyte membrane	Kondo et al.
1982	GSSG and GS-conjugate release from Isolated perfused rat liver to bile	Akerboom et al.
1984	ATP-dependent transport of GS-conjugate in erythrocyte membrane	Labelle et al.
1984	GSSG and GS-conjugate release from isolated perfused rat heart	Ishikawa and Sies
1986	Energy dependent GSSG transport in rat heart measured by in-vivo NMR	Ishikawa et al.
1987	Discovery of transport-deficient rat that lack transport of bilirubin-glucuronide conjugates	Jansen et al
1987	Deficient hepatobiliary transport of cysteinyl leukotriens in TR$^-$ rats	Huber et al.
1989	Deficient hepatobiliary transport of GSH, GSSG, and GS-conjugates in TR$^-$ rats	Elferink et al.
1989	ATP-dependent transport of GS-conjugate in plasma membrane vesicles of rat heart	Ishikawa
1990	ATP-dependent transport of GS-conjugate in plasma membrane vesicles of rat liver	Kobayashi et al.
1990	ATP-dependent transport of leukotrine C_4 in rat liver and heart membrane vesicles	Ishikawa et al.
1991	lacking hepatobiliary transport of GS-conjugate	Takikawa et al.
1992	Definition of GS-X pump and phase III system for xenobiotic metabolism	Ishikawa
1992	Cloning of MRP1 cDNA from doxorubicin- resistant human lung cancer cell line	Cole et al.
1994	Discovery of leukotrine C_4 and GS-DNP transport by MRP1	Leier et al. Muller et al
1996	Cloning of Mrp2/cMOAT cDNA from the liver cDNA library of TR$^-$ rats	Paulusma et al.
1996	Cloning of Mrp2/cMOAT cDNA from the liver cDNA library of EHBR rats	Buchler et al.
1996	Cloning of human MRP2/cMOAT cDNA from the cisplatin-resiatnt human cancer	Taniguchi et al.
1997	Identification of MRP3,4 and 5 in human cancer cell lines	Kool et al.
1998	Identification of MRP6 in human tissues and cancer cell lines	Kool et al.

The discovery of two strains of jaundiced mutant Wistar and Sprague-Dawley rats, *i.e.*, transport-deficient (TR⁻) and (Eisai-hyperbilirubinemic (EHBR), greatly enhanced the study of the hepatic GS-X pump. The mutant rats manifest predominantly conjugated hyperbilirubinemia and are defective in the biliary secretion of GSH, GSSG, GS-conjugates (Elferink et al., 1989; Oude Elferink et al., 1990; Takikawa et al., 1991), GSH-metal complexes (Houven et al., 1990), bilirubin-glucuronide conjugates (Jansen et al., 1987a), cysteinyl leukotrienes (Huber et al., 1987; Ishikawa et al., 1990), as well as organic anions, *e.g.*, bromosulphthalein, indocyanine green, and dibromosulfophthalein (Jansen et al., 1987b). These findings suggested that the hepatobiliary *GS-X* pump has broad substrate specificity toward different organic anions. Thus, the hepatic *GS-X* pump is also called "canalicular multispecific organic anion transporter (cMOAT)". The functional defect of the hepatic *GS-X* pump or cMOAT is inherited with characteristics of an autosomal recessive abnormality, and those mutant rats are regarded as animal models of the Dubin-Johnson syndrome in humans. Interestingly, erythrocyte membranes from patients with Dubin-Johnson syndrome and from TR⁻ mutant rats exhibited ATP-dependent transport of GS-DNP and GSSG are normal (Board et al., 1992). These results suggested for the first time that GS-X pumps may be encoded by a multiple gene family and erythrocyte and hepatic GS-X pumps are encoded by distinct genes. This turned out to be true, as will be discussed below, the hepatic GS-X pump (encoded by the *MRP2* gene) is not expressed in erythrocytes which express MRP1.

The GS-X pump transports hydrophobic substrates with two negative charges (Oude Elferink et al., 1989; Ishikawa et al., 1990; Kitamura et al., 1990). Transport can be inhibited by orthovanadate and an onic organic substrates but not be neutral amphophilic compounds that are known substrates of P-glycoprotein (P-gp) encoded by MDR1 (Heijn et al., 1992; Ishikawa, 1989, 1992). Moreover, photoaffinity labeling of membrane protein from mastocytoma cells with [³H]LTC₄ revealed a 190-kDa protein (Leier et al., 1994), that differed from the 175-kDa of P-gp. These results suggest that GS-X pumps are functionally distinct from the well-known P-glycoprotein.

III. MOLECULAR CLONING AND IDENTIFICATION OF GS-X PUMP, THE MULTIDRUG-RESISTANT PROTEIN (MRP)

While function of GS-X pumps as transporters for endogenous metabolites was clearly demonstrated early on. Its role as transporter of xenobiotics was more difficult to demonstrate, although early studies had shown that GSH and GST are directly involved in cellular resistance to antitumor agents such as cisplatin, alkylating agents (Godwin et al., 1992; Perez et al., 1990) and anthracyclines (Lee et al., 1989). Ishikawa and Ali-Osman (1993) demonstrated that conjugation of cisplatin and GSH were eliminated by a GS-X pump(s), but purification of the GS-X pump protein remained difficult because of the lack of a convenient in vitro assay system. In 1992, Cole et al., by using differential screening approach, cloned a cDNA encoding a message with deduced protein of 190 kDa, which they named MRP, that was overexpressed in doxorubicin-resistant cell line (Cole et al., 1992). Sequence analyses of MRP revealed it to be an ABC transporter, with closer similarity to that of cystic fibrosis transmembrane conductance regulator than to P-glycoprotein-encoded MDR1.

Further studies demonstrated that membrane vesicles prepared from MRP-transfected cells exhibited elevated transport activities for GSH-conjugates such as LTC_4 and GS-DNP (Leier et al., 1994; Muller et al, 1994) and steroid conjugate 17-beta-glucuronosyl [^{3}H]estradiol, bile salt conjugates 6-alpha-[^{14}C]glucuronosylhypodeoxy-cholate, and 3-alpha-sulfatolithocholyl [^{3}H]taurine (Jedlitschky et al., 1996; Deeley and Cole 2006). These studies demonstrated that the newly cloned cDNA was related to that long-sought GS-X pump that transports LTC_4 and GS-DNP.

The completion of the Human Genome project and advances in bioinformatics enabled researchers to identify a total of 48 ABC transporters in the human genome, classified into seven groups, ABCA through ABCG. It is now known that MPR belongs to the C group of ABC transporter superfamily. This group contains 13 members, of which nine are MRP-related, designed MRP1 through MRP9 (ABCC1-6, and ABCC10-12, respectively). The other three are CFTR (ABCC7), sulfonylurea receptor 1 (SUR1, ABCC8) and SUR2 (ABCC9). ABCC13, which is highly expressed in fetal liver, encodes an open reading frame of 325 amino acids. ABCC13 is most probably a pseudo gene (Yabuuchi et al. 2002).

All of the MRP proteins contain two ATP-binding cassettes in the intracellular part and two core membrane-spanning domains MSD_1 and MSD_2. In addition, MRP1-3, 6, and 7 contain one additional membrane-spanning domain (MSD_0) (Figure 2). Topologically, MSD_0 is not essential for the catalytic function of MRP1, because deleting this domain does not compromise its LTC4 transport activity (Bakos et al. 1998). However, mutations at certain Cys residues within MSD_0 drastically reduce LTC_4 transport activities (Yang, et al., 2002; Leslie et al, 2003), and photoaffinity labeling study demonstrated that MSD_0 interacts with photoreactive azido analogue of LTC_4 (Karwatsky et al., 2005), suggesting that MSD_0 may not be entirely functionless.

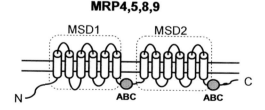

(A)

Figure 2. (Continued)

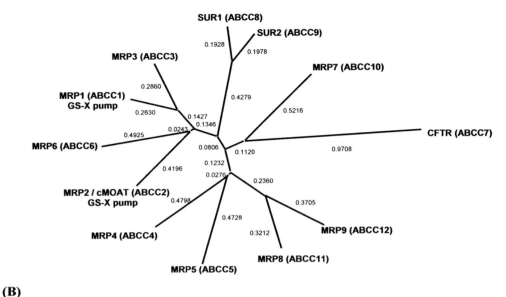

(B)

Figure 2. Structures of the MRPs (A) and phylogenic tree of the ABCC subfamily, including CFTR, SUR1, SUR2, and MRPs (B). MRP1, 2, 3, 6, and 7 have a total of 17 transmembrane regions (cylinders), clustered into three membrane-spanning domains (MSD0 to MSD2), and two intracellular ABCs. MRP4, 5, 8, and 9 have 12 transmembrane regions, as they lack MSD0. The phylogenic tree was modified from Ishikawa (2003).

As the MRPs have been reviewed in many recent articles (Borst et al, 2000; Kruh and Belinsky, 2003; Borst and Efferink, 2003; Borst et al., 2000, 2006; Deeley and Cole, 2006), we will only briefly review these MRPs here. We will focus our review on the role of GSH playing in MRP transport and regulation of MRP genes expression.

ROLES OF GLUTATHIONE IN DRUG TRANSPORT BY MRP GENE FAMILY

MRP1 (ABCC1)

The expression of MRP1 is ubiquitous. While MRP1-overexpressing cells exhibit resistance to many antitumor agents including doxorubicin, vincristine, etoposide, campathecin, and methotrexate, MRP1 transports GSH conjugates such as LTC_4, GS-prostaglandine A_2, glucuronide conjugates such as 17β-estradiol-17-□-glucuronide, and sulfate conjugates such as estron-3-sulfate and sulfatolithocholate. Mice lacking MRP1 are viable and fertile, but have a defective imflammatory response to LTC_4, which is an endogenous substrate of MRP1 (Wijnholds et al., 1997).

The roles of GSH in MRP1-mediated drug sensitivity in cultured cells were demonstrated that drug resistance in MRP1-overproducing cells can be partially reversed by exposing the cells to buthionine sulfoximine (BSO), an inhibitor of GSH synthesis. The effect of BSO on drug resistance was associated with a decreased GSH levels and an increased intracellular accumulation of daunorubicin owing to inhibition of the enhanced drug efflux. Increased GSH levels in BSO-treated cells by exposing cells in GSH ethyl ester restored the accumulation deficit of daunorubicin (Versantwoort et al, 1995).

MRP1 was initially shown to transport glutathionyl, glucuronide, and sulfate conjugates (Leier et al, 1994; Muller et al., 1994), suggesting that covalent conjugation reactions may be required. Later, it was found that GSH does not have to be covalently linked to substrates for transport. Uptake of vincristine into membrane vesicles prepared from MRP1- overproducing cells is poor; in the presence of GSH, the uptake can be greatly enhanced (Loe et al, 1996). Likewise, Loe et al. (2000) found that verapamil stimulates transport of GSH by MRP1 and no GSH transport was detectable in the absence of verapamil. This raises the possibilities as whether GSH functions as a co-transport or a factor that stimulates the transport of the others. The co-transporter mechanism was based on the findings that transport of substrates requires GSH and substrates can also increase the transport of GSH. However, such reciprocal stimulation of transport was not found in the transport of nitrosamine metabolite, NNAL-O-glucuronide (Leslie et al. 2001). Likewise, conjugated estrogen, estrone-3-sulfate, could be efficiently transported only in the presence of GSH; but there is no reciprocal increase in MRP1-mediated GSH transport (Qian et al., 2001). These findings support a regulatory role for GSH in MRP1 function.

Leslie et al (2003) investigated the GSH-binding domain of MRP1 using a variety of amino acid substitutions in the tripeptide and concluded that, while other factors are contributory to the overall interactions, the molecular volume of the tripeptide is most important for supporting MRP1 transport activity. Substituting the γ-Glu residues with Gly, β-Asp, and γ-Glu resulted in a complete loss of transport stimulation of MRP-mediated transport of estron 3-sulfate, whereas substitution with Cys residue had no effect. These observations suggest that stimulation of MRP1 transport activity by is dependent upon the stereospecificity of GSH.

How can GSH regulate the transport activity of MRP1? One model may be the allosteric effect induced by GSH. GSH may induce conformational changes of MRP1 that render more accessible to substrate binding, or enhance its affinity to the substrate binding. In supporting this view, conformational changes were detected by direct measurement of proteolytic accessibility of MRP1. Ren et al. (2005) observed that GSH inhibited the digestion of the L_o region which links MSD_0 and MSD_1 of MRP1 in purified membrane vesicle by trypsin. Using reconstituted lipid vesicles with an inside-out MRP1 configuration, Manciu et al. (2003) showed that GSH binding induces a conformational change of MRP1 that affects the structural organization of the cytosolic domains and enhances ATP binding and/or hydrolysis.

MRP2 (ABCC2)

MRP2 is mainly expressed in the liver and kidneys (Kuo, et al., 1996) which contain polarized cells. The MRP2 is localized in the apical surface, predominantly in the canalicular membrane of hepatocytes. The major physiological function of this protein is to transport conjugated metabolites into the bile canaliculus in the livers. Rats with impaired MRP2 expression show defects in hepatobiliary extrusion of bilirubin glucuronide and developed Dubin-Johnson syndrome (Karwatsky et al., 1996).

MRP2, like MRP1, actively transports LTC_4 and other glutathionyl derivative such as N-ethylmaleimide glutathione (NEM-GS). However, the relative affinity of MRP2 for these substrates was found to be significantly lower than that of MRP1. In contrast, methotrexate was actively transported by both proteins, although more efficiently by MRP2. NEM-GS transport by MRP2 was greatly stimulated by sulfinpyranzone, penicillin G, and indomethacin; but not by GSH. These results indicate that MRP1 is a more efficient transporter of glutathione conjugates and free glutathione than MRP2 (Bakos, et al. 2000).

Bodo et al (2003) found bile salt transport by MRP2 in membrane vesicle can be stimulated by $E_2 17\beta G$ and active $E_2 17\beta G$ transport by MRP2 can be reciprocally stimulated by several conjugates of bile acids. This suggested an allosteric cross-stimulation mechanism in which bile acids and glucuronide conjugates are co-transported. However, Zelcer et al. (2003) found that compounds that stimulate transport of substrates by MRP2 are not necessarily themselves transported by MRP2. In vesicular transport assays, these investigators found that taurocholate, penicillin G and pantoprazole are good stimulators of $E_2 17\beta G$ transport by MRP2, but these compounds are not transported by MRP2, suggesting that they allosterically stimulate transport may involve two distinct binding sites: one for drug transport and the other for allosteric regulation of the former.

MRP3 (ABCC3)

The general structural organization of MRP3 is similar to those of MRP1 and MRP2, but the substrate specificity of MRP3 is not entirely similar to those of MRP1 and MRP2. MRP3 transports $E_2 17\beta G$, LTC4, GS-DNP. However, unlike MRP1, transport of $E_2 17\beta G$ by MRP3 is not stimulated by GSH. Likewise, etoposide appears to be transported by MRP3 in unmodified form and requires no GSH (Zelcer et al., 2001), suggesting that the hypothetical co-transport mechanism for MRP1 is not valid for MRP3.

The other difference between MRP2 and MRP3 lies on their expression sites in polarized cells. In the livers, MRP2 is expressed in the canalicular compartment and is involved in the transport of organic anionic conjugated compounds into the bile. MRP3 is expressed in the basolateral membrane and seems to have a compensatory transport function by transport into the sinusoidal blood. Moreover, while organic anions that actively stimulate transport of $E_2 17\beta G$ by MRP2, these compounds inhibit its transport by MRP3. And there is no cross-stimulation of bile acid transport by MRP3.

MRP3 may be the major transporter involved in basolateral transport of organic anions in the liver, because animals deficient in MRP3 have defects in transport of morphine-3-glucuronide in the liver into the blood stream (Zelcer et al, 2005). It may be of relevance that another transporters that also located at the basolateral side of hepatocyte is the organic anion transporting peptide Oatp1 (SLC21A1) which transport GSH in exchange for organic anions (Li et al., 1998).

MRP4 (ABCC4) and MRP5 (ABCC5)

Perhaps because of the absence of MSD_0 domains in MRP4 and MRP5 these transporters display distinct substrate specificities and drug resistance profiles from those of MRP1, MRP2, and MRP3. MRP4 and MRP5 are capable of transporting organic anionic compounds, such as glucuronide, and sulfate conjugates of steroids, such as $E_217\beta G$ and DHEAS, MRP4 and MRP5 are important transporters of cAMP and cGMP (Guo, et al., 2003; Chen et al., 2001; Jedlitschky et al., 2000).

The roles of GSH in MRP4- and MRP5-mediated cyclic nucleotide transport have not been well-established. Intracellular GSH levels are reduced in MRP4- and MRP5-transfected cells, suggesting that GSH is a substrate of these transporters (Lai and Tan, 2002; Wijnholds et al., 2000), but the requirements of GSH for cyclic nucleotide transports are low. Using membrane vesicles prepared from MRP4-transfected Chinese hamster cells in transport assay, Rius et al. (2003) reported that mono-anionic bile salt taurocholate is transported by MRP4 in the presence of GSH and its analogs, methyl-SG and ophthalmic acid. More recently, these authors reported that human MRP4 has a high affinity for the taurine and glycine conjugates of the common natural bile acids and for the unconjugated bile acid cholate in the presence of physiological concentrations of GSH. Chenodeoxycholyltaurine and chenodeoxycholylglycine were the GSH co-substrates with the highest affinities for MRP4 (Ruis et al. 2006). These results are consistent with GSH being required for the co-transport of these organic anions. However, no depletion of GSH levels was found in MRP4-transfected HEK293 cells and no requirement for GSH in MRP4-mediated transport of steroid and bile-acid conjugates was observed in transport assays using membranes prepared from MRP4- or MRP5- overexpressing cells (Wielinga et al, 2003). The requirements of GSH in MRP4 and MRP5 mediated transport remains to be investigated. MRP4 is also expressed in the basolateral membrane of the choroid plexus epithelium and in the brain capillary endothelium. Laggars et al. (2004) showed that *Mrp4* (-/-) animals effectively limit the movement of topotecan from the blood into the brain tissue and cerebrospinal fluid, resulting in accumulation of topotecan in the brain. These results suggest that MRP4 transports not only cyclic nucleotides but also antitumor agents.

MRP6 (ABCC6) and MRP7 (ABCC10)

Like MRP2, MRP6 is expressed in the liver and kidneys. Animals with ablated MRP6 by knockout technology develop mineralization in connective skin, a phenotype resembling pseudoxanthoma elasticum syndrome (Klement et al., 2005). Expression of MRP7 is ubiquitous but high in pancreas among the adult and fetal tissues. Increased MRP7 expression was detected in doxorubicin-treated MCF7 cells, suggesting that it may be involved in resistance to antitumor agents (Takayanagi et al., 2004). Belinsky et al. (2002) demonstrated that MRP6 transports GS-conjugates such as LTC_4 and GS-DNP but not glucuronide conjugates such as $E_217\beta G$, suggesting that MRP6 is also a GS-X pump. On the other hand, MRP7 can transport $E_217\beta G$, and by comparison only modest transport LTC_4 (Chen et al., 2003). The roles of GSH for the function of these transporters have not been as well characterized as other MRP transporters.

MRP8 (ABCC11)

MRP8 (ABCC11) as well as MRP9 (ABCC12) were cloned from a cDNA library of human adult liver (Yabuuchi et al. 2001). These two genes are located in a tandem tail-to-head orientation on human chromosome 16q12.1. The predicted amino acid sequences of both gene products show a high similarity to those of MRP4 and MRP5 (Figure 2B). However, it appears that no putative mouse orthologous gene corresponding to human *ABCC11* (Shimizu et al. 2003).

Because of these structural similarities, it would anticipate that the substract specificities would be related to MRP4 and MRP5. This indeed has been the case. Ectopic expression of MRP8 in mammalian cells enhances cellular efflux of cyclic nucleotides and confers resistance to certain anticancer and antiviral nucleotide analogs (Guo et al., 2003). Interestingly, a single nucleotide polymorphism in MRP8 (G538A) is associated with dry earwax phenotype in humans, and GA and GG to wet type. Functional assay demonstrated that cells with allele A show a lower excretory activity for cGMP than those with allele G, consistent with its roles as cGMP transporter (Yoshiura et al., 2006). In addition, MRP8 is able to transport a range of glutathione and glucuronate conjugates, monoionic bile acids, and other amphipathic anionic compounds (Chen et al., 2005).

MRP9 (ABCC12)

Like MRP8, the predicted amino acid sequence of MRP9 shows a similarity with those of MRP4 and MRP5 (Figure 2B). MRP9 is expressed in many normal human tissues. However, its biological role, substrate specificity, and requirement of GSH, is not known. Shimizu et al. (2003) recently cloned and characterized Mrp9 (*Abcc12*), a mouse orthologue of human MRP9 (*ABCC12*). The cloned *Abcc12* cDNA was 4511-bp long, comprising a 4,101-bp open reading frame. The deduced peptide consists of 1367 amino acids and exhibits high sequence identity (84.5%) with human MRP9. The mouse *Abcc12* gene consists of at least 29 exons and is located on the mouse chromosome 8D3 locus where conserved linkage homologies have hitherto been identified with human chromosome 16q12.1 (Shimizu et al., 2003). The mouse *Abcc12* gene was expressed at high levels exclusively in the seminiferous tubules in the testis. The function of MRP12 remains to be elucidated.

Questions Remaining to be Elucidated

So what have we learned from these studies? It is clear that the roles of GSH in MRP transports vary among different members of the MRP family. Moreover, in members which require GSH for enhancement, the extents of enhancement vary from one to others; and in some cases, it appears that GSH is involved in co-transport; but in others, in allosteric stimulation. Even more complex is that some members of MRP prefer glucuronide conjugates to GSH conjugates for transports. These observations underscore the diversity of MRP transport systems.

The question, then, is why such complex transport systems exist. For one thing, animals without many of these MRP transporters, including MRP1 (Wijhholds et al., 1997), MRP3

(Zelcer, et al., 2005) and MRP4 (Laggas, et al., 2004), are apparently normal and fertile, suggesting that these transporters exert no selection pressure during evolution because of functional redundancy. For the other, there are transporters such as ABCB1 which encodes P-glycoprotein that transports unmodified xenobiotic compounds without GSH. However, one should not downplay the importance of GS-X pumps. Perhaps animals need these many different GS-X pumps to share the task of transporting enormous amounts of diverse endogenous metabolites and to handle the constant challenges of exogenous insults by xenobiotics.

V. REGULATION OF γ-GLUTAMYLCYSTEINE SYNTHETASE GENE EXPRESSION

To learn how GSH regulates expression of the MRP gene family, it is helpful to understand mechanisms that regulate biosynthesis of GSH. *De novo* synthesis of GSH is regulated by the rate-limiting enzyme, γ-glutamylcysteine synthetase (γ-GCS). The mammalian γ-GCS is a heterodimer consisting of one 73-kDa heavy or catalytic subunit (γ-GCSh) (Huang et al., 1993a; Gipps et al., 1992) and one 28-kDa light (regulatory) subunit (Huang et al., 1993b; Gipps et al. 1995). Hereditary γ-GCSh deficiency is associated with anemia, jaundice, and neurological abnormalities (Hamilton et al., 2003; Ristoff et al., 2000), whereas totally γ-GCSh deficient in knockout mice is embryonic lethal (Shi et al., 2000; Dalton et al., 2002).

We previously demonstrated that expression of γ-GCSh can be induced by many cytotoxic agents, including antitumor agents (Gomi et al., 1997; Ishikawa et al., 1996), heavy metals (Ishikawa et al., 1996), carcinogens (Yamane et al., 1998) and prooxidants (Yamane et al., 1998; Tatebe et al., 2002; Ikegami et al., 2000). Furthermore, enhanced expression of γ-GCSh mRNA was found in colorectal cancers (Kuo et al., 1996; Tatebe et al, 2002). All these inducers, at the concentrations used, exert various extents of oxidative stresses. These observations strongly suggested that GSH/γ-GCS system is a molecular sensor of oxidative stress conditions. While elevated expression of γ-GCSh catalyzes the enhanced expression of GSH, importantly, we observed that increased GSH levels feedback and downregulate the steady-state γ-GCSh mRNA level (Yamane et al., 1998) in addition to suppressing γ-GCSh enzymatic activities as reported previously (Huang et al. 1993; Meister, 2000). This feedback mechanism underscores the importance of γ-GCSh as a major redox regulator.

Transcriptional Regulation

Previous studies of γ-GCSh gene regulation have mainly focused on transcriptional regulation. Transcriptional upregulation of γ-GCSh expression is mediated by an antioxidant response element (ARE) located at -3802 bp (Mulcahy et al., 1997; Wild et al., 1999), although other investigators also reported the involvement of an AP-1 binding site (Tomonari et al., 1997; Urata et al., 1999; Rahman et al., 1996) at the 5' side of the γ-GCSh gene. The ARE contains a consensus sequence 5'-TGAGTCA which is a target of the transcription factor, NF-E2-related factors (Nrf2). That Nrf2 is involved in γ-GCS expression in vivo is supported by the northern blot analyses of liver γ-GCSh and γ-GCSl mRNA that show 58% and 65%, respectively, reduction in Nrf2(-/-) cells as compared with the wild-type control cells (Chan et al. 2001).

The transcription factor Nrf2 is a member of the "cap 'n' collar" family of basic leucine zipper transcription factors. The mechanisms by which Nrf2 upregulates antioxidant enzyme genes have been intensively studied in the recent years (for reviews, see refs in Jaiswal, 2004; Nguyen et al. 2004; Giudice and Montella, 2006). Nrfs bind to ARE and regulate ARE-mediated antioxidant enzyme genes both at the basal levels and under conditions where upregulation is stimulated by a variety of antioxidants. Nrf2 is an unstable protein, and whose stability can be enhanced by proteasome inhibitor lactacystin. Treatment with lactacystin resulted in increased steady-state levels of γ-GCSh mRNA (Sekhar et al., 2000). Under normal conditions, Nrf2 is bound to Keap1, a cytosolic actin-associated protein (Itoh et al., 1999; Wakabayashi et al., 2004). Oxidative stress disrupts Keap1-Nrf2 interactions allowing Nrf2 to heterodimerize with small Maf proteins, Mafk or MafG co-activativator (Nguyen et al., 2000; Moran et al., 2001; Zipper and Mulcahy 2002) and binds to ARE whereby transactivates γ-GCSh expression. Similar mechanism are involved in the regulation of expression of many so called Phase II detoxifying enzymes, including NQO1, GSTA1, HO-1, etc. that have been extensively studying in the recent years (Nguyen et al., 2004).

Several dynamic mechanisms have been proposed to account for the dissociation of Keap1 from Nrf2 induced by oxidative stress that activates Nrf2 for transcriptional regulation of ARE-dependent genes: (i) First, oxidative stress activates several protein kinases including protein kinase C (Huang et al. 2000; Bloom et al., 2003), p38 mitogen-activated protein kinase (Yu et al., 2000; Zipper and Mulcahy, 2000) and PI-3 kinase (Lee et al., 2001) which phosphorylate Nrf2 and enhance transactivatiion of ARE-containing genes. (ii) Second, oxidative stress disrupts Keap1-Nrf2 interactions by modifying the two crucial cysteine residues of Keap1, resulting in the release of Nrf2, which subsequently translocates into the nucleus (Dinkova-Kostova et al., 2002; Itoh et al., 1999; Wakabayashi et al., 2004) (Figure 3). (iii) Third, Nrf2 is mainly a nuclear protein that supports constitutive basal transcription of genes encoding phase II enzymes. Under normal physiological conditions, Nrf2 is the target for Keap1-induced proteasome-mediated degradation. Oxidative stress prevents Keap1 from targeting Nrf2, resulting in further nuclear accumulation of Nrf2 and transactivation ARE-mediated gene expression (Nguyen et al., 2005).

Recently, Benassi et al. (2006) reported another signal transduction pathway that is involved in the transcriptional activation of both γ-GCS light and heavy subunit genes. These genes contain c-Myc binding sites at their respective promoter regions. Cultured cells exposed to H_2O_2 enhance c-Myc recruitments to these sites by phosphorylating c-Myc at the Ser-62 through ERK-dependent signal. These results identified a new role for c-Myc as an oxidative stress responsive transcription factor, in addition to its roles in the regulation of cell growth, differentiation, and apoptosis.

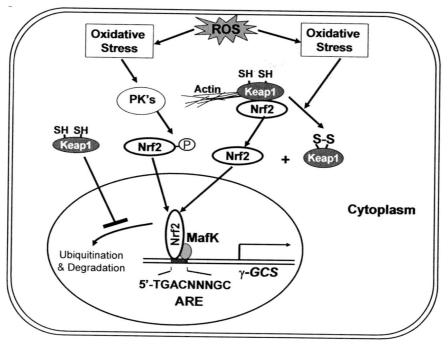

Figure 3. Oxidative stress-induced transcriptional activation of □-GCS expression. Activation of □-GCS involves transcription factor Nrf2, which is complexed with Keap1 and bound by cytoplasmic actin. Oxidative stress induces dissociation of Keap1 from Nrf2, either by phosphorylation of Nrf2 or by conformational changes in Keap1. The released Nrf2 translocates into nucleus, heterodimerizes with MafK, and activates the expression of □-GCS. Alternatively, oxidative stress may activate Keap1, which suppresses the ubiquitination and degradation of Nrf2. These mechanisms result in nuclear accumulation of Nrf2 and subsequent transcriptional activation.

Posttranscriptional Regulation

While oxidative stress-induced gene regulation can be at the translational levels, other studies demonstrated that posttranscriptional mechanisms also involved in oxidative stress-related gene regulation. Oxidative stress induced by glucose deprivation in cultured cells increases vascular endothelial growth factor mRNA stability (Yun et al., 2005) but reduces insulin growth factor-1 mRNA stability (Wang et al., 2000). Increased stability of extracellular superoxide dismutase mRNA, but not manganese superoxide dismutase mRNA, is associated with changes of cellular redox conditions by the treatment of 17β-estradiol (Strehlow et al., 2003).

Oxidative stress-induced posttranscriptional regulation of γ-GCSh expression was previously suggested by nuclear run-on assay (Gomi et al., 1997). However, mechanisms underlying the posttranscriptional regulation by enhancing mRNA stabilization was not known until recent. Song et al. (2005) reported that oxidative stress-inducing agents, e.g., sulindac, pyrrolidinediethiocarbamate, tert-butylhydroquinone, induced γ-GCSh mRNA stabilization by the p38 MAP kinase pathways. The p38 MAP kinase activates. MAPKAPK2 which promotes cytoplasmic translocation of mRNA stabilizing factor HuR from the nucleus to cytoplasm where it interacts with the AU-rich sequence located at the 3' untranslated region of γ-GCSh mRNA. The accumulated γ-GCSh mRNA produces elevated levels of GSH which in turn suppresses oxidative stress and also feedback to suppress γ-GCSh mRNA stabilization.

VI. ROLE OF GLUTATHIONE IN REGULATION OF MRP EXPFRESSION

Several lines of evidence suggest that MRP1 expression is also regulated by oxidative stress. (i) Our laboratories have demonstrated that the many cytotoxic agents that induce γ-GCSh expression also induce MRP1 expression (Yamane et al., 1996; Gomi et al., 1997; Kuo et al., 1998; Lin-Lee et al., 2001, Tatebe et al., 2002, 2003). The coexpression between γ-GCSh and MRP1 pattern also found in human malignant tissues. Kuo et al. (1996) reported that among 32 cases of human colorectal cancer biopsies, 78% of cases showed co-elevated expression of MRP1 and γ-GCSh in tumor samples as compared with their corresponding adjacent naïve normal samples (Figure 4). (ii) Overexpression of reduced GSH can be achieved by transfecting expression γ-GCSh cDNA into cultured cell. γ-GCSh transfected cells exhibit reduced intracellular redox conditions and concomitant downregulation of endogenous γ-GCS and MRP1 mRNA. The observations that γ-GCSh and MRP1 are often co-expressed strongly support the initial belief of GS-X pump for the detoxification mechanism of xenobiotics (Figure 1). When cells are under oxidative stress conditions, as reflected by elevated intracellular ROS levels, GSH provides a front line defense mechanism by chelating H_2O_2 which oxidizes GSH into GSSG. GSSG is then eliminated by GS-X pump transporter. As the GS-X pump is also involved in the elimination of cytotoxic glutathionyl agents, this requires upregulation of γ-GCS expression to supply the needed GSH. Thus, from a toxicological point of view, the coexpression between γ-GCSh and GS-X pump seen in many inducible systems is entirely understandable.

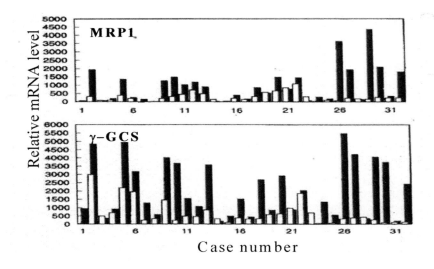

A

Figure 4. Continued.

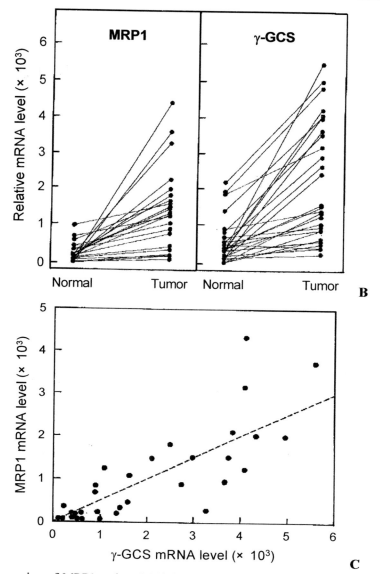

Figure 4. Coexpression of MRP1 and □-GCSh in coloctrectal cancer. A. RNase protection assay to detect MRP1 and □-GCSh mRNA in human colorectal cancer tissues. Both malignant tissues and their corresponding naïve normal tissues were corrected from 32 patients. Levels of mRNA were normalized to those of 28S ribosomal RNA. Relative mRNA levels of MRP1 and γ-GCSh were determined from the corresponding signals in autoradiograms by densitometric measurement. B. Association between relative mRNA levels of MRP1 and γ-GCSh in malignant tissues and their corresponding naïve normal tissues for each sample. C. Correlation between MRP1 and □-GCSh mRNA in the specimens shown in B (see Kuo et al. 1996).

The co-expression profiles between γ-GCSh and the GS-X pump extends to other members of the MRP family. Lin-Lee et al. (2001) investigated the expression profiles of MRP1, MRP2, MRP3, MRP4, MRP5, and MRP6 in HCT116 colorectal cancer cells treated with tert-butylhydroquinone and pyrrolidinedithiocarbamate, and reported that besides MRP1, expression of MRP2 and MRP3 are also induced by these oxidative stress-inducing agents;

wheras no induction was observed with MRP4 and MRP5. Levels of MRP6 were too low to be detected in these cell lines. Interestingly, GSH is not as important for MRP4 and MRP5 transport (Kruh and Belinsky, 2003) as it is for for MRP1, MRP2, and MRP6. These observations are consistent with the evolution of the GS-X pump as discussed above.

The observations that γ-GCSh and MRP1 are co-expressed in many systems suggest that these two genes are coordinately regulated. The MRP1 promoters of human (Zhu and Center, 1994, 1996; Kurz et al., 2001), and mouse and rat (Muredda et al., 2003) have been cloned, and several cis-acting elements for the basal transcription of these genes have been identified. While ARE/AP-1 like sequences have been found upstream from the transcription start sites of these genes, but these sequences do not response to the induced expression of MRP1 in transient transfection assays using reporter constructs (Kurz et al., 2001; Kauffmann et al., 2002).

Despite the inability of identifying authentic ARE sequence for MRP1, Nrf2 is thought to be involved in its regulation. Hayashi et al. (2003) reported that the constitutive expression levels of murine MRP1 mRNA are significantly lower in Nrf2(-/-) cells than that in the wild-type cells. Induction levels of MRP1 expression by diethyl maleate in Nrf2(-/-) cells were significantly reduced, suggesting a role of Nrf2 in the regulation of murine MRP1 by oxidative stress. However, whether Nrf2 is involved in the regulation of human MRP1 expression remains to be demonstrated.

Likewise, an ARE sequence in the mouse *Mrp2* gene promoter that responses to chemical-induced oxidative stress has been identified. This ARE contains an Nrf2-binding site and expression of Nrf2 up-regulates Mrp2 expression (Vollrath et al., 2006). However, no ARE sequence has been identified in the human MRP2 promoter (Kauffmann et al., 2002; Tanaka et al., 1999). Regulation of other MRP genes remains to be investigated.

CONCLUSIONS

The discovery of GS-X pump that requires GSH as a cofactor for transporting a group of endogenous substrates and exogenous xenobiotics has resulted in the cloning of the MRP transporter family. It is now known that the MRP transporter family consists of nine members. While, as a while, members of MRP share structural and functional similarities, i.e., they all contain multiple membrane spanning domains and two intracellularly localized ATP-binding cassettes (ABC) and function as energy-dependent efflux transporters. However, no two members have exactly the same tissue-specific expression patterns and substrate specificities. The requirements of GSH for transport also differ among the MRPs. Thus, the initially described GS-X pump has evolved into a multiple gene family with a broad transport spectrum that are involved in a wide range of physiological functions including cytotoxical defense mechanisms against everlasting insults by cytotoxic xenobiotics.

Many members of the MRP family require GSH for transports. However, the complexity that why in some cases GSH serves as a cotransporter; but an allosteric cofactor by altering substrate binding affinities to MRPs in others remains a challenge in understanding the roles of GSH in the activities of MRP transporters. Future studies are needed to delineate the molecular bases as how GSH is required for the transports by some MRP but not by the others; and why it is needed by some substrates but not by the others for the same transporter.

GSH not only functions as a cofactor for MRP transport, but also plays important roles in regulating the expression of some members in the MRP gene family, especially MRP1, MRP2 and MRP3. In many examples, expression of these genes is often coordinated with γ-GCSh. While substantial advance in understanding γ-GCSh gene regulation under oxidative stress has been learned, mechanisms that regulate MRP genes remains largely unknown. As the intimate relationships between GSH and GS-X pump/MRP has been established, understanding molecular bases how GSH levels regulate MRP gene expression is deemed to be necessary.

REFERENCES

Akerboom TPM; Bilzer M; Siev s H. Competition between transport of glutathione disulfide (GSSG) and glutathione S-conjugates from perfused rat liver into bile. *FEBS Lett.* 1982; 140: 73-76.

Bakos, E; Evers, R; Sinko, E; Varadi, A; Borst, P; Sarkadi, B. Interactions of the human multidrug resistance proteins MRP1 and MRP2 with organic anions. *Mol. Pharmacol* 2000; 57:760-768.

Bakos, E; Evers, R; Szakacs, G;Tusnady, GE; Welker, E; Szabo, K; de Haas, M; van Deemter, L; Borst, P; Varadi, A; Sarkadi, B.l. Functional multidrug resistance protein (MRP1) lacking the N-terminal transmembrane domain. *J Biol Chem* 1998; 273:32167-32175.

Belinsky, MG; Chen, ZS; Shchaveleva, I; Zeng, H; Kruh, GD. Characterization of the drug resistance and transport properties of multidrug resistance protein 6 (MRP6, ABCC6). *Cancer Res.* 2002; 62:6172-6177.

Benassi, B; Fanciulli, MF; Fiorentino, F; Porrello, A; Chiorino, G; Loda, M; Zupi, G; Biroccio, A. c-Myc phosphorylation is required for cellular response to oxidative stress. *Mol. Cell* 2006; 21: 509-519.

Bloom DA; Jaiswal AK. Phosphorylation of Nrf2 at Ser 40 by protein kinase C in response to antioxidants leads to the release of Nrf2 from INrf2, but is not required for Nrf2 stabilization/accumulation in the nucleus and transcriptional activation of antioxidant response element-mediated NAD(P)H:quinine oxidoreductase-1 gene expression. *J. Biol. Chem.* 2003; 278:44675-44682, 2003.

Board P. Transport of glutathione S-conjugate from human erythrocytes. *FEBS Lett.* 1981; 124: 163-165.

Board P; Nishida T; Gatmaitan Z; Che M; Arias IM. Erythrocyte membrane transport of glutathione conjugates and oxidized glutathione in the Dubin-Johnson syndrome and in rats with hereditary hyperbilirubinemia. *Hepatology* 1992; 15: 722-725.

Bodo, A; Bakos, E; Zseri, F; Varadi, A; Sarkadi, B. Differential modulation of the liver conjugate transporters MRP2 and MRP3 by bile acids and organic anions. *J. Biol. Chem.,* 2003; 278: 23529-23537.

Borst, P.; Evers, R; Kool, M; Wijnholds, J. A family of drug transporters: the multidrug resistance-associated proteins. *J. Natl. Natl. Inst.* 2000; 92:1295-1302.

Borst, P; Elferink, RO. Mammalian ABC transporters in health and disease. *Annu. Rev. Biochem.* 2002; 71:537-592.

Borst, P; Zelcer, N; van de Wetering, K; Poolman, B. On the putative co-transport of drugs by multidrug resistance proteins. *FEBS Lett.* 2006 (in press)

Buchler, M; Konig, J; Brom, M; Kartenbeck, J; Spring, H; Horie, T; Keppler, D. cDNA cloning of the hepatocyte canalicular isoform of the multidrug resistance protein, cMRP, reveals a novel conjugate export pump. *J. Biol. Chem.* 1996: 271: 15091-15098.

Chan, K; Han X-D; Kan YW. An important function of Nrf2 in combating oxidative stress: Detoxification of acetaminophen. Proc. Natl. Acad. USA 2001; 98:4611-4616, 2001.

Chance B; Sies H; Boveris A. Hydroperoxide metabolism in mammalian organs. *Physiol. Rev.* 1979; 59, 527-605.

Chen, ZS; Guo, Y; Belinsky, MG; Kotova, E; Kruh, GD. Transport of Bile Acids, Sulfated Steroids, Estradiol 17-β-D-Glucuronide, and Leukotriene C4 by Human Multidrug Resistance Protein 8 (ABCC11). Mol. Pharmacol. 2005; 67:545-557.

Chen, ZS; Hopper-Borge, E; Belinsky, MG; Shchaveleva, I; Kotova, E; Kruh, GD. Characterization of the transport properties of human multidrug resistance protein 7 (MRP7, ABCC10). *Cancer Res.* 2003; 63:351-358.

Chen, ZS; Lee, K; Kruh, GD. Transport of cyclic nucleotides and estradiol 17-β-D-glucuronide by multidrug resistance protein 4, resistance to 6-mercaptopurine and 6-thiogluanine. *J. Biol. Chem.* 2001; 276:33747-33754.

Cole, SP; Bhardway, JH; Gerlach JE: Mackie JE; Grant CE: Almquist KC; Stewart AJ; Kruz, EU; Duncan, AM; Deeley RG. Overexpression of a transporter gene in a multidrug-resistant human lung cancer cell line. *Science* 1992; 258:1650-1654.

Dalton, TP; Dieter, MZ; Yang, Y; Schertzer, HG; and Nebert, DW. Knockout of the mouse glutamate cysteine ligase catalytic subunit (Gclc) gene: embryonic lethal when homozygous, and proposed model for moderate glutathione deficiency when heterozygous. *Biochem. Biophys. Res. Commun.* 2002; 279:324-329.

Deeley, RG, Cole, SPC. Substrate recognition and transport by multidrug resistance protein 1 (ABCC1). FEBS Lett. 2006 (in press).

Dinkova-Kostova, AT; Holtzclaw, WD; Cole, RN; Itoh K; Wakabayashi, N; Katoh, Y; Yamamoto, M; Talalay, P. Direct evidence that sufhydryl groups of keap1 are the sensors regulating induction of phase 2 enzymes that protect against carcinogens and oxidants. *Proc. Natl. Acad. Sci. USA.* 2002; 99: 11908-11913.

Droge, W. Free radicals in the physiological control of cell function. *Physiol. Rev.* 2002; 82:47-95, 2002.

Elferink RPO; Ottenhoff R; Liefting W.; de Haan J; Jansen PLM. Hepatobiliary transport of glutathione and glutathione conjugate in rats with hereditary hyperbilirubinemia. *J. Clin. Invest.* 1989; 84: 476-483.

Fahey RC; Sundquist AR. Evolution of glutathione metabolism. *Adv. Enzymol. Relat. Mol. Biol.* 1991; 64: 1-53.

Finkel, T. Oxidant signals and oxidative stress. Curr. Opin. Cell Biol. 2003; 15:247-254.

Gipps, JJ; Bailey, HH; Mulcahy, RT. Cloning and nucleotide sequence of a full-length cDNA for human liver gamma-glutamylcysteine synthetase. *Biochem. Biophys. Res. Commun.* 1992; 198:29-35.

Gipps, JJ; Chang, C; Mulcahy, RT. Cloning and sequencing of the cDNA for the light subunit of human liver gamma-glutamylcysteine synthetase and relative mRNA levels for heavy and light subunits in human normal tissues. *Biochem. Biophys. Res. Commun.* 1995; 206:584-589.

Giudice, A; Montella, M. Activation of the Nrf2-ARE signaling pathway: a promising strategy in Cancer Prevention. *BioEssays* 2006; 28:169-181.

Godwin, AK; Meister, A; O'Dwyer, PJ; Huang, CS; Hamilton, TC; Anderson, ME. High resistance to cisplatin in human ovarian cancer cell lines is associated with marked increase of glutathione synthesis. *Proc. Natl. Acad. Sci* USA 1992; 89:3070-3074.

Gomi, A; Shinoda, S; Masuzawa, T; Ishikawa, T; Kuo, MT. Transient inductionof the MRP-GS-X pump and g-glutamylcysteine synthetase by 1-(4-amino-2-methyl-5-pyrimidinyl)methyl-3-(2-chloroethyl)-3-nitrosourea in human glioma cells. *Cancer Res.* 1997; 57:5292-5299, 1997.

Guo, Y; Kotova, E; Chen, S-S; Lee, K; Hopper-Borge, E; Belinsky, MG; Kruh GD. MRP8, ATP-binding cassette C11 (ABCC11), is a cyclic nucleotide efflux pump and a resistance factor for fluoropyrimidines 2',3' dideoxycytidine and 9'-(2'phosphonylmethoxyethyl) adenine. *J. Biol. Chem.* 2003; 278:29509-29561.

Hamilton, D; Wu, JH; Alaoui-Jamali, M; Batist, G. A novel missense mutation in the g-glutamylcysteine synthetase catalytic subunit gene causes both decreased enzymatic activity and glutathione production. *Blood* 2003; 102:725-730.

Hayashi, A; Suzuki, H; Itoh, K; Yamamoto, M; Sugiyama, Y. Transcription factor Nrf2 is require for the constitutive and inducible expression of multidrug resistance-associated protein 1 in mouse embryo fibroblasts. *Biochem. Biophys. Res. Commun.* 2003; 30:824-829.

Hayes, JD; Flanagan; JU; Jowsey IR. Glutathione transferases. *Annu. Rev. Pharmaco. Toxicol.* 2005; 45:51-88.

Heijn, M; Oude Elferink, RPJ; Jansen, PLM. ATP-dependent multispecific organic anion transport system in rat erythrocyte membrane vesicles. *Am. J. Physiol.* 1992; 262: C104-110.

Houven R; Dijkstra M; Kuipers F; Smit EP; Havinga R; Vonk, RJ. Two pathways for biliary copper excretion in the rat. The role of glutathione. *Biochem Pharmacol.* 1990; 6: 1039-1044.

Huang, CS; Chang, LS; Anderson, ME; Meister A. Catalytic and regulatory properties of the heavy subunit of rat kidney gamma-glutamylcysteine synthetase. *J. Biol. Chem.* 1993a; 268:19675-19680.

Huang, CS; Anderson, ME; Meister, A. Amino acid sequence and function of the light subunit of rat kidney gamma-glutamylcysteine synthetase. *J. Biol. Chem.* 1993b;268:20578-20583.

Huang, HC; Nguyen, T; Pickett CB. Regulation of the antioxidant response element by protein kinase C-mediated phosphorylation of NF-E2 related factor 2. *Proc. Natl. Acad. Sci.* USA 2000; 97:12475-12480.

Huber M; Guhlmann A; Jansen PLM; Keppler D. Hereditary defect of hepatobiliary cysteinyl leukotriene elimination in mutant rats with defective hepatic anion excretion. *Hepatology* 1987; 7: 224-228.

Hwang, C; Sinskey, AJ; Lodish,HF. Oxidized redox state of glutathione in the endoplasmic reticulum. *Science* 1992; 257:1496-1502.

Ikegami, Y; Tatebe, S; Lin-Lee, Y-C; Xie, Q-W; Ishikawa, T; Kuo, MT. Induction of MRP1 and g-glutamylcysteine synthetase gene expression by interleukin 1b is mediated by nitric oxide-related signaling in human colorectal cancer cells. *J. Cell. Physiol.* 2000; 158:293-301.

Ishikawa, T. ATP/Mg^{2+}-dependent cardiac transport system for glutathione S-conjugates. A study uing rat heart sarcolemma vesicles. *J. Biol. Chem.* 1989; 264:17343-17348, 1989.

Ishikawa T. The ATP-dependent glutathione S-conjugate export pump. *Trends Biochem. Sci.* 1992; 17:463-468.

Ishikawa T. Multidrug resistance in cancer: Genetics of ABC transporters. In: *Nature Encyclopedia of the Human Genome,* Nature Publishing Group, London. 2003; vol.4, pp. 154-160.

Ishikawa T; Akimaru K; Nakanishi M; Tomokiyo K; Furuta K; Suzuki M; Noyori R. Anti-cancer prostaglandin-induced cell cycle arrest and its modulation by an inhibitor of the ATP-dependent glutathione S-conjugate export pump (GS-X pump). *Biochem. J.* 1998; 336: 569-576.

Ishikawa, T; Ali-Osman, F. Glutathione-associated cis-diamminedichloroplatinum (II) metabolism and ATP-dependent efflux from leukemia cells. Molecular characterization of glutathione-platinum complex and its biological significance. *J. Biol. Chem.* 1993; 268:20116-20125, 1993.

Ishikawa, T; Bao, J-J; Yamane, Y; Akimaru, K; Frindrich, K; Wright, CD; Kuo, MT. Coordinated induction of MRP/GS-X pump and g-glutamylcysteine synthetase by heavy metals in human leukemia cells. *J. Biol. Chem.* 1996; 271:14981-14988.

Ishikawa T; Esterbauer H; Sies H. Role of cardiac glutathione transferase and of the glutathione S-conjugate export system in biotransformation of 4-hydroxynonenal in the heart. *J. Biol. Chem.* 1986a; 261: 1576-1581.

Ishikawa T; Kobayashi K.; Sogame Y; Hayashi K. Evidence for leukotriene C4 transport mediated by an ATP-dependent glutathione S-conjugate carrier in rat heart and liver plasma membrane vesicles. *FEBS Lett.* 1989; 259: 95-98.

Ishikawa T; Li Z-S; Lu Y-P; Rea PA. The GS-X pump in plant, yeast, and animal cells: structure, function, and gene expression. *Biosci. Rep.* 1997; 17: 189-207

Ishikawa, T; Muller, M; Klunemann, C; Schaub, T; Keppler, D. ATP-dependent primary active transport of cysteinyl leukotrienes across liver canalicular membrane. Role of the ATP-dependent transport system for glutathione S-conjugate. *J. Biol. Chem.* 1990; 265:19279-19286, 1990.

Ishikawa T; Sies H. Cardiac transport of glutathione disulfide and S-conjugate: studies with isolated perfused rat heart during hydroperoxide metabolism. *J. Biol. Chem.* 1984; 259: 3838-3843.

Ishikawa T; Zimmer M; Sies H. Energy-linked cardiac transport system for glutathione disulfide. *FEBS Lett.* 1986b; 200: 128-132.

Itoh, K; Wakabayashi, N; Katoh, Y; Ishii, T; Igarash, K; Yamamoto, M. Keap1 represses nuclear activation of antioxidant responsive elements by Nrf2 through binding to the amino-terminal Neh2 domain. *Genes Dev.*1999; 13:76-86.

Jaiswal AK. Nrf2 signaling in coordinated activation of antioxidant gene expression. *Free Rad Biol Medicine* 2004; 36:1199-1207.

Jansen PLM; Peters WHM; Meijer DKF. Hepatobiliary excretion of organic anions in double-mutant rats with a combination of defective canalicular transport and uridine 5'-diphosphate-glucuronyltransferase deficiency. *Gastroenterology 1987a*; 93: 1094-1103.

Jansen PLM; Groothuis GMM; Peters WHM; Meijer DFM. Selective hepatobiliary transport defect for organic anions and neutral steroids in mutant rats with hereditary-conjugated hyperbilirubinemia. *Hepatology* 1987b; 7: 71-76.

Jedligtschky, G; Burchell, G; Keppler, D. The multidrug resistance protein 5 functions as an ATP-dependent export pump for cyclic nucleotides. *J. Biol. Chem.* 2000; 275:30069-30074, 2000.

Jedlitschky G, Leier I, Bchholz U, Barmouin K, Kurz G, Keppler D. Transpor of glutathione, glucuronate and sulfate conjugates by MRP gene encoded conjugate export pump. *Cancer Res* 56:988-994, 1996.

Karwatsky, J; Leimanis, M; Cai, J; Gros, P; Georges, E. The leucotriene C4 binding sites in multidrug resistance protein 1 (ABCC1) include the first membrane multiple spanning domain. *Biochemistry* 2005; 44:340-351.

Karwatsky, J; Leuschner, U, Maver, R; Keppler, D. Absence of the canalicular isoform of the MRP gene-encoded conjugate export pump from the hepatocytes in Dubin-Johnson syndrome. *Hepatology* 1996; 23:1061-1066.

Kauffmann, H-M; Pfannschmidt, S; Zoller, H., Benz, A; Vorderstemann, B; Webster, JL; Schrenk, D. Influence of redox-active compounds and PXR-activators on human MRP1 and MRP2 gene expression. *Toxicology* 2002; 171:137-146.

Kitamura, T; Jansen, PLM; Hardenbrook, C; Kamimoto, Y; Gatmaitan, Z; Arias, IM. Defective ATP-dependent bile canalicular transport of organic anions in mutant (TR-) rats with conjugated hyperbilirubinemia. *Proc. Natl. Acad. Sci.* USA 1990; 87:3557-3561.

Klement, JF; Matsuzaki, Y; Jiang, Q-J; Terlizzi, J; Choi, HY; Fujimoto, N; Li, K; Pulkkine, L; Birk, DE; Sundberg, JP; Uitto, J. Targeted ablation of the abcc6 gene results in ectopic mineralization of connective tissue. *Mol. Cell. Biol.* 2005; 25:8299-8310.

Kobayashi K; Komatsu S; Nishi T; Hara H; Hayashi K. ATP-dependent transport for glucuronides in canalicular plasma membrane vesicles. *Biochem. Biophys. Res. Commun.* 1991; 176: 622-626.

Kobayashi K; Sogame Y; Hara H; Hayashi K. Mechanism of glutathione S-conjugate transport in canalicular and basolateral rat liver plasma membranes. *J. Biol. Chem.* 1990; 265: 7737-7741.

Kondo T; Dale G; Beutler E. Glutathione transport by inside-out vesicles from human erythrocytes. *Proc. Natl. Acad. Sci.* USA 1980; 77: 6359-6362.

Kondo T; Murao M; Taniguchi N. Glutathione S-conjugate transport using inside-out vesicles from human erythrocytes. *Eur. J. Biochem.* 1982; 125: 551-554.

Kool, M; de Haas, M; Scheffer, GL; Scheper, RJ; van Eijk, ML; Juijn, JA; Baas, F; Borst, P. Analysis of expression of cMOAT (MRP2), MRP3, MRP4, and MRP5,homologues of the multidrug resistance-associated protein gene (MRP1), in human cancer cell lines. *Cancer Res.* 1997: 57: 3537-3547.

Kool, M; van der Linden, M; de Haas, M; Baas, F; Borst, P. Expression of human MRP6, ahomologue of the multidrug resistance protein gene MRP1, in tissues and cancer cells. *Cancer Res.* 1999: 59: 175-182.

Kruh, GD; Belinsky, MG. The MRP family of drug efflux pumps. *Oncogene* 2003; 22:7537-7552.

Kuo, MT; Bao, J-J; Curley, SA; Ikeguchi, M; Johnston, DA; Ishikawa, T. Frequent coordinated overexpression of the MRP/GS-X pump and g-glutamylcysteine synthetase genes in human colorectal cancers. *Cancer Res.* 1996; 56:3642-3644.

Kuo, MT; Bao, J;Furuichi, M; Yamane, Y; Gomi, A; Savaraj, N; Masuzawa, T; Ishikawa, T. Frequent coexpression of MRP/GS-X pump and gamma glutamylcysteine synthase mRNA in drug-resistant cells, untreated tumors, and normal mice tissues. *Biochem. Pharmacol.* 1998; 55:605-615.

Kurz, EU; Cole, SP, Deeley RG. Identification of DNA-protein interactions in the 5' flanking and 5'-untranslated regions of the human multidrug resistance protein (MRP1) gene: evidence of a putative antioxidant response element/AP-1 binding site. *Biochem. Biophys. Res. Commun.* 2001; 285:981-990.

Labelle EF; Singh SV; Srivastava SK; Awasthi YC. Dinitrophenyl glutathione efflux from human erythrocytes is primary active ATP-dependent transport. *Biochem. J.* 1986; 238: 443-449.

Lai, L; Tan, TM. Role of glutathione in the multidrug resistance protein 4 (MRP4/ABCC4)-mediated efflux of cAMP and resistance to purine analogues. *Biochem. J.* 2002; 361:497-503, 2002.

Lee, FY; Siemann, DW; Sutherlan, RM. Changes in cellular glutathione content during adriamycin treatment in human ovarian cancer-a possible indicator of chemosensitivity. *Br. J Cancer* 1989; 60:291-298.

Lee, J-M; Hanson JM; Chu, WA; Johnson JA. Phosphatidylinositol 3-kinase, not extracellular signal-regulated kinase, regulates activation of the antioxidant-responsive element in IMR-32 human neuroblastoma cells. *J. Biol. Chem.* 2001; 276:20011-20016.

Leggas, M; Adachi, M; Scheffer, GL; Sun, D; Wielinga, P; Du, G; Mercer, KE; Zhuang, Y; Panetta, JC; Johnston, B; Scheper, RJ; Stewart ,CF; Schuetz, JD. Mrp4 confers resistance to topotecan and protects the brain from chemotherapy. *Mol. Cell. Biol.* 2004; 24:7612-7621.

Leier, I; Jedlitschky, G; Buchholz, U; Cole, SPC; Deeley, RG; Keppler, D. The MRP gene encodes an ATP-dependent export pump of leukotriene C4 and structurally related conjugates. *J. Biol. Chem.* 1994; 269:27807-27810.

Leslie, EM; Bowers, RJ; Deeley, RG; Cole SPC. Structural requirements for functional interaction of glutathione tripeptide analogs with the human multidrug resistance protein 1 (MRP1). *J Pharmacol. Exper. Therap.* 2003; 204:643-653.

Leslie, EM; Ito, K-I; Upadhyaya, P; Hecht, SS; Deeley, RG; Cole, SPC. Transport of the beta-O-glucuronide conjugate of the tobacco-specific carcinogen 4-(methylnitrosamino)-1-(3-pyridyl)-1-butanol (NNAL) by the Multidrug Resistance Protein 1 (MRP1). Requirement for glutathione or a non-sulfur-containing analog. *J. Biol. Chem.*, 2001; 276: 27846 – 27854

Leslie, EM; Letoumeau, IJ; Deeley, RG; Cole, SP. Functional and structural consequences of cysteine substitutions in the NH2 proximal region of he human multidrug resistance protein (MRP1/ABCC1). *Biochemistry* 2003; 42:5214-5224.

Li, L; Lee, TK; Meier, PJ; Ballatori, N: Identification of glutathione as a driving force and leukotriene C4 as a substrate for oatp1, the hepatic sinusoidal organic solute transporter. *J. Biol. Chem.* 1998; 273:16184-16191.

Li Z-S; Zhao Y; Rea PA. Magnesium adenosine 5'-triphosphate-energized transport of glutathione S-conjugates by plant vacuolar membrane vesicles. *Plant Physiol.* 1995; 107: 1257-1268.

Lin-Lee, Y-C; Tatebe, S; Savaraj, N; Ishikawa, T; and Kuo, MT. Differential sensitivities of MRP gene family and g-glutamylcysteine synthetase to prooxidants in human colorectal carcinoma cell lines with different p53 status. *Biochem. Pharmacol.* 2001; 61:555-563.

Loe, DW; Almquist, KC; Deeley, RG; Cole, SPC. Multidrug resistance protein (MRP)-mediated transport of leukotriene C4 and chemotherapeutic agents in membrane vesicles. Demonstration of glutathione-dependent vincristine transport. *J. Biol. Chem.* 1996; 271:9675-9682.

Loe, DW; Deeley, RG; Cole, SPC. Verapamil stimulates glutathione transport by the multidrug resistance protein1 (MRP1). *J. Pharmacol. Exp. Ther.* 2000; 293:530-538, 2000.

Manciu, L; Chang, X-B; Buyse, F; Hou, Y-X; Gustot, A; Riordan, JR; Ruysschaert, JM. Intermediate structural states involves in MRP1-mediated drug transport. *J. Biol. Chem.,* 2003; 278: 3347-3356.

Martinoia E; Grill E; Tommaini R; Kreuz K; Amrhein N. ATP-dependent glutathione S-conjugate 'export' pumps in the vacuolar membrane of plants. *Nature* 1993; 364: 247-249.

Meister, A. Glutathione metabolism. *Methods Enzymol.* 1995; 251: 3-7.

Meister, A. in Coenzymes and Cofactors. *Glutathione: Chemical, Biochemical and Medical Aspects* (Dolphin, D., Poulson, R., and Avramovic, O., eds) 2000; Vol. III, Part A, pp. 367-474, John Wiley & Sons, Inc., New York .

Meister A; Anderson M. Glutathione. *Annu. Rev. Biochem.* 1983; 52: 711-760.

Moran, JA; Dahl, EL; Mulcahy, RT. Differential induction of MafK, MafG, and MafF expression by electrophile-response-element activators. *Biochem. J.* 2001; 361:311-317.

Mulcahy, RT; Wartman, MA; Bailey, HH; Gipp, JJ. Constitutive and beta-naphthoflavone-induced expression of the human gamma-glutamylcysteine synthetase heavy subunit gene is regulated by a distal antioxidant response element/TRE sequence. *J. Biol. Chem.* 1997; 272:7445-7454, 1997.

Muller, M; Meijer, C; Zaman, GJR; Borst, P; Scheper, FJ; Mulder, N; de vries EGE,; Jansen, PLM. Overexpression of the gene encoding the multidrug resistance –associated protein results in increased ATP-dependent glutathione S-conjugate transport. *Proc. Natl. Acad. Sci.* USA 1994; 91:13033-13037.

Muredda, M; Nunoya, K-I; Burtch-Wriight, RA; Kurz, EU; Cole, SPC; Deeley, RG. Cloning and characterization of the murine and rat mrp1 promoter regions. *Mol. Pharmacol.* 2003; 64:1259-1269.

Nguyen, T; Huang, H C; Pickett, CB. Transcriptional regulation of the antioxidant response element. Activation by Nrf2 and repression by MafK. *J. Biol. Chem.* 2000; 275:15466-15473.

Nguyen, T; Sherratt, PJ; Nioi, P; Yang, CS; Pickett CB. Nrf2 controls constitutive and inducible expression of ARE-driven genes through a dynamic pathway involving nucleocytoplasmic shuttling by Keap1. *J. Biol. Chem.* 2005; 280:32485-32492.

Nguyen, T; Yang, CS; Pickett CB. The pathways and molecular mechanisms regulating Nrf2 activation in response to chemical stress. Free Rad. Biol. Med. 2004; 37:433-441, 2004.

Oude Elferink, RPJ; Ottenhoff, R; Liefting, W; De Haan, J; Jansen, PLM. Hepatobiliary transport of glutathione and glutathione conjugate in rats with hereditary hyperbilirubinemia. *J. Clin. Invest.* 1989; 84:478-483.

Oude Elferink RPJ; Ottenhoff R; Liefting WGM; Schoemaker B; Groen AK; Jansen PLM. ATP-dependent efflux of GSSG and GS-conjugate from isolated rat hepatocytes. *Am. J. Physiol.* 1990; 258: G699-G706.

Paulusma, CC; Kool, M; Bosma, PJ; Sheffer, GL; ter Borg, F; Scheper, RJ; Tytgat, GN; Borst, P; Baas, F; Oude Elferink, RP. Congenital jaundice in rats with a mutation in a multidrug resistance-associated protein gene. *Science* 1996; 271; 1126-1128.

Perez, RP; Hamilton, TC; Ozoles, RF. Resistance to alkylating agents and cisplatin: insights from ovarian carcinoma model systems. *Pharmacol. Ther.* 1990;48:19-27.

Qian, Y-M; Song, W-C; Cui, H; Cole, SPC; Deeley, RG. Glutathione stimulates sulfated estrogen transport by multidrug resistance protein 1. *J. Biol. Chem.* 2001; 276: 6404-6411.

Rahman, I; Smith, CA; Lawson, MF; Harrison, DJ; MacNee, W. Induction of gamma-glutamylcysteine synthetase by cigarette smoke is associated with AP-1 in human alveolar epithelial cells. *FEBS Lett.* 1996; 396:21-25.

Rea PA; Sanches-fernandez R; Chen S; Peng M; Klein M; Geisler M; Martinoia E. The plant ABC transporter superfamily: the functions of a few and identities of many. In: *ABC Proteins from Bacteria to Man* (Eds.: Holland, I.B., Cole, S.P.C., Kuchler, K., and Higgins, C.F.) Academic Press, Amsterdam, 2003; pp. 335-355.

Reed, DJ. Glutathione: toxicological implications. *Annu. Rev. Pharmacol. Toxicol.* 1990: 30, 603-631.

Ren, X-Q; Furukawa, T; Nakajima, Y; Takahashi, H; Aoki, S; Sumizawa,T; Haraguchi, M; Kobayashi, M; Chijiiwa, K; Akiyama, S-i. GSH inhibits trypsinization of the C-terminal half of human MRP1. *J. Biol. Chem.* 2005; 280:6231-6237.

Ristoff, E; Augustson, C; Geissler, J. A missense mutation in the heavy subunit of gamma-glutamylcysteine synthetase gene causes hemolytic anemia. *Blood* 2000; 95:2193-2196.

Ruis, M; Nies, NT; Hummel-Eisenbeiss, J; Jedlitschk, G; Keppler, D. Cotransport of reduced glutathione with bile salts by MRP4 (ABCC4) localized to the basolateral hepatocyte membrane. *Hepatology* 2003; 38:374-384.

Ruis, M; Hummel-Eisenbeiss, J; Hoffmann, AF; Keppler, D. Substrate specificity of human ABCC4(MRP4)-mediated cotransport of bile acids and reduced glutathione. *Am. J. Physiol. Gastrointest. Liver Physiol* 200t; (in press).

Sekhar, KR; Soltaninassab, SR; Borrelli, MJ; Xu, ZQ; Meredith, MJ; Domann, FE; Freeman, M:. Inhibition of the 26S proteasome induces expression of GLCLC, the catalytic subunit for gamma-glutamylcysteine synthetase. *Biochem. Biophys. Res. Commun.* 2000; 270:311-317.

Shi, Z Z; Osei-Frimpong, J; Kala, G; Kala, S; Barrios, RJ; Habib, GM; Lukin, DJ; Danney, CM; Matzuk, MM; and Lieberman, MW. Glutathione synthesis is essential for mouse development but not for cell growth in culture. *Proc. Natl. Acad. Sci.* USA 2000; 97:5101-5106.

Shimizu, H; Taniguchi, H; Hippo, Y; Hayashizaki, Y; Aubrata, H; Ishikawa, T. Characterization of the mouse Abcc12 gene and its transcript encoding an ATP-binding cassette transporter, an orthologue of human ABCC12. *Gene* 2003;310: 17-28.

Sies H. (Ed.) *Oxidative Stress.* 1985; Academic Press, Orlando.

Sies H; Ketterer B. (Eds.) *Glutathione Conjugation: Mechanisms and Biological Significance.* 1988; Academic Press, London.

Smith, CV; Jones, DP; Guenthner, TM; Lash, LH; Lauterbrug, BH. Compartmentation of glutathione: implications for the study of toxicity and disease. *Toxicol. Appl. Pharmacol.* 140: 1-13, 1996.

Song, I-M; Tatebe, S; Dai, W; Kuo, MT. Delayed mechanism for induction of gamma-glutamylcysteine synthetase heavy subunit mRNA stability by oxidative stress involving p38 mitogen-associated protein kinase signaling. *J. Biol. Chem.* 2005; 180:28230-28240.

Srivastava, SK; Beutler E. The transport of oxidized glutathione from human erythrocytes. J. Biol. Chem. 1969; 244: 9-16.

Strehlow, K; Rotter, S; Wassmann, S; Adam, O; Grohe, C; Laufs, K; Bohm, M; Nickenig, G. Modulation of antioxidant enzyme expression and function by estrogen. *Circ. Res.* 2003; 2003; 93, 170–177.

Suzuki M; Mori M; Niwa T; Hirata R; Furuta K; Ishikawa T; Noyori R. Chemical implications for antitumor and antiviral prostaglandins: Reaction of D^7-prostaglandin A1 and prostaglandin A1 methyl esters with thiols. *J. Am. Chem. Soc.* 1997; 119: 2376-2385.

Takayanagi, C; Kataoka, T; Ohara, O; Oishi, M; Kuo, MT; Ishikawa, T. Human ATP-binding cassette transporter ABCC10: expression profile and p53-dependent regulation. *J. Exp. Ther. Oncol.* 2004; 4:239-246.

Takikawa H; Sano N; Narita T; Uchida Y; Yamanaka M; Horie T; Mikami T; Tagaya O. Biliary excretion of bile acid conjugates in a hyperbilirubinemic mutant Sprague-Dawley rat. *Hepatology* 1991; 14: 352-360.

Tanaka, T; Uchiumi, T; Hinoshita, E; Inokuchi, A; Toh, S; Wada, M; Takano, H; Kohno, K; Kuwano, M. The human multidrug resistance protein 2 gene: functional characterization of the 5' flanking region and expression in hepatic cells. *Hepatology* 1999; 30:1507-1512.

Taniguchi, K; Wada, M; Kohno, K; Nakamura, T; Kawabe, T; Kawakami, M; Kagotani, K; Okumura, K; Akiyama, S; Kuwano, M. A human canalicular multispecific organic anion transporter (cMOAT) gene is overexpressed in cisplatin-resistant human cancer cell lines with decreased drug accumulation. *Cancer Res.* 1996: 56: 4124-4129.

Tatebe, S; Sinicrope, FA; Kuo, MT. Induction of multidrug resistance associated genes MRP1 and MRP3 and g-glutacysteine synthetase expression by the nonsteroidal anti-inflammatory drugs in human colon cancer cells. *Biochem. Biophys. Res. Commun.* 2002; 290:1427-1433, 2002.

Tatebe, S; Unate H; Sinicrope, FA;, Sakatani, T; sugamura, K; Makino, M; Ishikawa, T; Ito, H; Kaibara, N; Kaibara, N; Kuo, MT. Expression of heavy subunit of g-glutamylcysteine synthetase (g-GCSh) in human colorectal carcinoma. 2002; *Intern. J. Cancer* 97:21-27, 2002.

Tomonari, A; Nishio, K; Kurokawa, H; Arioka, H; Ishida, T; Fukumoto, H; Fukuoka, K; Nomoto, T; Iwamoto, Y; Heike, Y; Itakura, M; Saijo, N. Identification of cis-acting DNA elements of the human gamma-glutamylcysteine synthetase heavy subunit gene. Biochem. *Biophys. Res. Commun.* 1997; 232:522-527.

Townsend, DM; Tew, KD. The role of glutathione-S-transferase in anti-cancer drug resistance. *Oncogene* 2003; 22:7369-7375.

Urata, Y; Honma, S; Goto, S;Todoroki, S; Iida, T; Cho, S; Honma, K; Kondo, T. Melatonin induces gamma-glutamylcysteine synthetase mediated by activator protein-1 in human vascular endothelial cells. *Free Radic Biol. Med.* 1999; 27:838-837.

Versantvoort, CH; Broxterman, HJ; Bagrij, T; Scheper, RJ; Twentyman, PR. Regulation by glutathione of drug transport in multidrug-resistant human lun tumor cell lines overexpressing multidrug resistance-associated protein. *Br. J. Cancer* 1995; 72:82-89.

Vollrath, V; Wielandt, AM; Iruretagovena, M; Chianale, J. Role of Nrf2 in the regulation of Mrp2 (ABCC2) gene. *Biochem J* 2006: (in press).

Wakabayashi, N; Dinkova-Kostova, AT; Holtzclaw, WD; Kang, MI; Kobayashi, A; Yamamoto, M; Kensler, TW; Talalay, P. Protection against electrophile and oxidant stress by induction of the phase 2 response: fate of cysteines of the Keap1 sensor modified by inducers. *Proc Natl. Acad. Sci.* USA 2004; 101:2040-2045.

Wang, L; Yang, H; Admo, ML. Glucose starvation reduces IGF-I mRNA in tumor cells: Evidence for an effect on mRNA stability. *Biochem. Biophys. Res. Commun.* 2000; 269, 336–346

Wielinga, PR; van der Haijden, I; Reid, G; Beijnen, JH; Wijnholds, J; Borst, P. Characterization of the MRP4-and MRP5-mediated transport of cyclic nucleotide from intact cells. *J. Biol Chem.* 2003; 278:17664-17671.

Wijnholds, J; deLange, EC; Scheffer, GL; van den Berg, DJ; Mol, CA; van der Valk, M; Schinkel, AH; Scheper, RJ; Brimer, DD; Borst, P. Multidrug resistance protein 1 protects the choroids plexus epithelium and contributes to the blood-cerebrospinal fluid barrier. *J. Clin. Inv.* 2000; 105:279-285.

Wijnholds, J; Evers, R; van Leusden, MR; Mol CA, Zaman, CJ; Mayer, U; Beijnen, JH; van der Valk, M; Krimpenfort, P; Borst, P. Increased sensitivity to anticancer drugs and decreased inflammatory response in mice lacking the multidrug resistance-associated protein. *Nature Med.* 1997; 3:1275-1279.

Wild, AC; Moinova, HR; Mulcahy, RT. Regulation of gamma-glutamylcysteine synthetase subunit gene expression by the transcription factor Nrf2. *Biol. Chem.* 1999; 274:33627-33636.

Winvard, PG; Moody, CJ; Jacob, C. Oxidative activation of antioxidant defense. *Trends Biochem. Sci* 2005; 30:453-461.

Yabuuchi, H; Shimizu, H; Takayanagi, S-I; Ishikawa, T. Multiple splicing variants of new human ATP-binding cassette transporters, ABCC11 and ABCC12. *Biochem. Biophys. Res. Commun.* 2001;288:933-939.

Yabuuchi, K; Talauyanagi, S-I; Yoshinaga, K., Taniguchi, N; Aburatani, H; Ishikawa, T. ABC13, an unusual trancated ABC transporter, is highly expressed infetal human liver. *Biochem. Biophys. Res. Commu.* 2002; 299:410-417.

Yamane, Y; Furuichi, M; Song, R; Van, NT; Mulcahy, RT; Ishikawa, T; Kuo, MT. Expression of multidrug resistance protein/GS-X pump and g-glutamylcysteine synthetase genes. *J. Biol. Chem.* 1998; 20:31075-31085.

Yang, Y; Chen, Q; Zhang, JT. Structural and functional consequences of mutating cysteine residues in the amino terminus of human multidrug resistance-associated protein 1. *J. Biol. Chem.* 2002; 277:44268-44277.

Yoshiura, KI; Kinoshita, A, Ishida, T; Ninokata, A; Ishikawa, T; Kaname, T; et al. A SNP in the ABCC11 gene is the determinant of human earwax type. *Nature Genet.* 2006, (in press).

Yu, R; Chen, C; Moo, YY; Hebbar, V; Owuor, ED; Tan, T-H; Kong, ANAT. Activation of mitogen-activated protein kinase pathways induces antioxidant response element-mediated gene expression via a Nrf2-dependent mechanism. *J. Biol. Chem.* 2000; 275: 39907-39913.

Yun, H; Lee, M; Kim, S.-S; Ha, J. Glucose deprivation increases mRNA stability of vascular endothelial growth factor through activation of AMP-activated protein kinase in DU 145 prostate carcinoma. *J. Biol. Chem.* 2005; 280, 9963–9972.

Zelcer, N; Huisman, MT; Reid, G; Wielinga, P; Brfeedveld, P; Kuil, A; Knipscheer, P; Schellens, JHM; Schinkel, AH; Borst, P. Evidence for two interacting ligand binding sites in human multidrug resistance protein 2 (ATP binding cassette C2). *J. Biol. Chem.* 2003; 278: 23538-23544.

Zelcer, N; Saeki, T; Geid, G; Beijnen, JH; Beijnen, H; Borst, P. Characterization of drug transport by the human multidrug resistance protein 3 (ABCC3). *J. Biol. Chem.* 2001;276:46400-46407.

Zelcer, N; van de Wetering, K; Hillebrand, M; Sarton, E; Kuil, A; Wielinga, PR; Tephly, T; Dahan, A; Beijnen, JH; Borst, P. Mice lacking multidrug resistance protein 3 show altered morphine pharmacokinetics and morphine6-glucuronide antinociception. *Proc. Natl. Acad. Sci.* USA 2005; 102: 7274-7279.

Zhu, Q; Center MS. Cloning and sequence analysis of the promoter region of the MRP gene of HL60cells isolated for resistance to adriamycin. *Cancer Res.* 1994; 54:4488-4492.

Zhu Q; Center MS. Evidence that SP1 modulates transcriptional activity of the multidrug resistance-associated protein gene. *DNA Cell Biol* 1996; 15:105-111.

Zipper, LM; Mulcahy, RT. Inhibition of ERK and p38 MAP kinases inhibits binding of Nrf2 and induction of GCS genes. *Biochem. Biophys. Res. Commun.* 2000; 278: 484-492.

In: Multidrug Resistance-Associated Proteins
Editor: Christopher V. Aiello, pp. 31-48

ISBN 1-60021-298-0
© 2007 Nova Science Publishers, Inc.

Chapter 2

QUANTITATION OF O^6 – METHYLGUANINE – DNA METHYLTRANSFERASE GENE MESSENGER RNA IN GLIOMAS BY MEANS OF REAL-TIME RT-PCR

Satoshi Tanaka[1]*, Jiro Akimoto[2], Hidehiro Oka[3], Yoshihiro Muragaki[4], Hiroshi Ujiie[5] and Atsushi Kakimoto[6]

[1]Department of Neurosurgery, Kawasaki Hospital, Hitachiohta, Japan.
[2]Department of Neurosurgery, Tokyo Medical University, Tokyo, Japan
[3]Department of Neurosurgery, Kitasato University School of Medicine, Sagamihara, Japan
[4]Faculty of Advanced Techno-Surgery, Institute of Advanced Biomedical Engineering and Science ,Graduate School of Medicine, Tokyo Women's Medical University, Tokyo, Japan
[5]Department of Neurosurgery, Neurological Institute, Tokyo Women's Medical University, Tokyo, Japan
[6]Gene and Chromosome Center, SRL Inc., Hino, Japan

ABSTRACT

O^6-methylguanine-DNA methyltransferase (MGMT) is a drug-resistance gene for nitrosoureas. The level of MGMT varies widely according to the type of tumor, and even varies among tumors of the same histological classification. MGMT mRNA was measured in 65 neuroepithelial tumor specimens from 54 patients almost that had received 1- (4-amino-2-methyl-5-pyrimidynyl) methyl – 3 - (2-chloroethyl) – 3 - nitrosourea hydrochloride (ACNU) after the resection of the tumor by real-time reverse transcription-polymerase chain reaction (RT-PCR) using TaqMan probe and normalized to the level of the internal control.

* Correspondence to: Satoshi Tanaka, M.D., D.M.Sci., Department of Neurosurgery, Kawasaki Hospital, 2040 Kisaki-nicho, Hitachiohta, Ibaraki 313-8511, Japan; FAX +81-294-72-7056; E-mail address: stanaka-nsu@umin.net

The absolute value of MGMTmRNA normalized to the level of GAPDH in 65 neuroepithelial tumor specimens was $1.20 \times 10^4 \pm 1.19 \times 10^4$ copy/µg RNA(mean ± standard deviation). The mean value of 35 glioblastomas ($1.20 \times 10^4 \pm 1.00 \times 10^4$ copy/µg RNA) was not significantly different from that of 7 low grade gliomas ($1.13 \times 10^4 \pm 0.60 \times 10^4$ copy/µg RNA) ($P = 0.4241$ by Student's t-test). The mean value of 36 primary tumors ($1.01 \times 10^4 \pm 0.92 \times 10^4$ copy/µg RNA) was not significantly different from that of the recurrent 21 tumors after ACNU therapy ($1.46 \times 10^4 \pm 1.53 \times 10^4$) ($P = 0.0920$ by Student's t-test). Similarly, in 8 patients who had been measured of MGMTmRNA more than twice, no significant elevations of MGMTmRNA after ACNU treatment were observed.

The response rate, more than 50% tumor regression rate, to ACNU of 28 patients who had MGMTmRNA less than 6×10^3 copy/µg RNA was 58.3% and that of 37 patients who had it more than 6×10^3 copy/µg RNA was 23.1%. Significant difference was observed in the response rates of these two groups ($P = 0.0421$ by Fisher's exact probability test). The value normalized MGMTmRNA < 6000 copy/µg RNA was the only significant factor predicted the initial effect of therapy with ACNU among some prognostic factors such as age, Kernofsky's performance status, histological grading, surgical reduction rate, and combination therapy.

A hundred and twenty-four adjuvant therapy individualized by the results of RT-PCR has been used to treat 100 patients with neuroepithelial tumors since 1997. Immediate after the operation, the mRNA expression for drug-resistance genes was investigated in 124 frozen samples of tumors (10 astrocytomas, 2 oligodendrogliomas, 9 anaplastic oligodendrogliomas, 40 anaplastic astrocytomas, 56 glioblastoma multiformes, and 7 medulloblastomas) by conventional RT-PCR in 51 samples, semi-quantitative RT-PCR in 12 samples, real-time RT-PCR using SYBR Green I in 55 samples, and real-time RT-PCR using TaqMan probe in 6 samples, all with the specific primers for MGMT. Eighty-five tumors were treated with ACNU because relative low expression value of MGMTmRNA and residual 39 tumors who had had relatively high MGMTmRNA were treated with platinum-compounds. The response rate of the individual adjuvant therapy (IAT) was 40.0% for glioblastoma multiformes, 51.4% for anaplastic astrocytomas, and 50.0% for all evaluable therapies. Two years survival rate of 45 glioblastoma patients was 55.6% at present.

These results suggest that quantitation of MGMTmRNA is the excellent method for predicting for the effect of ACNU in glioma therapy. Our IAT based on the results of real-time RT-PCR may lead to a simple and beneficial glioma therapy. A prospective randomized multi-center study should be performed to confirm the efficacy of this new method for glioma therapy

INTRODUCTION

Drug-resistance genes are some of the most important elements of tumors themselves in determining drug-resistance. The multidrug-resistance gene 1 (MDR1) has been thought to be associated with resistance to vincristine (VCR), etoposide, and other drugs.[1-8] Recently, multidrug resistance-associated protein (MRP) also thought to be important in the resistance to these drugs.[9-12] As previously described, Some drug-resistance genes, such as glutathion-S transpherase (GST), glutathion, and methalothionein, are thought to be related to the sensitivity of Pt-compounds. Of these molecules, GST-π was reported to have the closest relationship to tumor resistance to Pt-compounds.[13-16]

Actually, O^6-methylguanine-DNA methyltransferase (MGMT) is a drug-resistance gene for nitrosoureas.[17,18] The cross-linking of double-stranded DNA by alkylating agents is inhibited by the cellular DNA-repair protein MGMT. MGMT rapidly reverses alkylation at the O^6 position of guanine, thereby averting lethal cross-linking.[19]This is the mechanism by which MGMT induces resistance to nitrosoureas.

Glioma is the most popular during brain tumors, and it is one of the worst malignant tumors. Difficulty in glioma therapy is due to the invasive growth that interferes with total removal of the tumors. Thus, adjuvant therapy, including radiation, various chemotherapeutic agents and biological-response modifiers such as interferon (IFN), is essential for treating malignant gliomas.[20, 21] Nitrosoureas are alkylating agents that cause cell death by binding to DNA. Among nitrosoureas, 1 – (4 – amino – 2 – methyl – 5 – pyrimidynyl) methyl – 3 – (2 – chloroethyl) – 3 -nitrosourea hydrochloride (ACNU) is widely used in Japan to treat gliomas because of its ability to permeate the blood-brain-barrier and its considerable clinical effects in combination with radiation and IFN-β.[22, 23] We think that the MGMT gene expression is the most important drug-resistance gene in the treatment of gliomas, since ACNU is the first choice for gliomas of all chemotherapeutic agents in Japan.[24-26]Pt-compounds such as cis-platinum (CDDP) and carboplatin (CBDCA) are used for primary and recurrent gliomas in some institutes instead of ACNU because of the severe myelosuppression caused by ACNU and the clinically obvious resistance to it.[27]

Although many clinical trials have been performed using adjuvant therapy for malignant gliomas, there has been little evidence based on prospective randomized trials other than an increase in survival by radiation therapy and tumor regression by with radiation in combination with nitrosoureas.[28] Protocol studies for malignant gliomas have not provided encouraging therapeutic results because of the heterogeneity and various drug-sensitivities of the tumors.[29] Individualization of glioma therapy is recommended. Since 1997, we have performed individual adjuvant therapy (IAT) that was individualized based on the results of reverse transcription-polymerase chain reaction (RT-PCR) for MGMT to treat malignant gliomas.[23]

The level of MGMT varies widely according to the type of tumor, and even varies among tumors of the same histological classification.[18, 23-26, 30] Approximately 30 to 50 percent of gliomas lack MGMT.[31] The fact that more than half of gliomas express MGMT limits the indications for ACNU. In our preliminary IAT, platinum (Pt)-compounds were used instead of ACNU even though Pt-compounds had not been accepted as being effective in gliomas. [23, 27, 32]

To ensure IAT for gliomas, absolute quantitation of MGMTmRNA is needed for a higher initial response and prolongation of survival. We performed the absolute quantitation of MGMTmRNA by using TaqMan probe and normalized to the level of the internal control in 64 glioma tissues from the patients who had received ACNU after the resection of the tumor.[26]

MATERIALS AND METHODS

Real-time RT-PCR Using TaqMan Probe

Sixty-five neuroepithelial tumor frozen tissues (3 astrocytomas, 3 oligoastrocytomas, 5 anaplastic oligoastrocytomas, 17 anaplastic astrocytomas, 35 glioblastoma multiforme, and a medulloblastoma) from 54 patients were used for this retrospective study. Total RNA was extracted from about 10 mg frozen specimen at -70℃ or fresh tissue stored in RNA*later* RNA Stabilization Reagentat (QIAGEN, Hilden, Germany) at 4℃ according to the guanidinium thiocyanate-phenol-chloroform extraction method using Isogen (WAKO junyaku, Osaka, Japan) and were collected from the precipitate in ethanol.[33] The cDNA synthesized from 1 µg total RNA with a random primer (Invitorogen, CA, USA), 40U M-MLV Reverse transcriptase (Invitorogen, CA, USA), 0.5mM dNTP (Takara BIO, Shiga, Japan), 24U RNase inhibitor(Takara BIO, Shiga, Japan), 10µM DTT(Sigma genosys, USA), 5x RT buffer at 37℃ for 60 min, and stored at -20℃ until used. The Real-time PCR reaction mixture was prepared using a TaqMan Universal Master Mix (Applied Biosystems, CA, USA), 120nM of each primer,[26] 200nM probe (5'-CGA GCA GTG GGA GGA GCA ATG AGA-3'), 2.5µL each cDNA samples. The PCR condition were performed denaturation step at 95 °C for 10 min and 50 cycles at 95 °C for 30 sec, 60 °C for 40 sec, 72 °C for 30 sec using a real-time PCR system (ABI PRISM 7700 Sequence Detection System : Applied Biosystems, CA, USA). We monitored glyceraldehyde-3-phosphate dehydrogenase (GAPDH) mRNA expression levels as the quantitative internal control. The standard curves for MGMT and GAPDH mRNA were generated using 10-fold serial diluted standard plasmid clones inserted by MGMT or GAPDH PCR products as template, and the amount of each mRNA expression levels was calculated from the standard curve. To quantify precisely, the MGMT mRNA expression level of each sample was normalized using the expression of GAPDH gene.

Individual Adjuvant Therapy Based on RT-PCR Results

Since April 1997, 124 adjuvant therapy individualized by the results of RT-PCR has been used to treat 100 patients with neuroepithelial tumors. Immediate after the operation to remove the tumor as much as possible, the mRNA expression for drug-resistance genes was investigated by conventional RT-PCR in 51 samples, [23]semi-quantitative RT-PCR in 12 samples, [24] real-time RT-PCR using SYBR Green I in 55 samples, [25] and real-time RT-PCR using TaqMan probe in 6 samples, [26] all with the specific primers for MGMT. A hundred and twenty-four frozen samples of tumors were consisted with 10 astrocytomas, 2 oligodendrogliomas, 9 anaplastic oligodendrogliomas, 40 anaplastic astrocytomas, 56 glioblastoma multiformes, and 7 medulloblastomas.

IAT was approved according to institutional policies of the ethical committee and written informed consent was obtained from each patient before entry into IAT study. According to our previously reported the retrospective analysis, tumors with relative low MGMTmRNA expression (negative by conventional RT-PCR, relative index compared with internal control

<1 by semi-quantitative RT-PCR or by real-time RT-PCR with SYBR Green I or <6000 copy/μgRNA by normalized real-time RT-PCR with TaqMan probe) were treated with 90~100 mg/m^2 of ACNU.[23-26] Tumors with relative high MGMTmRNA expression (positive by conventional RT-PCR, relative index compared with internal control □1 by semi-quantitative RT-PCR or by real-time RT-PCR with SYBR Green I or □ 6000 copy/μgRNA by normalized real-time RT-PCR with TaqMan probe) were treated with 5 serial day's administration of cis-platinum (20 mg/m^2) or 350-400 mg/m^2 of carboplatin, instead of ACNU. One mg/m^2 of vincristine with ACNU or 50 mg/m^2 of etoposide with platinum compounds were co-administrated in 62.1% of the therapy. Three times per a week of IFN-β (6 x 10^6 IU) was used in 92.7% of the therapy because it has less adverse effects than chemotherapeutic agents and an indirect anti-tumor effect is expected especially during maintenance therapy [11]. Radiation therapy (60 Gy for all patients) was also used in 60.5% of the therapy concurrently with chemotherapy. Maintenance therapy was performed as possible (65.0%) mainly by a weekly or bi-weekly IFN-β. ACNU or CBDCA was also used once 2 or 3 months for the patients with glioblastoma multiforme.

Statistical Analysis

The extent of the resection was calculated actually from contrast-enhanced images by computer-assisted tomography (CT) scan or magnetic resonance imaging (MRI) within 3 postoperative days by the previously reported methods.[34,35] Basically enhanced-lesion was compared. In non-enhancing tumors, the high signal-intensity areas on T2-weighted MR images were evaluated. Ninety-five to a hundred percent resections were defined as 95%. Seventy-five to 95 was defined as 75%. Fifty to 75 was as 50%. The effect of IAT was evaluated at least two months after the beginning of therapy. The results of the therapies were also judged in terms of a reduction of the tumor volume by 50% or more in contrast-enhanced images by CTscan or MRI. [34,35] If the tumor had not been enhanced with contrast mediums, the tumor size was evaluated by the high signal intensity area in T2 weighted image on MRI. The complete tumor regression was defined as complete response (CR), more than 50% tumor reduction as partial response (PR), less than 50% reduction as no change (NC), and the progressive disease as progressive disease (PD). When there is no residual tumor after the total removal, it was described as not evaluable (NE). Although our observation period was too short to evaluate the effect of therapy on survival, the analyses on survival period and the progression free survival period at present have performed.

Some independent prognostic factors regarding the results of therapy with ACNU, such as age, Karnofsky's performance scale (KPS), histological grade, tumor resection rate, combination drugs and therapies, the use of radiation, and mRNA expression, were statistically analyzed. All reported P values are two-tailed. Differences in the effect of therapy with ACNU according to the histological grade were calculated by the chi-square test. Fisher's exact probability test was used for binary variables that predicted the results of therapies with ACNU, including primary or recurrence, combination drugs, the use of radiation, and the absolute normalized value of MGMTmRNA expression. Student's t-test was used for continuous variables, including age, KPS, surgical resection rate, and dose of ACNU (mg/m^2). All statistical analyses were performed using Stat-View 5.0.

RESULTS

Real-time RT-PCR Using TaqMan Probe

The results of real-time RT-PCR using TaqMan probe in 65 neuroepithelial tumor specimens were shown in Table 1. The absolute value of MGMTmRNA normalized to the level of GAPDH in 65 neuroepithelial tumor specimens was $1.20 \times 10^4 \pm 1.19 \times 10^4$ copy/µg RNA(mean ± standard deviation). Although the more malignant tumors showed the tendency of higher MGMTmRNA value in general, the mean value of 35 glioblastomas ($1.20 \times 10^4 \pm 1.00 \times 10^4$ copy/µg RNA) was not significantly different from that of 7 low grade gliomas ($1.13 \times 10^4 \pm 0.60 \times 10^4$ copy/µg RNA) ($P = 0.4241$ by Student's t-test). No significant differences were observed between glioblastoma and other histological classification as shown in Table 1. In all 8 oligodendroglial tumors that had been known as chemosensitive,[37] the mean MGMTmRNA value ($0.91 \times 10^4 \pm 0.71 \times 10^4$ copy/µg RNA) was equivalent to that of anaplastic astrocytomas.

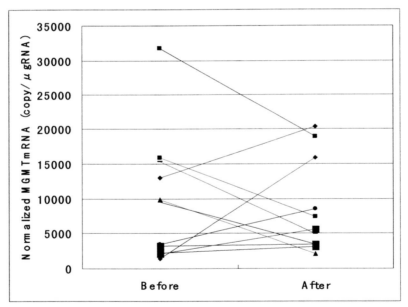

Figure 1. The changes of the absolute normalized values of MGMTmRNA in 11 measurement before and after the treatment with ACNU. MGMTmRNA was measured twice in 5 patients, three times in 3 patients. All these patients had reccurred after the treatments with ACNU. No significant elevations of MGMTmRNA after ACNU treatment were observed.

The mean value of 36 primary tumors ($1.01 \times 10^4 \pm 0.92 \times 10^4$ copy/µg RNA) was not significantly different from that of the recurrent 21 tumors after ACNU therapy ($1.46 \times 10^4 \pm 1.53 \times 10^4$) ($P = 0.0920$ by Student's t-test). MGMTmRNA was measured twice in 5 patients, three times in 3 patients. All these patients had recurred after the treatments with ACNU. The change of the absolute values of MGMTmRNA in these 11 measurement before and after the treatment with ACNU were described in Figure 1. No significant elevations of MGMTmRNA after ACNU treatment were observed.

Table 1. Summary of MGMTmRNA measurement in 65 neuroepithelial tumors

	N	Recurrent (%)	Age (Mean)	KPS (Mean)	MGMTmRNA* (x 10^3 copy/μ gRNA)	MPFS (mo.)	MST (mo.)	Effect# (CR+PR,%)
All neuroepithelial tumors	65	44.6	44.7	70.6	12.0± 11.9	7	25	40.0
Primary tumors	36	0.0	47.3	74.2	10.1± 9.2	7	18	57.1
Recurrent after ACNU therapy	21	100.0	43.0	62.4	14.6± 15.3	5	58	13.3
Medulloblastoma	1	100.0	10.0	30.0	71.9	2	102	0
Oligodendroglioma	3	66.7	28.7	83.3	10.8± 6.3	56	149	50.0
Anaplastic oligodendroglioma	5	80.0	46.0	62.0	8.1± 7.4	12	23	25.0
Astrocytoma	3	0.0	34.7	80.0	5.5± 2.6	17	62	100
Anaplastic astrocytoma	17	52.9	45.8	67.1	9.9± 8.2	8	28	53.8
Glioblastomas	35	37.1	47.3	72.0	12.0± 10.0	6	24	31.0

KPS, Karnofsky's performance scale; *mean ± standard deviation; MPFS, median progression-free survival; MST, median survival time;

*, #effect of the adjuvant therapy with ACNU; CR, complete response; PR, partial response.

Table 2. Comparison of the patients who had more and less than 6000 copy /μ gMGMTmRNA

	Normalized MGMTmRNA (copy/μ g RNA)		P value
	6000≦	6000>	-
N	37	28	-
Rate of recurrent tumor after ACNU (%)	40.0	30.8	0.7849[a]
Age (mean ± SD)	42.5 ± 14.9	47.6 ± 13.0	0.2221[b]
Karnofsky's performance scale (mean ± SD)	69.2 ± 19.6	72.5 ± 24.6	0.3070[b]
Histology (rate of Glioblastoma, %)	56.8	50.0	>0.9999[a]
Eloquent area (%)	62.2	57.1	0.6131[a]
Surgical reduction (mean ± SD, %)	65.1 ± 25.1	72.9 ± 19.1	0.2501[b]
Use of Vincristine (%)	73.0	71.4	>0.9999[a]
Radiation (%)	59.5	60.7	0.7999[a]
Dose of ACNU (mean ± SD, mg/m^2)	96.1 ± 7.2	97.2 ± 5.6	0.4843[b]
Initial effect (CR[c] +PR[d], %)	23.1	58.3	0.0421[a]

[a], Fisher's exact probability test; [b], Student's t-test; [c]CR, complete response; [d]PR, partial response (more than 50% tumor regression)

Table 3. Summary of 124 individual adjuvant therapy based on the results of RT-PCR

Histology	N	Recurrence (%)	Age*	KPS*	Surgical Reduction*(%)	Use of ACNU (%)	Results				Effect (CR+PR,%)	PFS (mo.)	MST (mo.)	2y survival rate (%)
							CR	PR	NC	PD				
All	124	43.5	45.6	66.3	65.8	68.5	7	47	25	29	50	12	20	60.7
Astrocytoma	10	10	28.9	64	59.5	50	0	6	3	0	66.7	20	31	66.7
Oligodendroglioma	2	50	30.5	95	50	100	0	1	1	0	50	34	88	100
Anaplastic oligodendroglioma	9	77.8	42.1	67.8	61.1	88.9	0	3	2	1	50	12	26	83.3
Anaplastic astrocytoma	40	50	47.4	64.3	60.5	70	3	15	9	8	51.4	10	18	57.5
Glioblastoma multiforme	56	39.3	53	66.3	70.1	67.3	4	16	10	20	40	6	22	55.6
Medulloblastoma	7	42.9	9.1	71.4	82.1	57.1	0	6	0	0	100	19	39	83.3

* = mean; KPS, Karnofsky performance scale; CR, complete response; PR, partial response; NC, no change; PD, progressive disease;

PFS, progression free survival period; MST, median survival time

The response rate, more than 50% tumor regression rate, to ACNU of 28 patients who had MGMTmRNA less than 6 x 10^3 copy/µg RNA was 58.3% and that of 37 patients who had it more than 6 x 10^3 copy/µg RNA was 23.1%. Significant difference was observed in the response rates of these two groups ($P = 0.0421$ by Fisher's exact probability test). The value normalized MGMTmRNA < 6000 copy/µg RNA was the only significant factor predicted the initial effect of therapy with ACNU among some prognostic factors such as age, Kernofsky's performance status, histological grading, surgical reduction rate, dose of ACNU, and combination therapy as shown in Table 2.

Individual Adjuvant Therapy

The patients' characteristics, therapy, and the results were described in Table 3. In 124 IAT, no lethal adverse events were happened among all therapies. Although the elevation of the body temperature more than 38°C had been observed in almost patients at the first administration of IFN-β, it was controlled well by the antipyretic agents. Eighty-five tumors (68.5%) were treated with ACNU because relative low expression value of MGMTmRNA and residual 39 tumors (31.5%) that had had relatively high MGMTmRNA were treated with platinum-compounds. The response rate of the IAT was 40.0% for glioblastoma multiformes, 51.4% for anaplastic astrocytomas, and 50.0% for all evaluable therapies. Although the median survival periods were relatively short because of the too short follow-up periods, the two year survival rate of 45 glioblastoma patients was 55.6% at present.

DISCUSSION

Drug-resistance genes are some of the most important elements of the tumors themselves for determining drug-resistance. [15] For the individualization of chemotherapy based on the evaluation of drug-resistance, many drug-resistance genes have recently been examined. Multidrug-resistance genes (MDRs) have been thought to be associated with resistance to vincristine, etoposide, and other drugs. [2, 4, 5, 8] Recently, multidrug resistance-associated proteins (MRPs) have also been considered to be important in resistance to these drugs. [9] Some drug-resistance genes, such as glutathion-S transferase (GST), glutathion, and methalothionein, are thought to be related to the sensitivity to Pt-compounds. Of these molecules, GST-π has been reported to be the most closely related to tumor resistance to Pt-compounds. [13, 14] The significance of MDRs, MRPs, and GST-πexpression in brain tumors is also controversial. [2, 4, 8, 9] No evidence on the correlation of MDR1, MRP, and GST-π expression with the clinical response to applicable drugs has been reported for brain tumors, in contrast to other tumors. [2] Even with other tumors, the correlation between MDR1 and MRP expression and a clinical response to an applicable drug is controversial. MGMT is one of the most important genes for ACNU resistance.[18, 19, 30, 37] According to our results, the tumor with compensated MGMTmRNA value greater than 6000 copy/µgRNA in real-time quantitative RT-PCR should not be treated by ACNU.

As previously mentioned, MGMT expression is closely related to resistance to ACNU. [18, 37] Some authors, including us, have reported that MGMT expression is closely correlated with the clinical or experimental resistance of brain tumors to ACNU. [25, 38] There are at least two possible approaches to increase the effectiveness of nitrosoureas in the presence of MGMT; i.e., avoid using nitrosoureas in MGMT active tumors as in our approach, and overcome the resistance of MGMT to nitrosoureas. MGMT is different from other enzymes because it is consumed. Some authors have tried to repair alkylated DNA by MGMT using this specificity. Excessive alkylating agents, such as high-dose ACNU or 5-(3-3,-dimethyl-1-triazeno) imidazole-4-carboxamate, which can waste MGMT, have been used for this purpose. [39, 40] However, the results of these therapies were disappointing due to severe side effects and a low response rate. Antisense MGMTmRNA and some other drugs may reduce the ability of MGMT to repair the effects of alkylation. [41] Although O^6-benzylguanine and streptozocin have been expected to modulate the resistance to nitrosoureas, favorable clinical results with large numbers of patients have not yet been reported. [42, 43]

Recently, the inactivation of MGMT by promoter hypermethylation has been reported to be a common event in primary human neoplasm. [44] Esteller *et al.* reported that hypermethylation of the MGMT promoter in gliomas was a useful predictor of the responsiveness of the tumors to alkylating agents. [31] Our results of quantitative RT-PCR for MGMT showed a close relationship between MGMTmRNA expression and the prognosis of patients treated with ACNU. This does not contradict the promoter methylation theory of MGMT inactivation because promoter hypermethylation resulted in a decrease or disappearance of MGMT expression in real-time quantitative RT-PCR. This hypermethylation in the promoter region of MGMT may be useful for clinically overcoming MGMT function and for making ACNU effective in gliomas.

A large randomized trial by European Organization for Research and Treatment of Cancer of newly diagnosed patients with glioblastoma comparing radiation alone with radiation plus temozolomide has published.[45] Since MGMT is an enzyme thought to confer resistance to temozolomide as well as nitrosoureas, our technique of ascertaining MGMT activity by real-time RT-PCR may have applicable for the use of temozolomide.[47]

In our presented results, down-regulation of MGMTmRNA by the administration of ACNU has not been observed. We recently reported that platinum compounds might be able to reduce MGMTmRNA expression with a subsequent high response rate compared to nitrosoureas in chemotherapy for recurrence.[47] Platinum compounds may provide a longer useful life for patients with malignant gliomas than nitrosoureas.

Evidence-based medicine (EBM) now seems to be widely accepted.[48] In adjuvant glioma therapy, there is no confirmed evidence that any treatment other than radiation or radiation plus chemotherapy with nitrosoureas prolongs patient survival.[28] A major prospective randomized controlled study is currently impossible because there are no control therapies that are widely performed.

One of the major reasons why glioma therapy has been difficult is the heterogeneity of the tumor. Histological features, biological behavior, and the response to therapy all vary in such cases. Histological grading does not always coincide with the sensitivity of the tumor. A new grouping that indicates the appropriate therapeutic modality is needed for gliomas. Some recent molecular biological studies have shown new classifications of gliomas, which include the concept of primary and secondary glioblastoma.[49] Our previous report also showed that secondary glioma has a better therapeutic response than primary glioblastomas.[24]

The individualization of tumor therapy, such as "made-to-order therapy", is now widely recommended for many kinds of malignant tumors.[50] Gliomas seem to be suitable for made-to-order therapy based on the heterogeneity of the tumor as described above. In this study, we addressed individualization mainly based on a molecular biological analysis of the tumor itself. Some independent factors regarding the patient and tumor, such as age, KPS, histological grade, combined use of radiation and other anti-cancer drugs, varied between individuals. Since our study has been preliminary, our results cannot be compared to those with other protocols, even to historical controls, since the therapies applied were heterogeneous. This fact makes it difficult to evaluate the efficacy of any made-to-order therapy, including our IAT.

Studies on made-to-order therapies can be grouped into two types: investigations of drug-sensitivity and evaluations of drug-resistance. Investigations of the sensitivity of a tumor prior to use of a drug seem to be ideal for tumor therapy. Primary cell cultures have been used to test sensitivity in tumor therapy.[51] However, these methods have often failed in the first primary cell culture, despite the high cost and time needed. In addition, the *in vitro* and *in vivo* sensitivities often do not agree with the clinical effectiveness because of problems with the drug-delivery system or for other reasons.

In our results of the overall IAT described above, the response rate was more higher than the other any previously reported result of the protocol therapy for glioma.[22] In contrast, the median survival period of the patients was relatively short, because the follow-up periods of the patients were too short to compare with other series. [28] In spite of the relatively short follow-up periods, more than 50% two years survival rate of the patients with glioblastoma is further excellent therapeutic results than the previous reports. A prospective randomized multi-center study should be performed to confirm the efficacy of this new method for glioma therapy.

Essentially, PCR is not suitable for quantification.[52] However, because it is easy, rapid, and sensitive, quantification by PCR has been attempted. Competitive PCR is one of the most popular methods: it requires new primers to be made and the results vary according to differences in the amplification efficacy.[53, 54] Furthermore, the ratio of the products may not remain constant throughout amplification. Additionally, the dynamic range of competitive PCR is limited to a target ratio-to-competitor ratio of about 1:10 or 10:1. Before the introduction of real-time PCR, some manual quantitative RT-PCR that had been theoretically equivalent to real-time PCR were performed.[55-59] The real-time PCR methods we used are based on a kinetic analysis of the amplification curve.[60] At present, real-time PCR seems to be the most sensitive and rapid method for the quantitation of DNA and RNA.

Real-time PCR systems can be improved by the probe-based, rather than intercalator-based, detection of PCR product. Fluorescently labeled probes for detecting amplified products have been used in most reports on real-time PCR for diagnostic purposes.[61] However, labeled probes introduce an additional complexity to both the design and parameters of the amplification reaction. Despite the use of specific probes, artifacts can occur, especially beyond the 30th amplification cycle. In previous study, we used SYBR Green dye, which binds to double-stranded DNA and provides a fluorescent signal.[62] This approach is simpler and more sensitive, since many fluorescent labels, instead of just one molecule, are incorporated into an amplified fragment. The disadvantage of fluorescence dye is that both specific and non-specific products generate signal. At present, our presented methods are seemed to be most accurate measurement of mRNA because of the absolute value measurement by the comparison with the control DNA and the normalization by the internal control.

CONCLUSION

Our presented results suggest that quantitation of MGMTmRNA is the excellent method for predicting for the effect of ACNU in glioma therapy. IAT by means of absolute value quantitation of MGMTmRNA normalized to the level of GAPDH seems to be the effective for glioma therapy. The primary results of the overall IAT based on the results of RT-PCR of MGMTmRNA since 1997 is encouraging. A prospective randomized multi-center study should be performed to confirm the efficacy of this new method for glioma therapy.

REFERENCES

[1]   Becker I, Becker KF, Meyermann R, Hollt V: The multidrug resistance gene MDR1 is expressed in human glial tumors. *Acta Neuropathol Berl 82:* 516-519, 1991.

[2]   Kartner N, Riordan JR, Ling V: Cell surface P-glycoprotein associated with multidrug resistance in mammalian cell lines. *Science 221:* 1285-1288, 1983.

[3]   Kirches E, Oda Y, Von Bossanyi P, Diete S, Schneider T, Warich Kirches M, Dietzmann K: Mdr1 mRNA expression differs between grade III astrocytomas and glioblastomas. *Clin Neuropathol 16:* 34-36, 1997.

[4]   Nabors MW, Griffin CA, Zehnbauer BA, Hruban RH, Phillips PC, Grossman ST, Brem H, Colvin M: Multudrug resistance gene (MDR1) expression in human brain tumors. *J Neurosurg 75:* 941-946, 1991.

[5]   Noonan KE, Beck C, Holzmayer TA, Chin JE, Wunder JS, Andrulis IL, Gazdar AF, Willman CL, Griffith B, von Hoff DD, Roninson IB: Quantitative analysis of MDR1 (multidrug resistance) gene expression in human tumors by polymerase chain reaction. *Proc Natl Acad Sci USA 87:* 7160-7164, 1990.

[6]   Riordan JR, Deuchars K, Kartner N, Alon N, Trent J, Ling V : Amplification of P-glycoprotein genes in multidrug-resistant mammalian cell lines. *Nature 316:* 817-819, 1985 .

[7]   Tishler DM, Weinberg KI, Sender LS, Nolta JA, Raffel C: Multidrug resistance gene expression in pediatric primitive neuroectodermal tumors of the central nervous system. *J Neurosurg 76*: 507-512, 1992.

[8]   Toth K, Vaughan MM, Peress NS, Slocum HK, Rustum YM : MDR1 P-glycoprotein is expressed by endothelial cells of newly formed capillaries in human gliomas but is not expressed in the neovasculature of other primary tumors. *Am J Pathol 149:* 853-858, 1996.

[9]   Abe T, Hasegawa S, Taniguchi K, Yokomizo A, Kuwano T, Ono M, Mori T, Hori S, Kohno K, Kuwano M: Possible involvement of multidrug-resistance-associated protein (MRP) gene expression in spontaneous drug resistance to vincristine, etoposide and adriamycin in human glioma cells. *Int J Cancer 58 :*860-864, 1994 .

[10] Endo K, Maehara Y, Kusumoto T, Ichiyoshi Y, Kuwano M, Sugimachi K: Expression of multidrug-resistance-associated protein (MRP) and chemosensitivity in human gastric cancer. *Int J Cancer 68*: 372-377, 1996.

[11] Narasaki F, Matsuo I, Ikuno N, Fukuda M, Soda H, Oka M: Multidrug resistance-associated protein (MRP) gene expression in human lung cancer. *Anticancer Res 16:* 2079-2082, 1996.

[12] Tomonaga M, Oka M, Narasaki F, Fukuda M, Nakano R, Takatani H, Ikeda K, Teranishi K, Matsuo I, Soda H, Cowan KH, Kohno S: The multidrug resistance-associated protein gene confers drug resistance in human gastric and colon cancers. *Jpn J Cancer Res 87:* 1263-1270, 1996.

[13] Hara A, Sakai N, Yamada H, Tanaka T, Kato K, Mori H, Sato K: Induction of glutathion S-transferase, placental type in T9 glioma cells by dibutyryladenosine 3',5'-cyclic monophosphate and modification of its expression by naturally occurring isothiocyanates. *Acta Neuropathol (Berl) 79 :*144-148, 1989 .

[14] Hara A, Yamada H, Sakai N, Hirayama H, Tanaka T, Mori H: Immunohistochemical demonstration of the placental form of glutathione S-transferase, a detoxifying enzyme in human gliomas. *Cancer 66 :*2563-2568, 1990 .

[15] Kim W-J, Kakehi Y, Kinoshita H, Arao S, Fukumoto M, Yoshida O: Expression patterns of multidrug-resistance (MDR1), multidrug resistance-associated protein (MRP), glutathion-S-transferase-π (GST-π) and DNA topoisomerase□ (TOPO□) genes in renal cell carcinomas and normal kidney. *J Urol 156:* 506-511, 1996.

[16] Silvani A, Milanesi I, Munari L, Broggi G, Botturi M, Boiardi A: Intratumoral beta interferon and systemic chemotherapy. Preliminary data in GBM patients. *J Neurosurg Sci 34:* 257-259, 1990.

[17] Tano K, Shiota S, Collier J, Foote RS, Mitra S: Isolation and structural characterization of a cDNA clone encoding the human DNA repair protein for O^6-alkylguanine. *Proc Natl Acad Sci USA 87:* 686-690, 1990.

[18] Nagane M, Asai A, Shibui S, Nomura K, Matsutani M, Kuchino Y: Expression of O^6-methylguanine-DNA methyltransferase and chloroethylnitrosourea resistance of human brain tumors. *Jpn J Clin Oncol 22:* 143-149, 1992.

[19] Wu Z, Chan CL, Eastman A, Bresnick E: Expression of human O^6-methylguanine-DNA methyltransferase in Chinese hamster ovary cells and restoration of cellular resistance to certain N-nitroso compounds. *Mol Carcinog 4:* 482-488, 1991 .

[20] Hori T, Muraoka K, Saito Y, Sasahara K, Inagaki H, Inoue Y, Adach S, Anno Y: Influence of mode of ACNU administration on tissue and blood drug concentration in malignant tumors. *J Neurosurg 66:* 372-378, 1987.

[21] Tanaka S, Tabuchi S, Watanabe K, Takigawa H, Akatsuka K, Numata H, Hokama Y, Hori T: Preventive effects of interleukin 1β for ACNU-induced myelosuppression in malignant brain tumors: the experimental and preliminary clinical studies. *J Neuro-Oncology 14:* 159-168, 1992.

[22] Yoshida J, Kajita Y, Wakabayashi T, Sugita K. Long-term follow up results of 175 patients with malignant glioma: importance of radical tumor resection and postoperative adjuvant therapy with interferon, ACNU and radiation. *Acta Neurochir (Wien) 127:* 55-59, 1994.

[23] Tanaka S, Kamitani H, Amin MR, Watanabe T, Oka H, Fujii K, Nagashima T, Hori T: Preliminary individual adjuvant therapy for gliomas based on the results of molecular biological analyzes for drug-resistance genes. *J Neuro-Oncology 46:* 157-171, 2000.

[24] Tanaka S, Kobayashi I, Oka H, Fujii K, Watanabe T, Nagashima T, Hori T: Drug-resistance gene expression and progression of astrocytic tumors. *Brain Tumor Pathol 18*: 131-137, 2001.

[25] Tanaka. S, Kobayashi I, Oka H, Fujii K, Watanabe T, Nagashima T Hori T: O^6-methylguanine-DNA methyltranspherase gene expression in gliomas by quantitative real-time RT-PCR and clinical response to nitrosoureas. *Int J Cancer 103:* 67-72, 2003.

[26] Tanaka S, Oka H, Fujii K, Watanabe K, Nagao K, Kakimoto A: Quantitation of O^6 – Methylguanine - DNA Methyltransferase Gene Messenger RNA in Gliomas by Means of Real-Time RT-PCR and Clinical Response to Nitrosoureas. *Cell Mol Neurobiol 25:* 1067-1071, 2005.

[27] Boiardi A, Silvani A, Milanesi I, Botturi M, Broggi G: Primary glial tumor patients treated by combining cis-platin and etoposide. *J Neurooncol 11:* 165-170, 1991.

[28] Walker MD, Green SB, Byar DP, Alexander E Jr, Batzdorf U, Brooks WH, Hunt WE, MacCarty CS, Mahaley MS Jr, Mealey J Jr, Owens G, Ransohoff J 2nd, Robertson JT, Shapiro WR, Smith KR Jr, Wilson CB, Strike TA: Randomized comparisons of radiotherapy and nitrosoureas for the treatment of malignant glioma after surgery. *N Engl J Med 303:* 1323-1329, 1980.

[29] Arcicasa M, Roncadin M, Bortolus R, Bassignano G., Boz G., Franchin G., De Paoli A, Trovo MG.: Results of three consecutive combined treatments for malignant gliomas. Ten-year experience at a single institution. *Am J Clin Oncol 17*: 437-443, 1994.

[30] Mineura K, Izumi I, Watanabe K, Kowada M: Influence of O^6-methylguanine-DNA methyltransferase activity on chloroethylnitrosourea. *Int J Cancer 55:* 76-81, 1993.

[31] Esteller M, Garcia-Foncillas J, Andion E, Goodman SN, Hidalgo OF, Vanaclocha V, Baylin SB, Herman JG.: Inactivation of the DNA-repair gene MGMT and the clinical response of gliomas to alkylating agents. *New Engl J Med 343:* 1350-1354, 2000.

[32] Boiardi A, Silvani A, Milanesi I, Botturi M, Broggi G.: Carboplatin combined with carmustine and etoposide in the treatment of glioblastoma. *Ital J Neurol Sci 13:* 717-722, 1992..

[33] Chomczynski P, Sacchi N: Single-step methods of RNA isolation by acid guanidinium thiocyanate-phenol-chloroform extraction. *Anal Biochem 162:*156-159, 1987.

[34] Mogami H, Ushio Y, Sano K, Takakura K, Handa H, Yamashita J, Ueki K, Tanaka R, Hatanaka H, Nomura K: Criteria for evaluation treatment regimens for patients with brain tumor. *Neurol Med Chir (Tokyo) 26:* 191-194, 1986.

[35] Gebel JM, Sila CA, Sloan MA, Granger CB, Weisenberger JP, Green CL, Topol EJ, Mahaffey KW: Comparison of the ABC/2 estimation technique to computer-assisted volumetric analysis of intraparencymal and subdural hematomas complicating the GUSTO-1 trial. *Stroke 29:* 1799-1801, 1998.

[36] Ueki K: Oligodendroglioma: impact of molecular biology on its definition, diagnosis and management. Review. *Neuropathology 25:* 247-253, 2005 .

[37] Mineura K, Yanagisawa T, Watanabe K, Kowada M, Yasui N: Human brain tumor O(6)- methylguanine-DNA methyltransferase mRNA and its significance as an indicator of selective chloroethylnitrosourea chemotherapy. *Int J Cancer 69:* 420-426, 1996.

[38] Nagane M, Shibui S, Oyama H, Asai A, Kuchino Y, Nomura K: Investigation of chemoresistance-related genes mRNA expression for selecting anticancer agents in successful adjuvant chemotherapy for a case of recurrent glioblastoma. *Surg Neurol 44:* 462-468, 1995.

[39] Ikeda J, Aida T, Sawamura Y, Abe H, Kaneko S, Kashiwaba T, Kawamoto T, Mitsumori K, Saitoh H: Phase II study of DTIC, ACNU, and vincristine combined chemotherapy for supratentorial malignant astrocytomas. *Neurol Med Chir (Tokyo) 36:* 555-559, 1996.

[40] Nomura K, Watanabe T, Nakamura O, Ohira M, Shibui S, Takakura K, Miki Y: Intensive chemotherapy with autologous bone marrow rescue for recurrent malignant gliomas. *Neurosurg Rev 7:* 13-22, 1984.

[41] Nagane M, Asai A, Shibui S, Nomura K, Kuchino Y: Application of antisense ribonucleic acid complementary to O^6-methylguanine-deoxyribonucleic acid methyltransferase messenger ribonucleic acid for therapy of malignant gliomas. *Neurosurgery 41:* 434-441, 1997.

[42] Marathi UK, Dolan ME, Erickson LC: Anti-neoplastic activity of sequenced administration of O^6-benzylguanine, streptozotocin, and 1, 3-bis(2-chloroethyl)-1-nitrosourea *in vitro* and *in vivo*. *Biochem Pahrmacol 48:* 2127-2134, 1994.

[43] Zhao KM, Chen JM, Zuo HZ, Wu Y, Zhang YP: Modulation of O6-methylguanine-DNA methyltranspherase-mediated nimustine resistance in recurrent malignant gliomas by streptozotocin – a preliminary report. *Anticancer Res 15:* 645-648, 1995.

[44] Esteller M, Hamilton SR, Burger PC, Baylin SB, Herman JG.: Inactivation of the DNA repair gene O6-methylguanine-DNA methyltranspherase by promotor hypermethylation is a common event in primary human neoplasia. *Cancer Res 59:* 793-797, 1999.

[45] Ataman F, Poortmans P, Stupp R, Fisher B, Mirimanoff RO: Quality assurance of the EORTC 26981/22981; NCIC CE3 intergroup trial on radiotherapy with or without temozolomide for newly-diagnosed glioblastoma multiforme: the individual case review. *Eur J Cancer 40:* 1724-1730, 2004.

[46] Hegi ME, Diserens AC, Godard S, Dietrich PY, Regli L, Ostermann S, Otten P, Van Melle G, de Tribolet N, Stupp R: Clinical trial substantiates the predictive value of O-6-methylguanine-DNA methyltransferase promoter methylation in glioblastoma patients treated with temozolomide. *Clin Cancer Res 10:* 1871-1874, 2004.

[47] Tanaka S, Kobayashi I, Utsuki S, Oka H, Yasui Y, Fujii K: Down-regulation of O^6-methylguanine-DNA methyltransferase gene expression in gliomas by platinum compounds. *Oncology Reports 14:* 1275-1280, 2005.

[48] Sackett DL, Rosenberg WM: The need for evidence-based medicine. *J R Soc Med 88:* 620-624, 1995.

[49] James CD, Olson JJ: Molecular genetics and molecular biology advances in brain tumors. *Curr Opin Oncol 8:* 188-195, 1996.

[50] Ragnhammar P, Brorsson B, Nygren P, Glimelius B: A prospective study of the use of chemotherapy in Sweden and assessment of the use in relation to scientific evidence. *Acta Oncol 40:* 391-411, 2001.

[51] Kubota T, Sasano N, Abe O, Nakao I, Kawamura E, Saito T, Endo M, Kimura K, Demura H, Sasano H, Nagura H, Ogawa N, Hoffman RM: Potential of the histoculture drug-response assay to contribute to cancer patient survival. *Clin Cancer Res 1:* 1537-1543, 1995.

[52] Saiki RK, Gelfand DH, Stoffel S, Scharf SJ, Higuchi R, Horn GT, Mullis KB, Erlich HA: Primer-directed enzymatic amplification of DNA with a thermostable DNA polymerase. *Science 239:* 487-491, 1988.

[53] Gilliland G, Perrin S, Blanchard K, Bunn HF: Analysis of cytokine mRNA and DNA: detection and quantitation by competitive polymerase chain reaction. *Proc Natl Acad Sci USA 87:* 2725-2729, 1990.

[54] Siebert PD, Larrick JW: Competitive PCR. *Nature 359:* 557-558, 1992.

[55] Kinoshita T, Imamura J, Nagai H, Shimotohno K: Quantification of gene expression over a wide range by the polymerase chain reaction. *Anal Biochem 206:* 231-235, 1992.

[56] Nakayama H, Yokoi H, Fujita J: Quantification of mRNA by non-radioactive RT-PCR and CCD imaging system. *Nucleic Acid Res 220:* 4939, 1992.

[57] Yokoi H, Natsuyaa S, Iwai M, Noda Y, Mori T, Mori KJ, Fujita K, Nakayama H, Fujita J: Non-radioisotopic quantitative RT-PCR to detect changes in mRNA levels during early mouse embryo development. *Bioochem Biophys Res Comm 195:* 769-775, 1993.

[58] Kojima K, Kanzaki H, Iwai M, Hatayama H, Fujimoto M, Inoue T, Horie K, Nakayama H, Fujita J, Mori T: Expression of leukemia inhibitory factor in human endometrium and placenta. *Biol Reprod 50:* 882-887, 1994.

[59] Schwartz SJr, Caceres C, De Torres I, Morote J, Rodriguez-Vallejo JM, Gonzalez J, Reventos J: Over-expression of epidermal growth factor receptor and erbB2/neu but not of int-2 genes in benign prostatic hyperplasia by means of semi-quantitative PCR. *Int J Cancer 76:* 464-467, 1998.

[60] Heid CA, Stevens J, Livak KJ, Williams PM: Real time quantitative PCR. *Genome Res 6:* 986-994, 1996.

[61] Mullah B, Livak K, Andrus A, Kenney P: Efficient synthesis of double dye-labeled oligodeoxyribonucleotide probes and their application in a real time PCR assay. *Nucleic Acids Res 26:* 1026-1031, 1998.

[62] Aldea C, Alvarez CP, Folgueira L, Delgado R, Otero JR: Rapid detection of herpes simplex virus DNA in genital ulcers by real-time PCR using SYBR green I dye as the detection signal. *J Clin Microbiol 40:* 1060-1062, 2002.

In: Multidrug Resistance-Associated Proteins
Editor: Christopher V. Aiello, pp. 49-79

ISBN 1-60021-298-0
© 2007 Nova Science Publishers, Inc.

Chapter 3

PREDICTION OF THERAPEUTIC RESPONSES TO CHEMOTHERAPY AND MONITOR OF EFFECTS OF MDR-MODULATION WITH RADIOTRACERS IN MALIGNANT TUMORS

Seigo Kinuya*, Xiao-Feng Li, Jingming Bai, Kunihiko Yokoyama, Takatoshi Michigishi and Norihisa Tonami

Department of Biotracer Medicine, Kanazawa University Graduate School of Medical Sciences, Kanazawa, Japan

ABSTRACT

Lipophilic cationic nuclear tracers, technetium-99m-sestamibi (^{99m}Tc-MIBI) and technetium-99m-tetrofosmin (^{99m}Tc-TF), have been investigated as tumor imaging agents in various kinds of malignancy. They may not only delineate lesions but also provide information pertaining to tumor characteristics. There is sufficient evidence that these tracers are substrates of cell surface molecules, P-glycoprotein (P-gp) and multi-drug resistance associated proteins (MRP); therefore, they may enable scintigraphic pre-therapeutic prediction of tumor responses to chemotherapy. That is, tumors that do not take up these tracers are likely to fail to respond to chemotherapy. Furthermore, effectiveness of modulators to reverse the resistance attributable to these molecules may be monitored by changes in the tracer accumulation. In this paper, tracer kinetics of ^{99m}Tc-MIBI and ^{99m}Tc-TF in MRP-expressing tumor cell lines and their limitations to assess reversal effects of classical modulators on the function of MRP are demonstrated based on our experimental results. In addition, recent findings regarding the feasibility of scintigraphic monitoring on translational inhibition of mRNA coding MRP with antisense oligodeoxynucleotide are discussed.

* Correspondence to: Seigo Kinuya, M.D., Ph.D., Department of Biotracer Medicine (Nuclear Medicine), Kanazawa University Graduate School of Medical Sciences, 13-1 Takaramachi, Kanazawa, Ishikawa 920-8640, Japan. Tel:+81-76-265-2333; Fax:+81-76-234-4257; E-mail: kinuya@med.kanazawa-u.ac.jp

Key words: multidrug resistance; multidrug resistance-associated protein; p-glycoprotein; technetium-99m-tetrofosmin; technetium-99m-sestamibi; modulator; oligodeoxy-nucleotide; scintigraphy

INTRODUCTION

Intrinsic or acquired resistance of tumor cells to chemotherapeutic drugs, multi-drug resistance (MDR), is extremely complex and is mediated in most cases by a combination of multifactorial events caused by environmental difficulties in delivering drugs to tumors due to poor and heterogeneous vascularization in tissues and biochemical cellular mechanisms [1]. The latter includes enhanced drug detoxification by glutathione-S-transferase, changes in the levels or activity of nuclear targets such as topoisomerase II, alterations in the control of apoptosis and decreased intracellular cytotoxic drug accumulation [2]. Reduced accumulation of drugs most frequently results from the increased expression of cell surface molecules belonging to the adenosine triphosphate (ATP)-binding cassette (ABC) superfamily of transporters such as the P-glycoprotein/MDR1 (P-gp), a 170-kDa protein, and multi-drug resistance associated proteins (MRP) [3-6]. They are transmembrane pumps extruding drugs from the cells. Chemotherapeutic drugs, including the anthracyclines, taxanes, vinca alkaloids and epipodophyllotoxins are involved in this mechanism. Although these drugs possess diverse chemical features, they are generally hydrophobic and positively charged at neutral pH [7].

Technetium-99m-labeled cationic compounds, technetium hexakis 2-methoxyisobutylisonitrile (sestamibi or MIBI) and trans-dioxo-bis(disphosphine)-technetium (tetrofosmin or TF), were originally developed as agents that provide information on myocardial perfusion [2, 8, 9]. In 1987, Muller et al. [10] has first reported ^{99m}Tc-MIBI accumulation in lung tumors during cardiac imaging. ^{99m}Tc-TF has been also found to have tumor-avid properties [2, 8, 9]. It is now known that these tracers are taken up by various kinds of malignant tumors [2, 8, 9]. Previous works have indicated that these compounds may not only enable to delineate lesions but also provide information pertaining to tumor characteristics [2, 8, 9]. There is sufficient evidence suggesting that lesion response can be monitored during and at the conclusion of treatment including chemotherapy and radiotherapy [2, 8, 9, 11-24]. For instance, in breast cancer patients undergoing chemotherapy, reduction of ^{99m}Tc-MIBI accumulation in lesions after treatment is related with good therapeutic responses [12, 13, 16]. Similar results have been demonstrated in other types of malignant tumors such as small cell lung cancer [14, 15], non-small cell lung cancer [17-21], bone and soft tissue sarcomas [22] with ^{99m}Tc-MIBI and ^{99m}Tc-TF.

Depending on their lipophilic, cationic properties, they serve as substrates for ABC transporters [25, 26]. That is, ^{99m}Tc-MIBI and ^{99m}Tc-TF are cleared out from cells expressing ABC transporters, indicating that negative visualization of tumors with these tracers is a sign of poor response to chemotherapy [27-36]. Furthermore, potential utility of these radiotracers to assess the effects of agents that can reverse MDR functions of tumours has been documented [37-48]. Effects of translational inhibition of mRNA coding ABC transporters with antisense oligodeoxynucleotide (ODN) [49-52] or hammerhead ribozymes [53, 54] may be assessed by these tracers as well. The most recent report indicated that inhibition of the MDR1 expression by RNA interference may be monitored with ^{99m}Tc-MIBI [55].

Biopsy combined with molecular biological analysis such as Western blotting and Northern blotting or immunohistochemical techniques is beneficial for the detection of MDR ability of tumors; however, technical difficulties and possible sampling error may lead to incorrect diagnosis. In addition, because of the fact that distribution of P-gp and MRP is heterogeneous in many types of tumors, MDR determination by the small biopsy specimen may not reflect expression of these transporter proteins throughout tumor tissues [35]. In contrast, nuclear medicine imaging can non-invasively assess whole-tumor characteristics, so that it scan be a choice in terms of prediction of chemotherapeutic effects on malignancies. In this review, current status and future perspectives of scintigraphic monitoring of tumor characteristics with radiotracers are discussed.

EXPERIMENTAL EVIDENCE ON ^{99M}TC-MIBI AND ^{99M}TC-TF AS SUBSTRATES FOR P-GP AND MRP

The first results that have showed the relationship between P-gp function and ^{99m}Tc-MIBI accumulation were reported by Piwnica-Worms et al [56]. Numerous reports succeeded this one, demonstrating relationship between P-gp or MRP and ^{99m}Tc-MIBI or ^{99m}Tc-TF [25, 34, 37, 39, 41, 42, 57-62].

We observed ^{99m}Tc-MIBI accumulation in the P-gp expressing P388/R murine monocytic leukemia cell line and its parental P388 non-MDR cell line [63, 64]. Cells were incubated at 1 x 10^7 cell/ml with ^{99m}Tc-MIBI at 185 kBq/ml in 5% CO_2/95% air. At various time points, 200 μl aliquots were transferred to 4.5-mL plastic tubes containing 3 mL cold PBS and centrifuged for 5 min (1000 rpm). The pellets were washed twice with 3 mL cold PBS. ^{99m}Tc-MIBI accumulation in P388 cells increased with time, but it was steadily low in P388/R cells (Figure 1).

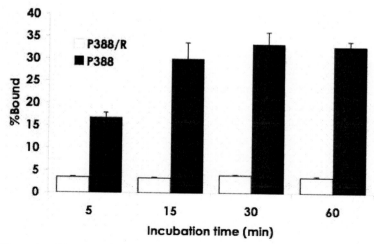

Figure 1. 99mTc-sestamibi accumulation in non-MDR P388 murine leukemia cells and P-gp expressing P388/R cells. Mean ± SD (n=3).

Similarly, the human leukemia cell line HL60/WT and its subclone, HL60/DOX that expresses MRP, but does not show P-gp expression, were incubated with ^{99m}Tc-TF [57]. ^{99m}Tc-TF uptake was initiated by adding to the cell suspension of 1 x 10[7] cells/ml at 4°C or 37°C. ^{99m}Tc-TF accumulation did not appreciably occur at 4°C in either HL60/WT cells or HL60/DOX cells (Figure 2). At 37°C, ^{99m}Tc-TF accumulated in HL60/WT cells, but not in HL60/DOX cells. These results indicate that cellular ^{99m}Tc-TF accumulation is an energy-dependent phenomenon, and ^{99m}Tc-TF is a substrate for MRP.

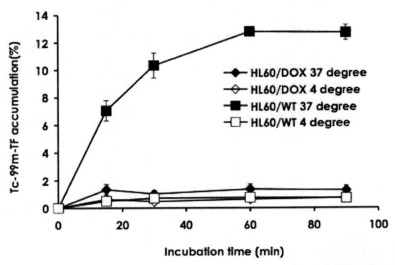

Figure 2. 99mTc-TF accumulation in HL60/WT (□) and HL60/DOX (◇) cells at 37oC (closed symbol) and 4oC (open symbol). Mean ± SD (n=3).

Retention of tracers also diminished in MDR cells. HL60/DOX and HL60/WT cells were incubated with ^{99m}Tc-TF at 37°C. After incubated for 60 min, the cells were washed twice with cold PBS and then resuspended in tracer-free medium at 37°C. Sample aliquots of 200 µl were taken from the cell suspension at various time points, the efflux of ^{99m}Tc-TF was terminated by adding cold PBS, and the radioactivity in the cell pellets was measured. The washout of ^{99m}Tc-TF was much faster in HL60/DOX than in HL60/WT: the retention of ^{99m}Tc-TF was 18.20 ± 0.34% in HL60/DOX and 84.74 ± 0.65% in HL60/WT at 3 min after the initiation of the efflux (Figure 3). This type of time-dependent washout has been also found in the P388 and P388/R cell lines with ^{99m}Tc-MIBI.

Tracer kinetics similar to these results is reported in many other kinds of cells such as lung cancer cells, breast cancer cells, colon cancer cells, glioma cells and sarcoma cells [25, 34, 37, 39, 41, 42, 57-62]. Furthermore, there is clear evidence that the content of mRNA for MDR proteins is inversely correlated with tracer accumulation in cells [49, 50, 65-67]. We isolated Poly(A)[+]RNAs from subcutaneous tumors of P388 and P388/R cells in BALB/c nu/nu nude mice, and mdr1 mRNA expression was measured by Reverse Transcription-Polymerase Chain Reaction (RT-PCR) analysis [64]. P388/R cells intensely expressed mdr1 mRNA in comparison with P388 cells (Lanes 1, 2 in Figure 4), whereas ^{99m}Tc-MIBI accumulation in P388/R cells was mush lower than that in P388 cells (Figure 1). We similarly found approximately 6 times higher MRP1 mRNA content in the MCF7/VP human breast cancer cell line exhibiting MDR profile than that in the parental non-MDR MCF7 cell line

[50, 68]. ^{99m}Tc-MIBI accumulation in MCF7 cells was approximately 7 times higher than that in MCF7/VP cells.

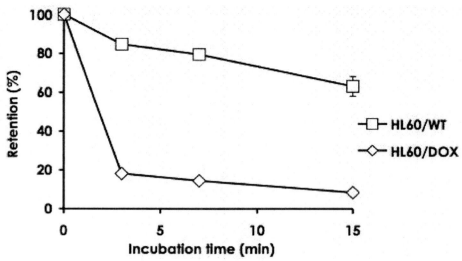

Figure 3. 99mTc-TF washout kinetics in HL60/DOX and HL60/WT cells. Retention of 99mTc-TF expressed as a percentage of initial cellular 99mTc-TF accumulation. Mean ± SD (n=3).

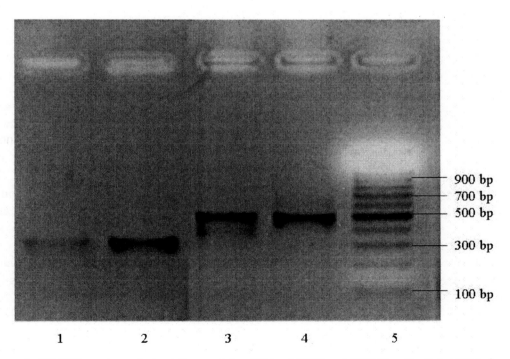

Figure 4. RT-PCR products derived from mdr1 mRNA of P388 and P388/R cells. Poly+RNA from P388 and P388/R cells was analyzed by RT-PCR with primers specific to mouse mdr1 mRNA and GAPDH mRNA. Lane 1, mdr1 in P388; lane 2, mdr1 in P388/R; lane 3, Glyceraldehyde-3-phosphate dehydrogenase (GAPDH) in P388/S; lane 4, GAPDH in P388/R; lane 5, size marker.GAPDH served as an internal reference to ensure integrity of the RNAs.

Clinical Results to Pretherapeutically Predict Efficacy of Chemotherapy

In terms of the pretherapeutic prediction of lesion responses to chemotherapy with ^{99m}Tc-MIBI and ^{99m}Tc-TF, numerous literatures are available in many kinds of malignant tumors such as small cell lung cancer, non-small lung cancer, breast cancer, malignant lymphoma, gastric cancer and hepatocellular cancer [27-36, 67, 69-73]. In general, number of reports supporting the feasibility in this issue is increasing. However, the clinical data remain to be somewhat conflicting [74-76].

Lack of standard imaging protocol may be responsible for this conflict [2]. For instance, time of imaging after administration varies among reports. Data acquisition is commonly performed at several time points after intravenous administration, based on in vitro experimental results suggesting that initial tracer accumulation and/or its washout from lesions would reflect transporter expression. Typically, so-called early images and delayed images are obtained. Early and delayed uptake ratios defined as target counts to background counts are usually obtained to express lesional signal intensities. In addition, retention index defined as (delayed ratio – early ratio)/early ratio is calculated to demonstrate washout kinetics of tracers from lesions. The problem is that there is a wide variation of acquisition time for both early imaging, 10-60 min after injection, and delayed imaging, 2-4 hours. Because tracer kinetics in tissues is extremely time-dependent, difficulty remains in comparing uptake ratios and retention indexes reported in different literatures.

These facts strongly suggest the necessity to make standard acquisition protocols to further validate the feasibility of scintigraphic evaluation of MDR functions of tumors. In addition, large variation of treatment regimens among reports including both agents possessing profiles of substrates for ABC transporters and others requires the assessment not only for each cell type but also for each therapeutic regimen [2]. Furthermore, it should be remembered that relatively low special resolution and related partial-volume effects of scintigraphic images may interfere with precise evaluation of functional status of transporters [2, 44].

Moorin, et al. [77] has pointed out that the limitation occurs because the SPECT acquisition data collection process will incorporate an error component which is directly proportional to the imaging time. Data acquisition by conventional methods takes up to 30 min. This time interval has been regarded as a discrete event which does not take into account the actual imaging time. Therefore, they aimed to reduce the overall imaging time, thereby reducing the statistical uncertainty in the efflux rate measurement of tracers, while maintaining adequate spatial resolution to allow lesion discrimination. They have concluded that 180° acquisition arcs are a practical option for accurate quantitative SPECT kinetic imaging for potential studies of chemotherapy response in patients.

Monitoring Effects of Reversing Agents and Approaches to Knockdown MDR

In order to overcome MDR functions of tumours, modulators for ABC transporters have been intensively investigated [3, 78]. Verapamil, cyclosporin A, diltiazem and FK-506 are classical modulators which competitively inhibit transport of antitumour drugs [3, 78]. However, utility of these non-specific inhibitors was limited because of their inability to achieve clinically effective plasma levels to inhibit transporters [78]. Second-generation agents such as the non-immunosuppresive cyclosporin PSC-833, a quinoline delivative, MS-209 and GG918, have been in clinical trials [79-83]. In an animal xenograft model of MCF7 breast cancer cells, effects of PSC833 has been successfully delineated in vivo with a SPECT system named FastSPECT, a dedicated SPECT for small animals [48]. However, these agents still shored undesirable pharmacokinetic interactions with chemotherapeutic drugs that often require dose reductions. A new agent, Tariquidar (XR9578), is currently investigated in patients with chemotherapy-resistant, advanced breast cancer [46, 84]. These agents have reportedly reversed the release of ^{99m}Tc-MIBI and ^{99m}Tc-TF from cells expressing ABC transporters; consequently, potential utility of these radiotracers to assess the effects of reversing agents in vivo has been documented [37-48]. For instance, a clinical study reported a patient who responded to docetaxel containing chemotherapy showed the greatest increase in ^{99m}Tc-MIBI uptake after Tariquidar treatment compared with that before treatment [46].

We observed uptake of ^{99m}Tc-MIBI and ^{99m}Tc-TF in MRP-expressing HL60/DOX cells in the presence of 10-200 μM verapamil [57]. Verapamil significantly increased the ^{99m}Tc-TF net accumulation in HL60/DOX: with 10 μM verapamil, the accumulation in HL60/DOX at 60 min was 302% of the control (Figure 5). In contrast, the effect of verapamil on HL60/WT was minimal, which was 125% of the control at 60 min. Figure 6 shows the comparison between ^{99m}Tc-TF and ^{99m}Tc-MIBI in terms of the reversal effect verapamil on HL60/DOX cells. The increase of net accumulation was approximately 2-fold higher with ^{99m}Tc-MIBI than in the concentration up to 200 μM (Figure 6A). However, when expressed as the accumulation relative to HL60/WT cell, the recovery was identical for these two tracers (Figure 6B).

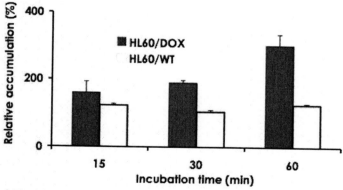

Figure 5. Effects of 10 μM verapamil on 99mTc-TF accumulation in HL60/WT and HL60/DOX cells. Each column represents 99mTc-TF accumulation relative to that of the non-treated control cells in HL60/WT (blank column) and HL60/DOX (hatched column). Mean ± SD (n=3).

Similarly, MCF7 breast cancer cells and etoposide-resistant MCF7/VP cells were incubated in the presence of increasing concentrations of verapamil [85]. ^{99m}Tc-TF was introduced to the medium at 1×10^{6} cells/185 kBq/ml in the presence of increasing concentrations of verapamil up to 200 μM at 37°C. Results of ^{99m}Tc-TF uptake in the absence of correction for viable cell numbers are displayed in Figure 7. When verapamil was not present, MCF7/VP cells exhibited significantly lower ^{99m}Tc-TF uptake than did MCF7 cells: $0.52 \pm 0.04\%$ in the former and $1.35 \pm 0.13\%$ in the latter, respectively. ^{99m}Tc-TF uptake increased with increasing concentrations of verapamil up to 50 μM in MCF7 cells; however, enhancement of ^{99m}Tc-TF uptake diminished at higher verapamil concentrations. Increased uptake in MCF7/VP cells was relatively constant at verapamil concentrations of 50-200 µM. In Figure 8, the effect of verapamil was expressed as values relative to those obtained in the absence of verapamil. Changes in tracer uptake were significant in MCF7/VP cells, displaying increases of approximately 100-150% at all verapamil concentrations up to 200 µM. In contrast, uptake in MCF7 cells increased 80% at 50 µM; however, significant effects of verapamil were not observed at high concentrations. That is, it appears that 100 µM verapamil exerted no effect on uptake in MCF7 cells, whereas it induced an increase of 150% in MCF7/VP cells. On the contrary, following correction of the results for viable cell numbers, ^{99m}Tc-TF uptake in MCF7 cells was approximately 2-fold greater than that in MCF7/VP cells irrespective of verapamil concentration (Figure 9). In addition, uptake in viable MCF7 cells was approximately 100% higher at all concentrations of verapamil in comparison with uptake in the absence of verapamil (Figure 10). Verapamil increased uptake in viable MCF7/VP cells by 100% at 50 µM and by 200% at higher concentrations. Verapamil affected the retention of ^{99m}Tc-TF in a dose-dependent manner in both cell lines (Figure 11). MCF7 cells consistently retained more radioactivity irrespective of verapamil concentration than did MCF7/VP cells. At lower concentration, effects on MCF7 cells were more apparent than those on MCF7/VP cells.

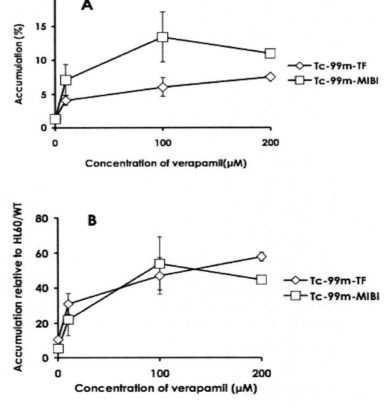

Figure 6. Effects of the increasing concentrations of verapamil on the net accumulation of 99mTc-TF and 99mTc-MIBI in HL60/DOX cells at 60 min. A, net accumulation (%); and B, % accumulation relative to that in parental HL60/WT cells. Mean ± SD (n=3).

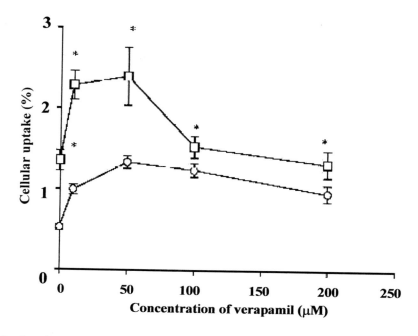

Figure 7. Uptake of 99mTc-tetrofosmin in MCF7 cells (square) and MCF7/VP cells (circle). The results were not corrected by viable cell numbers. Bars indicate s.d. *, p<0.05 between MCF7 and MCF7/VP.

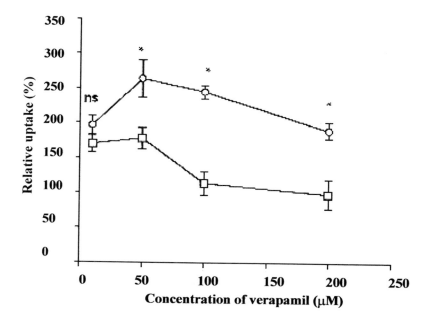

Figure 8. Effects of verapamil on uptake of 99mTc-tetrofosmin in MCF7/WT cells (square) and MCF7/VP cells (circle). Results demonstrated in Figure 7 are expressed as percentages relative to control values in the absence of verapamil. Bars indicate s.d. *, p<0.05 between MCF7/WT and MCF7/VP.

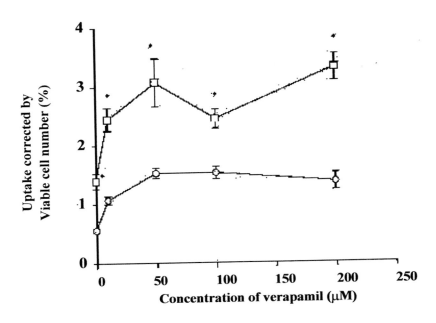

Figure 9. Uptake of 99mTc-tetrofosmin in 1 x 105 MCF7 cells (square) and MCF7/VP cells (circle). Results demonstrated in Figure 7 are corrected by viable cell numbers demonstrated in Figure 1. Bars indicate s.d. *, p<0.05 between MCF7 and MCF7/VP.

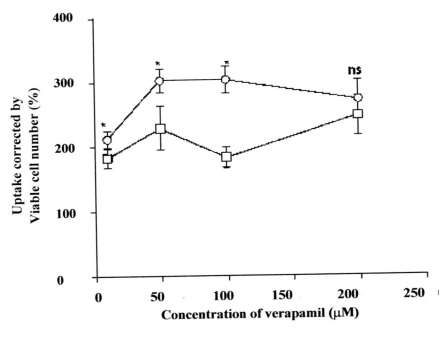

Figure 10. Effects of verapamil on uptake of 99mTc-tetrofosmin in 1 x 105 MCF7/WT cells (square) and MCF7/VP cells (circle). Results demonstrated in Figure 9 are expressed as percentages relative to control values in the absence of verapamil. Bars indicate s.d.

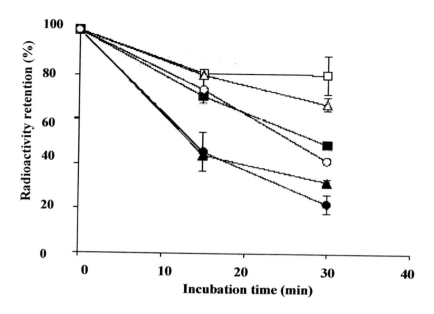

Figure 11. Washout kinetics of 99mTc-tetrofosmin from MCF7/WT cells (open symbols) and MCF7/VP cells (closed symbols) in the absence of verapamil (circle) and the presence of 10 μM (triangle) or 50 μM (square) of verapamil.

The fact that verapamil increased tracer uptake in both MCF7 cells and MCF7/VP cells indicate that cellular functions other than MRP1 expression play significant simultaneous roles in the verapamil-induced modulation of cellular uptake of ^{99m}Tc-TF; that is, cellular responses to verapamil regarding ^{99m}Tc-TF uptake would not necessarily reflect the modulation of MRP1-related chemoresistance of cells. In other words, observation of verapamil-induced alteration of ^{99m}Tc-TF uptake would not provide precise information regarding MRP1-related chemoresistance. Washout kinetics of ^{99m}Tc-cationic tracers is also believed to be associated with MDR function. However, verapamil induced prolongation of radioactivity retention in both MCF7 cells and MCF7/VP cells, suggesting that comparison of tracer retention in the absence and in the presence of verapamil would not lead to the correct diagnosis of chemoresistance.

Verapamil, functioning as a calcium antagonist and K^+ channel blocker [86], decreases intracellular Ca^{++} and K^+ concentrations; moreover, it subsequently increases intracellular Na^+ concentration. ^{99m}Tc-TF behaves in a manner somewhat similar to Na^+; furthermore, its accumulation is correlated with intracellular Na^+ concentration [87-90]. Therefore, the decrease in intracellular Ca^{++} and K^+ concentrations due to verapamil would induce $Na^+/^{99m}$Tc-TF accumulation in cells irrespective of MRP1 expression [87-90].

Other classical modulators, including cyclosporin A, diltiazem and FK-506, also affect ion channels in a manner identical to that of verapamil [91-93]; therefore, ^{99m}Tc-TF would exhibit drawbacks with respect to assessment of the reversal effect on MDR function similarly observed in the case of verapamil. PS-833 did not affect ^{99m}Tc-MIBI uptake in non-MDR breast cancer cells in vitro [37, 39, 41]. However, in chemosensitive rhinonasopharyngeal cancer cells, PSC-833 increased ^{99m}Tc-MIBI uptake; moreover, discrepant cellular responses to reversal agents, including verapamil, PSC-833 and S9788, have been documented for ^{99m}Tc-MIBI and ^{3}H-daunomycin [41]. These facts suggest the requirement of analogous compounds that would be handled by cells in a manner identical to chemotherapeutic agents in order to assess precisely the potential of reversal agents.

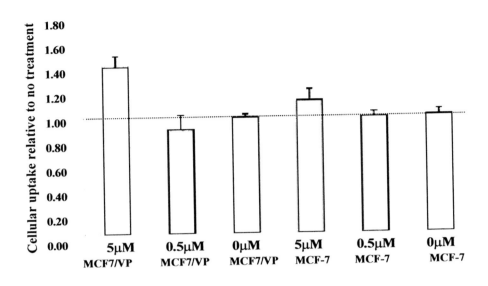

Figure 12. Effects of treatment with antisense ODN to MRP mRNA on 99mTc-MIBI uptake in MCF7/VP and MCF7 cells. Cells were treated for 4 consecutive days at various concentrations. NS, difference is not statistically significant.

Recently, approaches other than use of these types of modulators have been extensively investigated, including translational inhibition of mRNA coding ABC transporters with antisense (AS) ODN [49-52] or hammerhead ribozymes [53, 54]. We examined ^{99m}Tc-MIBI uptake in MCF7 breast cancer cells and MCF7/VP cells that express high levels of MRP1 following treatment with a 20-mer AS phosphorothioate ODN complementary to the mRNA sequences of MRP1 in comparison with sense (S) ODN treatment [50]. In the first experiment, cells were incubated in the presence of AS-ODN at 0.5 or 5 µM for 4 days (Figure 12). Administration of 0.5 µM AS-ODN failed to improve ^{99m}Tc-MIBI uptake in MCF7/VP cells. However, at 5 µM, uptake increased 43%. Uptake in MCF7 cells was not appreciably affected at either concentration. Based on these results, effects of treatment duration were observed in the presence of 5 µM AS-ODN (Figure 13). Five-day treatment afforded superior enhancement of ^{99m}Tc-MIBI uptake in MCF7/VP cells in comparison to 4-day treatment. Uptake in MCF7 cells was unchanged under these conditions. Five-day treatment with 25 µM AS-ODN provided no significant advantage in terms of ^{99m}Tc-MIBI uptake enhancement in MCF7/VP cells relative to that detected at 5 µM (Figure 14A). Uptake in MCF7/VP cells was not altered by S-ODN at any concentration. Neither AS-ODN nor S-ODN affected uptake in MCF7 cells (Figure 14B). These results confirmed the specificity of AS-ODN treatment in MCF7/VP cells. RT-PCR analyses demonstrated MRP mRNA expression in MCF7/VP cells (Figure 15). MRP mRNA was negligible in MCF7 cells. AS-ODN administration suppressed MRP mRNA expression in MCF7/VP cells in dose-dependent fashion: the intensity of the MRP mRNA band decreased partially at 5 μM. In contrast, the band was faintly recognizable at 25 μM. These results suggest that effects of AS-ODN treatment on MRP function in cells possessing MDR capability can be monitored via detection of cellular uptake of ^{99m}Tc-MIBI. In addition, changes in mRNA levels clearly affect cellular ^{99m}Tc-MIBI uptake. Previously, several reports documented the association between mRNA expression of MRP or Pgp and ^{99m}Tc-MIBI accumulation in a group of patients [65-67, 94]; however, as tracer uptake in vivo is a multifactorial event [93], such in vivo findings do not necessarily provide direct evidence regarding correlation between changes in ^{99m}Tc-MIBI accumulation and functional level of mRNA with respect to MDR.

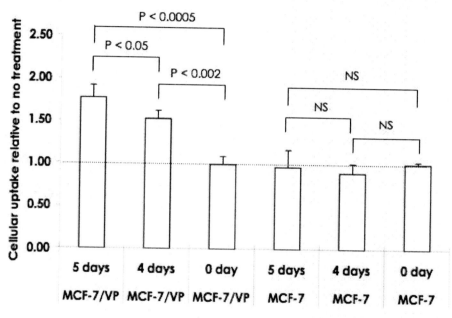

Figure 13. Effects of treatment with antisense ODN to MRP mRNA on 99mTc-MIBI uptake in MCF7/VP and MCF7 cells. Cells were treated for 4 or 5 consecutive days at 5 μM. NS, difference is not statistically significant.

Another selective blocking of mRNA of transporters to reverse MDR is explored with RNA interference (RNAi) [55]. RNAi relies on the sequence-specific interaction between small interfering RNA (siRNA) and mRNA. siRNAs are incorporated into a nuclease complex known as RNA-induced silencing complex where unwinding of the duplex siRNAs take place. The antisense strand binds in a highly sequence-specific manner to target mRNA, which is then endonucleolytically cleaved and degraded. Pichler et al. [55] demonstrated that short hairpin RNA interference (shRNAi) effectively inhibited *MDR1* expression and function in cultured cells and tumor implants, documenting the feasibility of this approach. In addition, ^{99m}Tc-MIBI accumulation in shRNAi cell lines was 8-10 times enhanced as compared with control cell lines, suggesting that ^{99m}Tc-MIBI and probably ^{99m}Tc-TF have the potential to monitor the effects of shRNAi targeted to ABC transporters in patients.

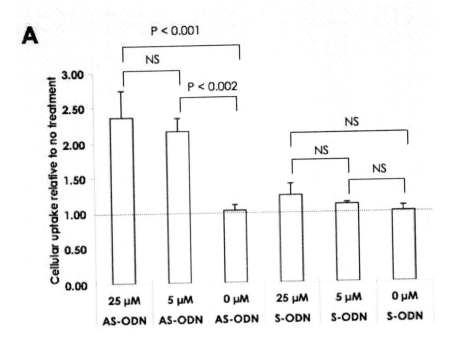

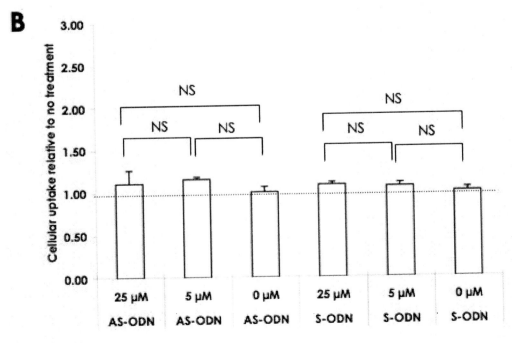

Figure 14. Effects of treatment with antisense ODN (AS-ODN) and sense ODN (S-ODN) to MRP mRNA on 99mTc-MIBI uptake in MCF-7/VP (A) and MCF-7 (B) cells. Cells were treated for 5 consecutive days at indicated concentrations. NS, difference is not statistically significant.

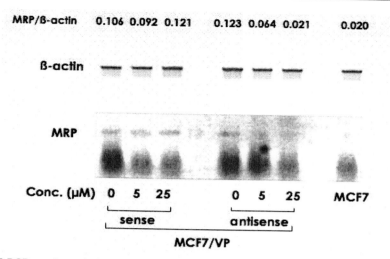

Figure 15. RT-PCR products derived from MRP mRNA of MCF7/VP treated with antisense ODN (AS-ODN) and sense ODN (S-ODN) to MRP mRNA at indicated concentrations. β-actin served as an internal reference. Results with parental MCF7 cells are also shown. Values indicated above PCR profiles indicate the density ratios of MRP/β-actin.

Limitations due to Mechanisms of Tumor Accumulation other than MDR Function

Accumulation of ^{99m}Tc-MIBI and ^{99m}Tc-TF in tumors would be regulated by many factors related with tissue conditions and cellular activities other than function of ABC transporters regarding MDR ability [8, 9]. First of all, their delivery to tumors and their extraction and retention there strongly depend on tissue blood flow [95-97]. Therefore, poor accessibility of tracers to tumors may simply inhibit tracer accumulation. Number of cells in tumors, cell viability and tissue necrosis may also significantly influence uptake of these tracers [95-97].

Cellular uptake of ^{99m}Tc-MIBI and ^{99m}Tc-TF is mediated by Na$^+$,K$^+$ pump and Na$^+$,H$^+$ antiport; however, passive diffusion through membranes also plays a major role [87-90]. The mitochondrion is primarily the localization site in cells [8, 97]. The cellular entry of these cationic tracers is related to the mitochondrial metabolism and the negative inner membrane potential of the mitochondria. Because of the charge and lipophilicity of the tracers, they are trapped in the organelle by the negative potential on the inner mitochondrial membrane. Therefore, mitochondrial conditions are crucial for accumulation of ^{99m}Tc-MIBI and ^{99m}Tc-TF. Most ^{99m}Tc-MIBI accumulates inside the mitochondria, but the smaller fraction of ^{99m}Tc-TF localizes there [87].

Recent observation indicated that apoptotic process is related with ^{99m}Tc-MIBI accumulation in tumor cells [97-99]. A decisive event in the apoptotic process is an early increase in the permeability of the mitochondrial membrane and release of cytochrome c and other soluble proteins that participate in the degradation phase of apoptosis [100, 101]. Changes in the permeability of mitochondrial membrane in response to death are under the control of the Bcl-2 protein family that includes both death antagonists such as Bcl-2 and Bcl-x and death agonist such as Bax and Bak [102]. Bcl-2 is overexpressed in many types of malignant cells. Bcl-2 is a protein of the outer mitochondrial membrane that protects cells from induction of apoptosis caused by variety of anticancer agents [102]. Bcl-2 prevents mitochondrial membrane permeabilization and cytochrome c release triggered by the death signals. Therefore, in cells overexpressing Bcl-2 gene products, ^{99m}Tc-MIBI may not accumulate in the mitochondria, and it is eventually effluxed from cells passively [97]. In breast cancer patients, a reduction in the apoptotic index and overexpression of Bcl-2 were accompanied with low ^{99m}Tc-MIBI accumulation [97-99]. This correlation is confirmed in transfected cells to overexpress Bcl-2. That is, breast cancer MCF7 cells and T47D cells transfected with the Bcl-2 gene took up ^{99m}Tc-MIBI 97% and 83% less than mock transfected cells did [103]. These facts suggest that, although ^{99m}Tc-MIBI may not differentiate resistant cells with Bcl-2 overexpression from cells expressing ABC transporters, ^{99m}Tc-MIBI may enable to assess the efficacy of agents that neutralize the effect of Bcl-2.

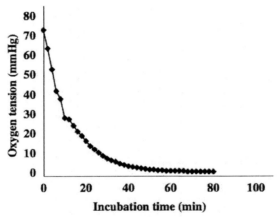

Figure 16. Change of oxygen tension (pO2) in the cell-suspended medium during N2 gas exposure at 37oC.

Aforementioned facts indicate that poor visualization of tumors with ^{99m}Tc-MIBI and ^{99m}Tc-TF is a sign of failure in responding to chemotherapy. Similarly, radiotherapeutic responses of tumors may be predicted by these tracers [19, 104]. However, expression of ABC transporters cannot explain the radioresistance of tumor cells. Consequently, factors other than transporter expression should be involved in the scintigraphic evaluation in this regard. Bcl-2 overexpression would be an important factor [97]. Another possible factor is tissue oxygenation in tumors. The occurrence of hypoxic cells in tumors is one of the major causes of therapeutic failure in both chemotherapy and radiotherapy [105]. Hypoxia affects a number of tumor cell functions [105], thereby resulting in the interference of cellular uptake of radiotracers. Therefore, we attempted to determine the effect of hypoxia on ^{99m}Tc-MIBI and ^{99m}Tc-TF accumulation in human cancer cells in vitro and in vivo [68, 94]. Oxygen tension in culture medium and tumors was measured with microelectrodes. A hypoxic marker, ^{99m}Tc-HL91, was employed as a reference for the hypoxic condition [106-111]. LS180 human colon cancer cells were incubated at $37^{\circ}C$ in 95% air and 5% CO_2. Cells were gassed continuously at $37^{\circ}C$ with a mixture of 95% N_2 and 5% CO_2 in order to generate hypoxic conditions. Subsequently, one of the ^{99m}Tc-compounds was introduced to the medium at 2×10^6 cells/370 kBq/ml after achieving equilibrium of oxygen tension measured with O_2 microelectrodes (Figure 16). ^{201}Tl chloride was simultaneously added as a comparison at 185 kBq/ml because this tracer is often used in the diagnosis of various malignant lesions [11, 19, 28, 30, 71, 112]. Similar in vitro procedures were performed with T24 human bladder cancer cells to ascertain whether hypoxic effects on tracer uptake would be a common phenomenon among tumor cell lines. Figure 16 shows a representative curve of pO_2 in the incubation medium with LS180 colon cancer cells under an N_2 gas flow. pO_2 in the medium gradually decreased and attained equilibrium at 1-2 mmHg approximately 60 min following the initiation of exposure to N_2 gas. Cellular uptake of ^{99m}Tc-MIBI in LS180 cells decreased approximately 30% in N_2 gas in comparison to that in air throughout the study (Figure 17A). The influence of hypoxia was more prominent on ^{201}Tl uptake, which displayed reduction of approximately 60% in N_2 gas at 120 min, than on ^{99m}Tc-MIBI uptake (Figure 17B). In contrast, N_2 gas induced an increase of 170% in ^{99m}Tc-HL91 uptake at 120 min that confirmed hypoxia of the cells under these assay conditions (Figure 17C). The results of in vitro assays employing the T24 cell line, which demonstrated reductions of approximately 40% and 50% in ^{99m}Tc-MIBI and ^{201}Tl uptake in N_2 gas, respectively, were similar to those obtained with the LS180 cell line (Figure 18A and B).

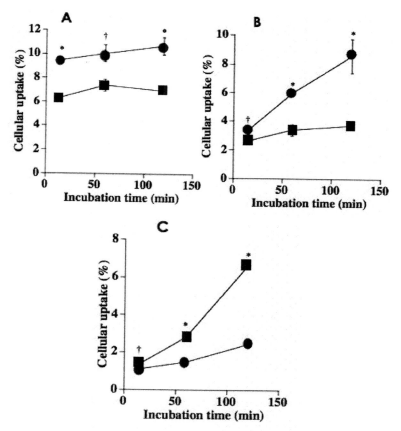

Figure 17. Cellular uptake of 99mTc-MIBI (A), 201Tl chloride (B) and 99mTc-HL91 (C) in LS180 colon cancer cells (n=3). Tracer uptake studies were conducted twice, and one set of data is presented as a representative example. Bars indicate the s.d., which are omitted where the range is within the symbol. J, in air; B, in N2 gas. *, p<0.01; †, p<0.05.

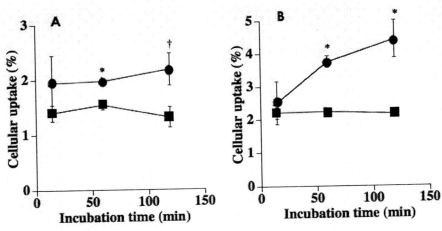

Figure 18. Cellular uptake of 99mTc-MIBI (A) and 201Tl chloride (B) in T24 bladder cancer cells (n=3). Tracer uptake studies were conducted twice, and one set of data is presented as a representative example. Bars indicate the s.d., which are omitted where the range is within the symbol. J, in air; B, in N2 gas. *, p<0.01; †, p<0.05.

Effects of tissue hypoxia were also examined in Balb/c nu/nu mice subcutaneously xenografted with LS180 cells in the thigh [94]. The animals were utilized when tumors attained a diameter of 5-6 mm. Tumor oxygenation was chemically reduced by hydralazine [113]. Tracer accumulation of 1.85 MBq of ^{99m}Tc-MIBI and ^{99m}Tc-HL91 in xenografts was determined. A dose of 185 kBq of ^{201}Tl chloride was simultaneously injected with ^{99m}Tc-MIBI. Administration of hydralazine decreased tumor pO_2 to 7.56 ± 6.18 mmHg from 14.5 ± 6.62 mmHg in non-treated control tumors (p<0.0001) (Figure 19). Hydralazine treatment markedly reduced ^{99m}Tc-MIBI and ^{201}Tl accumulation in tumors (Table 1); tumor accumulation of ^{99m}Tc-MIBI decreased 27% and 35% relative to control values at 30 min and 90 min, respectively, whereas tumor accumulation of ^{201}Tl decreased 57% at 30 min and 39% at 90 min. In contrast, the treatment increased accumulation of ^{99m}Tc-HL91 by 86% and 41% at 30 min and 90 min, respectively, which indicated the induced hypoxia of the tumors.

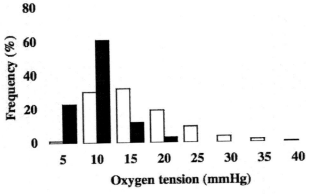

Figure 19. Frequency distribution of pO2 in LS180 colon cancer xenografts. Open columns, injected with 0.1 ml saline; solid columns, injected with 50 mg/kg hydralazine.

Table 1. Effect of hydralazine-induced hypoxia on tracer accumulation within LS180 colon cancer xenografts

(n=6-10)	^{201}Tl chloride (n=6)		^{99m}Tc-MIBI (n=6)		^{99m}Tc-HL91	
	30 min	90 min	30 min	90 min	30 min	90 min
Control	5.84± 1.05	5.80± 0.72	1.81± 0.47	0.71± 0.35	2.00± 0.22	1.19± 0.35
Hydralazine	2.52± 0.99*	3.51± 1.10†	1.32± 0.20‡	0.46± 0.16‡	3.72± 0.29*	1.68± 0.48‡
%change	-57%	-39%	-27%	-35%	+86%	+41%

Control, injected with 0.1 ml saline; hydralazine, injected with 50 mg/kg hydralazine.
% change, change in tumor accumulation induced by hydralazine injection.
*, p<0.001; †, p<0.01; ‡, p<0.05 versus control group.

The results of these in vitro and in vivo experiments proved our hypothesis that tissue hypoxia would interfere with the accumulation of ^{99m}Tc-MIBI in tumor cells. The uptake mechanisms of ^{99m}Tc-MIBI and ^{201}Tl differ [87, 89, 114]; consequently, the decrease in uptake of these tracers in hypoxic cells would be caused by the alteration of several cellular activities. ^{201}Tl uptake is related to cell membrane potential, Na$^+$,K$^+$ pump activity and Na$^+$,K$^+$,2Cl$^-$ co-transport [89]. ^{99m}Tc-MIBI uptake is mediated by Na$^+$,K$^+$ pump and Na$^+$,H$^+$ antiport; however, passive diffusion through membranes also plays a major role [89, 114]. ^{99m}Tc-MIBI localizes inside mitochondria, whereas ^{201}Tl remains in the cytosolic compartment [86, 88, 114]. Hypoxia is known to reduce the O$_2$ consumption rate and ATP production; thereby, hypoxia leads to a pO$_2$-dependent inhibition of Na$^+$,K$^+$ pump and Na$^+$,K$^+$,2Cl$^-$ co-transport and causes depolarization of membranes [105]. These functional changes appear to be responsible for the reduced uptake of these radiotracers in the LS180 colon cancer cell and T24 bladder cancer cell lines.

^{201}Tl chloride exhibited larger reduction of tumor accumulation in response to hypoxia than did ^{99m}Tc-MIBI in both in vitro and in vivo studies. Susceptibility to hypoxia-induced inhibition varies among the aforementioned tracer uptake mechanisms [105]. For instance, pO$_2$ critical for a constant level of cellular ATP is approximately 10 mmHg [105]. On the other hand, mitochondria, in which ^{99m}Tc-MIBI localizes, may physiologically function above the threshold of 0.5 mmHg [105]. Therefore, the retention mechanism of ^{99m}Tc-MIBI is relatively maintained in the hypoxic condition as compared to the function of cell membrane channels, which may be responsible for the differences observed between ^{99m}Tc-MIBI and ^{201}Tl.

The influence of hypoxia on the function of p-GP or MRP was not considered in this investigation. Because the LS180 cell line weakly expresses p-GP [115] and the T24 cell line weakly expresses MRP [116], it is possible that hypoxia-induced modulation of transporter expression is involved in mechanisms of reduced ^{99m}Tc-MIBI accumulation in hypoxic cells. Therefore, we further aimed to determine influence of hypoxic conditions on tracer uptake with respect to function of cell membrane transporters [68]. Uptake of ^{99m}Tc-MIBI and ^{99m}Tc-TF was examined in MCF7 cells and MCF7/VP cells under normoxic and hypoxic conditions. In addition, MRP1 expression of cells was detected by anti-MRP1 antibody. Hypoxia reduced cellular uptake of these two tracers in both parental MCF7 and MRP1-expressing MCF7/VP cells (p<0.05 at 30 min and 60 min) (Figure 20). Hypoxia tended to reduce ^{99m}Tc-TF uptake more significantly than ^{99m}Tc-MIBI uptake under both normoxic and hypoxic conditions (Table 2). Cell binding assay with ^{125}I-anti-MRP1 antibody demonstrated specific binding to MCF7/VP cells, which increased with increasing cell number (Figure 21). Hypoxia did not affect the amount of antibody bound to MCF7/VP cells. Radioactivity associated with parental MCF7 cells did not vary with increasing cell number under normoxic and hypoxic conditions. These results clearly indicate that hypoxia-induced reduction of ^{99m}Tc-MIBI and ^{99m}Tc-TF accumulation in the MCF7 breast cancer cell line is a phenomenon independent of MRP function.

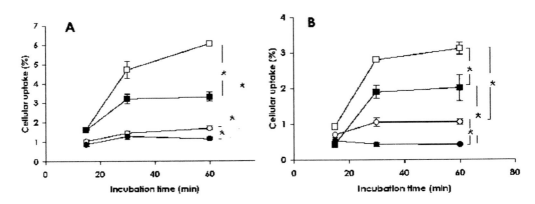

Figure 20. Cellular uptake of 99mTc-MIBI (A) and 99mTc-TF (B) in MCF7/WT breast cancer cells (square) and MRP1-expressing MCF7/VP cells (circle) under normoxic (open symbols) or hypoxic conditions (closed symbols). Mean ± s.d. of triplicate samples. Bars indicate the s.d., which are omitted where the range is within the symbol. *, p<0.05.

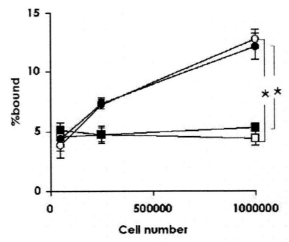

Figure 21. Cell binding assay with 125I-anti-MRP1 antibody in MCF7/WT breast cancer cells (square) and MRP1-expressing MCF7/VP cells (circle) under normoxic (open symbols) or hypoxic conditions (closed symbols). Mean ± s.d. of triplicate samples. *, p<0.05.

Table 2. Hypoxia-induced reduction of cellular uptake (%)

Min	^{99m}Tc-sestamibi		^{99m}Tc-tetrofosmin	
	WT	VP	WT	VP
15	0	16	55	23
30	32	12	33	60
60	45	32	36	60

Expressed as (normoxic uptake – hypoxic uptake)/normoxic uptake x 100
WT, parental MCF7 cells; VP, MRP-expressing subclonal MCF7/VP cells.

New Radiopharmaceuticals for Assessment of MDR

^{99m}Tc-MIBI and ^{99m}Tc-TF have already shown to be beneficial in the evaluation of functional activity of ABC transporters in human tumors in vivo. Other types of ^{99m}Tc-compounds and ^{67}Ga-compounds have been developed as alternatives for this purpose, such as ^{99m}Tc-furifosmin, one of nonreducible Tc(III) monocationic compounds known as Q-complexes, tris(carbonyl)tris(2-methoxyisobuthylisonitrile)technetium(I) ([[99m]Tc(CO)$_3$(MIBI)$_3$]$^+$), and ^{67}Ga-ENBDMPI, a Schiff-base Ga(III) complex [117].

In addition to single photon (SPECT) tracers, positron (PET) tracers have been extensively investigated [117]. Among organic scaffolds that coordinate both SPECT and PET radionuclides, two validated examples make use of the PET radionuclides, [94m]Tc and [68]Ga. [94m]Tc-sestamibi and ^{68}Ga-ENBPI have been reported to retain properties as substrates for ABC transporters [118, 119]. Several kinds of ^{64}Cu tracers that show P-gp targeting profiles have been also developed [120]. Incorporation of conventional PET radionuclides such as ^{11}C and ^{18}F into small organic drugs belonging to substrates or inhibitors know to interact with transporters has been attempted as follows: ^{11}C-colchicine, ^{11}C-verapamil, ^{11}C-daumomycin and ^{11}C/^{18}F-paclitaxel [121-127]. Although these ^{11}C/^{18}F compounds may enable MDR assessment, modest radiochemical yields, rapid metabolism in vivo and, furthermore, necessity for the in-house production facilitated with cyclotrons restrict the usage of these compounds [117].

Consequent to its specific characteristics in targeting, single strand ODN may be a potential candidate for future clinical imaging. Several studies have demonstrated accumulation of ^{111}In-ODN in tumor cells via various types of targets [128, 129]. We examined the feasibility of intracellular *mdr*1 mRNA expression detection with radiolabeled antisense ODN in the murine leukemia cell line, P388/S, and its subclonal, adriamycin-resistant cell line, P388/R [64]. A 15-mer phosphorothioate antisense ODN complementary to the sequences locating at –1 to 14 of *mdr*1 mRNA and its corresponding sense ODN were conjugated with the cyclic anhydride of diethylenetriaminepentaacetic acid (cDTPA) via an amino group linked to the terminal phosphate at the 5' end at pH 8-9. Furthermore, enhancing effects of synthetic lipid carriers (Transfast[TM]) on transmembrane delivery of ODN were assessed. Hybridization affinity of antisense ^{111}In-ODN was preserved at approximately 85% irrespective of specific activity. Cellular uptake of antisense ^{111}In-ODN did not differ from that of sense ^{111}In-ODN in either P388/S cells or P388/R cells. However, lipid carrier incorporation significantly increased transmembrane delivery of ^{111}In-ODN; moreover, specific uptake of antisense ^{111}In-ODN was demonstrated in P388/R cells (Table 3). Because the target mRNA copy usually ranges between 1 and 1,000 per cell at steady state [130], it cannot be expected that ^{111}In-ODN can enter into cells and bind with the target mRNAs in a great amount within a short time. Accordingly, ^{111}In-ODN with high specific radioactivity should be necessary to delineate lesions for in vivo imaging. This study has achieved radiolabeling with high specific radioactivity up to 1,634MBq/nmol, which is much higher than documented previously [131-133]. Compounds possessing high specific activity can afford a high signal intensity in targeted lesions, which surely improves the signal-to-background ratios, enhancing lesion delineation. Specific uptake of antisense ^{111}In-ODN in drug-resistant cells may facilitate future gene imaging of *mdr*1 mRNA.

Table 3. Intracellular uptake of vectorized ^{111}In-S-ODN and ^{111}In-AS-ODN

ODNs	Cell lines	Incubation time (hr.)			
		0.5	1	2	4
[111]In-S-ODN	P388	1.84±0.18*	1.58±0.10*	1.22±0.10*	1.39±0.11*
	P388/R	2.27±0.18	1.87±0.11	1.89±0.19	1.86±0.10
^{111}In-AS-ODN	P388	1.67±0.33*	1.43±0.03*	1.23±0.11*	1.49±0.19*
	P388/R	3.51±0.17**	2.58±0.43**	2.77±0.46**	2.87±0.25**

Expressed as % total dose/10^3 cells (mean ± SD)
*$P<0.05$ versus ^{111}In-S-ODN or ^{111}In-AS-ODN in p388/R cells.
**$P<0.05$ versus ^{111}In-S-ODN in P388/R cells.

CONCLUSION

A noninvasive method to determine MDR ability of tumors mediated by ABC-transporters is surely beneficial in guiding therapeutic choices. The feasibility of scintigraphic detection of MDR functions with cationic, lipophilic radiotracers, ^{99m}Tc-MIBI and ^{99m}Tc-TF, is supported by in vitro and in vivo experimental results in many cell types. Clinical results with these radiotracers also suggest their role in this regard; however, standard protocols should be established to determine their feasibility. Given that delineation of tumors with these tracers is a multi-factorial phenomenon, development of an imaging method specific to transporter function is required to assess precisely MDR of tumors related to transporter proteins.

ACKNOWLEDGMENTS

This study was partly supported by a Grant-in-Aid for Scientific Research from the Ministry of Education, Science and Culture, Japan. We are grateful to Dr. Hui Li, associate professor Hideto Yonekura and professor Hiroshi Yamamoto of the Second Department of Biochemistry, Kanazawa University, for their technical assistance.

REFERENCES

[1] Simon SM, Schindler M. Cell biological mechanisms of multidrug resistance in tumors. *Proc Natl Acad Sci U S A* 1994;91(9):3497-3504.

[2] Van de Wiele C, Rottey S, Goethals I, et al. 99mTc sestamibi and 99mTc tetrofosmin scintigraphy for predicting resistance to chemotherapy: a critical review of clinical data. *Nucl Med Commun* 2003;24(9):945-950.

[3] Kuwano M, Uchiumi T, Hayakawa H, et al. The basic and clinical implications of ABC transporters, Y-box-binding protein-1 (YB-1) and angiogenesis-related factors in human malignancies. *Cancer Sci* 2003;94(1):9-14.

[4] Bates SF, Chen C, Robey R, Kang M, Figg WD, Fojo T. Reversal of multidrug resistance: lessons from clinical oncology. *Novartis Found Symp* 2002;243:83-96.

[5] Wang RB, Kuo CL, Lien LL, Lien EJ. Structure-activity relationship: analyses of p-glycoprotein substrates and inhibitors. *J Clin Pharm Ther* 2003;28(3):203-228.

[6] Fojo T, Bates S. Strategies for reversing drug resistance. *Oncogene* 2003;22(47):7512-7523.

[7] Ford JM, Hait WN. Pharmacology of drugs that alter multidrug resistance in cancer. *Pharmacol Rev* 1990;42(3):155-199.

[8] Pauwels EK, McCready VR, Stoot JH, van Deurzen DF. The mechanism of accumulation of tumour-localising radiopharmaceuticals. *Eur J Nucl Med* 1998;25(3):277-305.

[9] Giannopoulou C. The role of SPET and PET in monitoring tumour response to therapy. *Eur J Nucl Med Mol Imaging* 2003;30(8):1173-1200.

[10] Muller S G-TB, Creutzig H. Imaging of malignant tumors with Tc-99m-MIBI SPECT [abstract]. *J Nucl Med* 1987;28(5):562.

[11] Kostakoglu L, Uysal U, Ozyar E, et al. Monitoring response to therapy with thallium-201 and technetium-99m-sestamibi SPECT in nasopharyngeal carcinoma. *J Nucl Med* 1997;38(7):1009-1014.

[12] Maini CL, Tofani A, Sciuto R, et al. Technetium-99m-MIBI scintigraphy in the assessment of neoadjuvant chemotherapy in breast carcinoma. *J Nucl Med* 1997;38(10):1546-1551.

[13] Ohira H, Kubota K, Ohuchi N, Harada Y, Fukuda H, Satomi S. Comparison of intratumoral distribution of ^{99m}Tc-MIBI and deoxyglucose in mouse breast cancer models. *J Nucl Med* 2000;41(9):1561-1568.

[14] Kao CH, ChangLai SP, Chieng PU, Yen TC. Technetium-99m methoxyisobutylisonitrile chest imaging of small cell lung carcinoma: relation to patient prognosis and chemotherapy response--a preliminary report. *Cancer* 1998;83(1):64-68.

[15] Kao A, Shiun SC, Hsu NY, Sun SS, Lee CC, Lin CC. Technetium-99m methoxyisobutylisonitrile chest imaging for small-cell lung cancer. Relationship to chemotherapy response (six courses of combination of cisplatin and etoposide) and p-glycoprotein or multidrug resistance related protein expression. *Ann Oncol* 2001;12(11):1561-1566.

[16] Mankoff DA, Dunnwald LK, Gralow JR, Ellis GK, Drucker MJ, Livingston RB. Monitoring the response of patients with locally advanced breast carcinoma to

neoadjuvant chemotherapy using [technetium 99m]-sestamibi scintimammography. *Cancer* 1999;85(11):2410-2423.

[17] Ceriani L, Giovanella L, Bandera M, Beghe B, Ortelli M, Roncari G. Semi-quantitative assessment of ^{99m}Tc-sestamibi uptake in lung cancer: relationship with clinical response to chemotherapy. *Nucl Med Commun* 1997;18(11):1087-1097.

[18] Sasaki M, Kuwabara Y, Ichiya Y, et al. Prediction of the chemosensitivity of lung cancer by ^{99m}Tc-hexakis-2-methoxyisobutyl isonitrile SPECT. *J Nucl Med* 1999;40(11):1778-1783.

[19] Nishiyama Y, Yamamoto Y, Fukunaga K, et al. Evaluation of radiotherapeutic response in non-small cell lung cancer patients by technetium-99m MIBT and thallium-201 chloride SPET. *Eur J Nucl Med* 2000;27(5):536-541.

[20] Koukourakis MI, Koukouraki S, Giatromanolaki A, Skarlatos J, Georgoulias V, Karkavitsas N. Non-small cell lung cancer functional imaging: increased hexakis-2-methoxy-isobutyl-isonitrile tumor clearance correlates with resistance to cytotoxic treatment. *Clin Cancer Res* 1997;3(5):749-754.

[21] Yuksel M, Cermik TF, Doganay L, et al. ^{99m}Tc-MIBI SPET in non-small cell lung cancer in relationship with Pgp and prognosis. *Eur J Nucl Med Mol Imaging* 2002;29(7):876-881.

[22] Taki J, Sumiya H, Tsuchiya H, Tomita K, Nonomura A, Tonami N. Evaluating benign and malignant bone and soft-tissue lesions with technetium-99m-MIBI scintigraphy. *J Nucl Med* 1997;38(4):501-506.

[23] Le Jeune N, Perek N, Denoyer D, Dubois F. Influence of glutathione depletion on plasma membrane cholesterol esterification and on Tc-99m-sestamibi and Tc-99m-tetrofosmin uptakes: a comparative study in sensitive U-87-MG and multidrug-resistant MRP1 human glioma cells. *Cancer Biother Radiopharm* 2004;19(4):411-421.

[24] Pace L, Catalano L, Del Vecchio S, et al. Washout of [^{99m}Tc] sestamibi in predicting response to chemotherapy in patients with multiple myeloma. *Q J Nucl Med Mol Imaging* 2005;49(3):281-285.

[25] Ballinger JR. Imaging multidrug resistance with radiolabeled substrates for P-glycoprotein and multidrug resistance protein. *Cancer Biother Radiopharm* 2001;16(1):1-7.

[26] Del Vecchio S, Ciarmiello A, Salvatore M. Scintigraphic detection of multidrug resistance in cancer. *Cancer Biother Radiopharm* 2000;15(4):327-337.

[27] Bom HS, Kim YC, Song HC, Min JJ, Kim JY, Park KO. Technetium-99m-MIBI uptake in small cell lung cancer. *J Nucl Med* 1998;39(1):91-94.

[28] Yamamoto Y, Nishiyama Y, Satoh K, et al. Comparative evaluation of Tc-99m MIBI and Tl-201 chloride SPECT in non-small-cell lung cancer mediastinal lymph node metastases. *Clin Nucl Med* 2000;25(1):29-32.

[29] Kao CH, Hsieh JF, Tsai SC, Ho YJ, Lee JK. Quickly predicting chemotherapy response to paclitaxel-based therapy in non-small cell lung cancer by early technetium-99m methoxyisobutylisonitrile chest single-photon-emission computed tomography. *Clin Cancer Res* 2000;6(3):820-824.

[30] Nishiyama Y, Yamamoto Y, Satoh K, et al. Comparative study of Tc-99m MIBI and TI-201 SPECT in predicting chemotherapeutic response in non-small-cell lung cancer. *Clin Nucl Med* 2000;25(5):364-369.

[31] Shih WJ, Rastogi A, Stipp V, Magoun S, Coupal J. Functional retention of Tc-99m MIBI in mediastinal lymphomas as a predictor of chemotherapeutic response demonstrated by consecutive thoracic SPECT imaging. *Clin Nucl Med* 1998;23(8):505-508.

[32] Moretti JL, Azaloux H, Boisseron D, Kouyoumdjian JC, Vilcoq J. Primary breast cancer imaging with technetium-99m sestamibi and its relation with P-glycoprotein overexpression. *Eur J Nucl Med* 1996;23(8):980-986.

[33] Fuster D, Vinolas N, Mallafre C, Pavia J, Martin F, Pons F. Tetrofosmin as predictors of tumour response. *Q J Nucl Med* 2003;47(1):58-62.

[34] Ballinger JR. 99mTc-tetrofosmin for functional imaging of P-glycoprotein modulation in vivo. *J Clin Pharmacol* 2001;Suppl:39S-47S.

[35] Kawata K, Kanai M, Sasada T, Iwata S, Yamamoto N, Takabayashi A. Usefulness of ^{99m}Tc-sestamibi scintigraphy in suggesting the therapeutic effect of chemotherapy against gastric cancer. *Clin Cancer Res* 2004;10(11):3788-3793.

[36] Burak Z, Moretti JL, Ersoy O, et al. ^{99m}Tc-MIBI imaging as a predictor of therapy response in osteosarcoma compared with multidrug resistance-associated protein and P-glycoprotein expression. *J Nucl Med* 2003;44(9):1394-1401.

[37] Ballinger JR, Hua HA, Berry BW, Firby P, Boxen I. ^{99m}Tc-sestamibi as an agent for imaging P-glycoprotein-mediated multi-drug resistance: in vitro and in vivo studies in a rat breast tumour cell line and its doxorubicin-resistant variant. *Nucl Med Commun* 1995;16(4):253-257.

[38] Luker GD, Fracasso PM, Dobkin J, Piwnica-Worms D. Modulation of the multidrug resistance P-glycoprotein: detection with technetium-99m-sestamibi in vivo. *J Nucl Med* 1997;38(3):369-372.

[39] Ballinger JR, Muzzammil T, Moore MJ. Technetium-99m-furifosmin as an agent for functional imaging of multidrug resistance in tumors. *J Nucl Med* 1997;38(12):1915-1919.

[40] Muzzammil T, Ballinger JR, Moore MJ. ^{99m}Tc-sestamibi imaging of inhibition of the multidrug resistance transporter in a mouse xenograft model of human breast cancer. *Nucl Med Commun* 1999;20(2):115-122.

[41] Cayre A, Moins N, Finat-Duclos F, Maublant J, Verrelle P. Comparative ^{99m}Tc-sestamibi and ^{3}H-daunomycin uptake in human carcinoma cells: relation to the MDR phenotype and effects of reversing agents. *J Nucl Med* 1999;40(4):672-676.

[42] Muzzammil T, Moore MJ, Ballinger JR. In vitro comparison of sestamibi, tetrofosmin, and furifosmin as agents for functional imaging of multidrug resistance in tumors. *Cancer Biother Radiopharm* 2000;15(4):339-346.

[43] Nokihara H, Yano S, Nishioka Y, et al. A new quinoline derivative MS-209 reverses multidrug resistance and inhibits multiorgan metastases by P-glycoprotein-expressing human small cell lung cancer cells. *Jpn J Cancer Res* 2001;92(7):785-792.

[44] Tatsumi M, Tsuruo T, Nishimura T. Evaluation of MS-209, a novel multidrug-resistance-reversing agent, in tumour-bearing mice by technetium-99m-MIBI imaging. *Eur J Nucl Med Mol Imaging* 2002;29(3):288-294.

[45] Mubashar M, Harrington KJ, Chaudhary KS, Lalani el N, Stamp GW, Peters AM. Differential effects of toremifene on doxorubicin, vinblastine and Tc-99m-sestamibi in P-glycoprotein-expressing breast and head and neck cancer cell lines. *Acta Oncol* 2004;43(5):443-452.

[46] Pusztai L, Wagner P, Ibrahim N, et al. Phase II study of tariquidar, a selective P-glycoprotein inhibitor, in patients with chemotherapy-resistant, advanced breast carcinoma. *Cancer* 2005;104(4):682-691.

[47] Marian T, Balkay L, Szabo G, et al. Biphasic accumulation kinetics of [^{99m}Tc]-hexakis-2-methoxyisobutyl isonitrile in tumour cells and its modulation by lipophilic P-glycoprotein ligands. *Eur J Pharm Sci* 2005;25(2-3):201-209.

[48] Liu Z, Stevenson GD, Barrett HH, et al. Imaging recognition of inhibition of multidrug resistance in human breast cancer xenografts using ^{99m}Tc-labeled sestamibi and tetrofosmin. *Nucl Med Biol* 2005;32(6):573-583.

[49] Nakamura K, Kubo A, Hnatowich DJ. Antisense targeting of p-glycoprotein expression in tissue culture. *J Nucl Med* 2005;46(3):509-513.

[50] Kinuya S, Bai J, Shiba K, et al. ^{99m}Tc-sestamibi to monitor treatment with antisense oligodeoxynucleotide complementary to MRP mRNA in human breast cancer cells. *Ann Nucl Med* 2006;20(1):29-34.

[51] Liu C, Qureshi IA, Ding X, et al. Modulation of multidrug resistance gene (mdr-1) with antisense oligodeoxynucleotides. *Clin Sci* (Lond) 1996;91(1):93-98.

[52] Stuart DD, Kao GY, Allen TM. A novel, long-circulating, and functional liposomal formulation of antisense oligodeoxynucleotides targeted against MDR1. *Cancer Gene Ther* 2000;7(3):466-475.

[53] Kobayashi H, Dorai T, Holland JF, Ohnuma T. Reversal of drug sensitivity in multidrug-resistant tumor cells by an MDR1 (PGY1) ribozyme. *Cancer Res* 1994;54(5):1271-1275.

[54] Holm PS, Scanlon KJ, Dietel M. Reversion of multidrug resistance in the P-glycoprotein-positive human pancreatic cell line (EPP85-181RDB) by introduction of a hammerhead ribozyme. *Br J Cancer* 1994;70(2):239-243.

[55] Pichler A, Zelcer N, Prior JL, Kuil AJ, Piwnica-Worms D. In vivo RNA interference-mediated ablation of MDR1 P-glycoprotein. *Clin Cancer Res* 2005;11(12):4487-4494.

[56] Piwnica-Worms D, Chiu ML, Budding M, Kronauge JF, Kramer RA, Croop JM. Functional imaging of multidrug-resistant P-glycoprotein with an organotechnetium complex. *Cancer Res* 1993;53(5):977-984.

[57] Li XF, Kinuya S, Yokoyama K, et al. Technetium-99m-tetrofosmin would be a substrate for multidrug resistance-associated protein (MRP): comparison between a leukemia cell line with high MRP gene expression and its parental cell line. *Cancer Biother Radiopharm* 2001;16(1):17-23.

[58] Marian T, Szabo G, Goda K, et al. In vivo and in vitro multitracer analyses of P-glycoprotein expression-related multidrug resistance. *Eur J Nucl Med Mol Imaging* 2003;30(8):1147-1154.

[59] Marian T, Balkay L, Tron L, Krasznai ZT, Szabo-Peli J, Krasznai Z. Effects of miltefosine on membrane permeability and accumulation of [^{99m}Tc]-hexakis-2-methoxyisobutyl isonitrile, 2-[^{18}F]fluoro-2-deoxy-D-glucose, daunorubicin and rhodamine123 in multidrug-resistant and sensitive cells. *Eur J Pharm Sci* 2005;24(5):495-501.

[60] Ballinger JR, Bannerman J, Boxen I, Firby P, Hartman NG, Moore MJ. Technetium-99m-tetrofosmin as a substrate for P-glycoprotein: in vitro studies in multidrug-resistant breast tumor cells. *J Nucl Med* 1996;37(9):1578-1582.

[61] Cordobes MD, Starzec A, Delmon-Moingeon L, et al. Technetium-99m-sestamibi uptake by human benign and malignant breast tumor cells: correlation with mdr gene expression. *J Nucl Med* 1996;37(2):286-289.

[62] Rao VV, Chiu ML, Kronauge JF, Piwnica-Worms D. Expression of recombinant human multidrug resistance P-glycoprotein in insect cells confers decreased accumulation of technetium-99m-sestamibi. *J Nucl Med* 1994;35(3):510-515.

[63] Konishi S KS, Yokoyama K, Tonami N, Hisada K. Evaluation of multidrug-resistance of tumor cells with ^{99m}Tc-MIBI: in vitro evaluation (in Japanese). *Menneki-Syuyokakuigaku* 1995;10(2):64-65.

[64] Bai J, Yokoyama K, Kinuya S, et al. In vitro detection of mdr1 mRNA in murine leukemia cells with ^{111}In-labeled oligonucleotide. *Eur J Nucl Med Mol Imaging* 2004;31(11):1523-1529.

[65] Zhou J, Higashi K, Ueda Y, et al. Expression of multidrug resistance protein and messenger RNA correlate with ^{99m}Tc-MIBI imaging in patients with lung cancer. *J Nucl Med* 2001;42(10):1476-1483.

[66] Kunishio K, Morisaki K, Matsumoto Y, Nagao S, Nishiyama Y. Technetium-99m sestamibi single photon emission computed tomography findings correlated with P-glycoprotein expression, encoded by the multidrug resistance gene-1 messenger ribonucleic acid, in intracranial meningiomas. *Neurol Med Chir* (Tokyo) 2003;43(12):573-580.

[67] Wang H, Chen XP, Qiu FZ. Correlation of expression of multidrug resistance protein and messenger RNA with ^{99m}Tc-methoxyisobutyl isonitrile (MIBI) imaging in patients with hepatocellular carcinoma. *World J Gastroenterol* 2004;10(9):1281-1285.

[68] Kinuya S, Li XF, Yokoyama K, et al. Reduction of ^{99m}Tc-sestamibi and ^{99m}Tc-tetrofosmin uptake in MRP-expressing breast cancer cells under hypoxic conditions is independent of MRP function. *Eur J Nucl Med Mol Imaging* 2003;30(11):1529-1531.

[69] Fujii H, Nakamura K, Kubo A, et al. Preoperative evaluation of the chemosensitivity of breast cancer by means of double phase ^{99m}Tc-MIBI scintimammography. *Ann Nucl Med* 1998;12(6):307-312.

[70] Fujii H, Nakamura K, Kubo A, et al. ^{99m}Tc-MIBI scintigraphy as an indicator of the chemosensitivity of anthracyclines in patients with breast cancer. *Anticancer Res* 1998;18(6B):4601-4605.

[71] Yamamoto Y, Nishiyama Y, Satoh K, et al. Comparative study of technetium-99m-sestamibi and thallium-201 SPECT in predicting chemotherapeutic response in small cell lung cancer. *J Nucl Med* 1998;39(9):1626-1629.

[72] Kim YS, Cho SW, Lee KJ, et al. Tc-99m MIBI SPECT is useful for noninvasively predicting the presence of MDR1 gene-encoded P-glycoprotein in patients with hepatocellular carcinoma. *Clin Nucl Med* 1999;24(11):874-879.

[73] Kao CH, Tsai SC, Wang JJ, Ho YJ, Ho ST, Changlai SP. Technetium-99m-sestamethoxyisobutylisonitrile scan as a predictor of chemotherapy response in malignant lymphomas compared with P-glycoprotein expression, multidrug resistance-related protein expression and other prognosis factors. *Br J Haematol* 2001;113(2):369-374.

[74] Bhatnagar A, Vezza PR, Bryan JA, Atkins FB, Ziessman HA. Technetium-99m-sestamibi parathyroid scintigraphy: effect of P-glycoprotein, histology and tumor size on detectability. *J Nucl Med* 1998;39(9):1617-1620.

[75] Gorlick R, Liao AC, Antonescu C, et al. Lack of correlation of functional scintigraphy with [99m]technetium-methoxyisobutylisonitrile with histological necrosis following induction chemotherapy or measures of P-glycoprotein expression in high-grade osteosarcoma. *Clin Cancer Res* 2001;7(10):3065-3070.

[76] Leitha T, Glaser C, Lang S. Is early sestamibi imaging in head and neck cancer affected by MDR status, p53 expression, or cell proliferation? *Nucl Med Biol* 1998;25(6):539-541.

[77] Moorin RE, Davison A, Turner JH. Optimization of technetium-99m Sestamibi single-photon emission tomography to define multidrug resistance with confidence. *Nucl Med Commun* 2004;25(10):1039-1048.

[78] Raderer M, Scheithauer W. Clinical trials of agents that reverse multidrug resistance. A literature review. *Cancer* 1993;72(12):3553-3563.

[79] Boesch D, Gaveriaux C, Jachez B, Pourtier-Manzanedo A, Bollinger P, Loor F. In vivo circumvention of P-glycoprotein-mediated multidrug resistance of tumor cells with SDZ PSC 833. *Cancer Res* 1991;51(16):4226-4233.

[80] Pourtier-Manzanedo A, Boesch D, Loor F. FK-506 (fujimycin) reverses the multidrug resistance of tumor cells in vitro. *Anticancer Drugs* 1991;2(3):279-283.

[81] Hyafil F, Vergely C, Du Vignaud P, Grand-Perret T. In vitro and in vivo reversal of multidrug resistance by GF120918, an acridonecarboxamide derivative. *Cancer Res* 1993;53(19):4595-4602.

[82] Pierre A, Dunn TA, Kraus-Berthier L, et al. In vitro and in vivo circumvention of multidrug resistance by Servier 9788, a novel triazinoaminopiperidine derivative. *Invest New Drugs* 1992;10(3):137-148.

[83] Kaye SB. Multidrug resistance in breast cancer--is the jury in yet? *J Natl Cancer Inst* 1997;89(13):902-903.

[84] Mistry P, Stewart AJ, Dangerfield W, et al. In vitro and in vivo reversal of P-glycoprotein-mediated multidrug resistance by a novel potent modulator, XR9576. *Cancer Res* 2001;61(2):749-758.

[85] Kinuya S, Li XF, Yokoyama K, et al. Limitations of ^{99m}Tc tetrofosmin in assessing reversal effects of verapamil on the function of multi-drug resistance associated protein 1. *Nucl Med Commun* 2004;25(6):585-589.

[86] DeCoursey TE. Mechanism of K^+ channel block by verapamil and related compounds in rat alveolar epithelial cells. *J Gen Physiol* 1995;106(4):745-779.

[87] Arbab AS, Koizumi K, Toyama K, Arai T, Araki T. Technetium-99m-tetrofosmin, technetium-99m-MIBI and thallium-201 uptake in rat myocardial cells. *J Nucl Med* 1998;39(2):266-271.

[88] Arbab AS, Koizumi K, Toyama K, Arai T, Araki T. Effects of ion channel modulators in the influx and efflux of Tc-99m-MIBI. *Ann Nucl Med* 1999;13(1):27-32.

[89] Arbab AS, Koizumi K, Toyama K, Araki T. Uptake of technetium-99m-tetrofosmin, technetium-99m-MIBI and thallium-201 in tumor cell lines. *J Nucl Med* 1996;37(9):1551-1556.

[90] Arbab AS, Ueki J, Koizumi K, Araki T. Effects of extracellular Na^+ and Ca^{2+} ions and Ca^{2+} channel modulators on the cell-associated activity of ^{99m}Tc-MIBI and ^{99m}Tc-tetrofosmin in tumour cells. *Nucl Med Commun* 2003;24(2):155-166.

[91] Hart J, Wilkinson MF, Kelly ME, Barnes S. Inhibitory action of diltiazem on voltage-gated calcium channels in cone photoreceptors. *Exp Eye Res* 2003;76(5):597-604.

[92] Su Z, Sugishita K, Li F, Ritter M, Barry WH. Effects of FK506 on $[Ca^{2+}]i$ differ in mouse and rabbit ventricular myocytes. *J Pharmacol Exp Ther* 2003;304(1):334-341.

[93] Thami GP, Bhalla M. Erythromelalgia induced by possible calcium channel blockade by ciclosporin. *Bmj* 2003;326(7395):910.

[94] Kinuya S, Yokoyama K, Li XF, et al. Hypoxia-induced alteration of tracer accumulation in cultured cancer cells and xenografts in mice: implications for pre-therapeutic prediction of treatment outcomes with ^{99m}Tc-sestamibi, ^{201}Tl chloride and ^{99m}Tc-HL91. *Eur J Nucl Med Mol Imaging* 2002;29(8):1006-1011.

[95] Mankoff DA, Dunnwald LK, Gralow JR, et al. [Tc-99m]-sestamibi uptake and washout in locally advanced breast cancer are correlated with tumor blood flow. *Nucl Med Biol* 2002;29(7):719-727.

[96] Wackers FJ, Berman DS, Maddahi J, et al. Technetium-99m hexakis 2-methoxyisobutyl isonitrile: human biodistribution, dosimetry, safety, and preliminary comparison to thallium-201 for myocardial perfusion imaging. *J Nucl Med* 1989;30(3):301-311.

[97] Moretti JL, Hauet N, Caglar M, Rebillard O, Burak Z. To use MIBI or not to use MIBI? That is the question when assessing tumour cells. *Eur J Nucl Med Mol Imaging* 2005;32(7):836-842.

[98] Aloj L, Zannetti A, Caraco C, Del Vecchio S, Salvatore M. Bcl-2 overexpression prevents 99mTc-MIBI uptake in breast cancer cell lines. *Eur J Nucl Med Mol Imaging* 2004;31(4):521-527.

[99] Del Vecchio S, Zannetti A, Aloj L, Caraco C, Ciarmiello A, Salvatore M. Inhibition of early 99mTc-MIBI uptake by Bcl-2 anti-apoptotic protein overexpression in untreated breast carcinoma. *Eur J Nucl Med Mol Imaging* 2003;30(6):879-887.

[100] Green DR, Reed JC. Mitochondria and apoptosis. *Science* 1998;281(5381):1309-1312.

[101] Gross A, McDonnell JM, Korsmeyer SJ. BCL-2 family members and the mitochondria in apoptosis. *Genes Dev* 1999;13(15):1899-1911.

[102] Cory S, Adams JM. The Bcl2 family: regulators of the cellular life-or-death switch. *Nat Rev Cancer* 2002;2(9):647-656.

[103] Rutledge SE, Chin JW, Schepartz A. A view to a kill: ligands for Bcl-2 family proteins. *Curr Opin Chem Biol* 2002;6(4):479-485.

[104] Fukumoto M, Yoshida D, Hayase N, Kurohara A, Akagi N, Yoshida S. Scintigraphic prediction of resistance to radiation and chemotherapy in patients with lung carcinoma: technetium 99m-tetrofosmin and thallium-201 dual single photon emission computed tomography study. *Cancer* 1999;86(8):1470-1479.

[105] Hockel M, Vaupel P. Tumor hypoxia: definitions and current clinical, biologic, and molecular aspects. *J Natl Cancer Inst* 2001;93(4):266-276.

[106] Cook GJ, Fogelman I. Tumor hypoxia: the role of nuclear medicine. *Eur J Nucl Med* 1998;25(4):335-337.

[107] Cook GJ, Houston S, Barrington SF, Fogelman I. Technetium-99m-labeled HL91 to identify tumor hypoxia: correlation with fluorine-18-FDG. *J Nucl Med* 1998;39(1):99-103.

[108] Tatsumi M, Yutani K, Kusuoka H, Nishimura T. Technetium-99m HL91 uptake as a tumour hypoxia marker: relationship to tumour blood flow. *Eur J Nucl Med* 1999;26(2):91-94.

[109] Yutani K, Kusuoka H, Fukuchi K, Tatsumi M, Nishimura T. Applicability of ^{99m}Tc-HL91, a putative hypoxic tracer, to detection of tumor hypoxia. *J Nucl Med* 1999;40(5):854-861.

[110] Honess DJ, Hill SA, Collingridge DR, et al. Preclinical evaluation of the novel hypoxic marker ^{99m}Tc-HL91 (Prognox) in murine and xenograft systems in vivo. *Int J Radiat Oncol Biol Phys* 1998;42(4):731-735.

[111] Iyer RV, Haynes PT, Schneider RF, Movsas B, Chapman JD. Marking hypoxia in rat prostate carcinomas with beta-D-[^{125}I]azomycin galactopyranoside and. *J Nucl Med* 2001;42(2):337-344.

[112] Nishiyama Y, Kawasaki Y, Yamamoto Y, et al. Technetium-99m-MIBI and thallium-201 scintigraphy of primary lung cancer. *J Nucl Med* 1997;38(9):1358-1361.

[113] Lewis JS, Sharp TL, Laforest R, Fujibayashi Y, Welch MJ. Tumor uptake of copper-diacetyl-bis(N(4)-methylthiosemicarbazone): effect of changes in tissue oxygenation. *J Nucl Med* 2001;42(4):655-661.

[114] Arbab AS, Koizumi K, Toyama K, Arai T, Araki T. Ion transport systems in the uptake of ^{99m}Tc-tetrofosmin, ^{99m}Tc-MIBI and ^{201}Tl in a tumour cell line. *Nucl Med Commun* 1997;18(3):235-240.

[115] Schuetz E, Beck, WT, Schuetz, JD. Modulators and substrates of p-glycoprotein and cytochrome P4503A coordinately up-regulate these proteins in human colon carcinoma cells. *Mol Pharmacol* 1996;49:311-318.

[116] Naito S, Hasegawa S, Yokomizo A, et al. Non-P-glycoprotein-mediated atypical multidrug resistance in a human bladder cancer cell line. *Jpn J Cancer Res* 1995;86(11):1112-1118.

[117] Sharma V. Radiopharmaceuticals for assessment of multidrug resistance P-glycoprotein-mediated drug transport activity. *Bioconjug Chem* 2004;15(6):1464-1474.

[118] Sharma V, Beatty A, Wey SP, et al. Novel gallium(III) complexes transported by MDR1 P-glycoprotein: potential PET imaging agents for probing P-glycoprotein-mediated transport activity in vivo. *Chem Biol* 2000;7(5):335-343.

[119] Bigott HM, Prior JL, Piwnica-Worms DR, Welch MJ. Imaging multidrug resistance P-glycoprotein transport function using microPET with technetium-94m-sestamibi. *Mol Imaging* 2005;4(1):30-39.

[120] Packard AB, Kronauge JF, Barbarics E, Kiani S, Treves ST. Synthesis and biodistribution of a Lipophilic ^{64}Cu-labeled monocationic Copper(II) complex. *Nucl Med Biol* 2002;29(3):289-294.

[121] Elsinga PH, Franssen EJ, Hendrikse NH, et al. Carbon-11-labeled daunorubicin and verapamil for probing P-glycoprotein in tumors with PET. *J Nucl Med* 1996;37(9):1571-1575.

[122] Hendrikse NH, Franssen EJ, van der Graaf WT, Vaalburg W, de Vries EG. Visualization of multidrug resistance in vivo. *Eur J Nucl Med* 1999;26(3):283-293.

[123] Hendrikse NH, de Vries EG, Eriks-Fluks L, et al. A new in vivo method to study P-glycoprotein transport in tumors and the blood-brain barrier. *Cancer Res* 1999;59(10):2411-2416.

[124] Hendrikse NH, Vaalburg W. Imaging of P glycoprotein function in vivo with PET. *Novartis Found Symp* 2002;243:137-145.

[125] Levchenko A, Mehta BM, Lee JB, et al. Evaluation of ^{11}C-colchicine for PET imaging of multiple drug resistance. *J Nucl Med* 2000;41(3):493-501.

[126] Luurtsema G, Molthoff CF, Windhorst AD, et al. (R)- and (S)-[11C]verapamil as PET-tracers for measuring P-glycoprotein function: in vitro and in vivo evaluation. *Nucl Med Biol* 2003;30(7):747-751.

[127] Kiesewetter DO, Jagoda EM, Kao CH, et al. Fluoro-, bromo-, and iodopaclitaxel derivatives: synthesis and biological evaluation. *Nucl Med Biol* 2003;30(1):11-24.

[128] Dewanjee MK, Ghafouripour AK, Kapadvanjwala M, et al. Noninvasive imaging of c-myc oncogene messenger RNA with indium-111-antisense probes in a mammary tumor-bearing mouse model. *J Nucl Med* 1994;35(6):1054-1063.

[129] Urbain JL, Shore SK, Vekemans MC, et al. Scintigraphic imaging of oncogenes with antisense probes: does it make sense? Eur J Nucl Med 1995;22(6):499-504.

[130] Gambhir SS, Barrio JR, Herschman HR, Phelps ME. Imaging gene expression: principles and assays. *J Nucl Cardiol* 1999;6(2):219-233.

[131] Fujibayashi Y, Yoshimi E, Waki A, et al. A novel ^{111}In-labeled antisense DNA probe with multi-chelating sites (MCS-probe) showing high specific radioactivity and labeling efficiency. *Nucl Med Biol* 1999;26(1):17-21.

[132] Karamychev VN, Panyutin IG, Kim MK, et al. DNA cleavage by ^{111}In-labeled oligodeoxyribonucleotides. *J Nucl Med* 2000;41(6):1093-1101.

[133] Karamychev VN, Reed MW, Neumann RD, Panyutin IG. Distribution of DNA strand breaks produced by iodine-123 and indium-111 in synthetic oligodeoxynucleotides. *Acta Oncol* 2000;39(6):687-692.

In: Multidrug Resistance-Associated Proteins
Editor: Christopher V. Aiello, pp. 81-118

ISBN 1-60021-298-0
© 2007 Nova Science Publishers, Inc.

Chapter 4

MULTIDRUG RESISTANCE-ASSOCIATED PROTEINS PROFILES IN CHILDHOOD AND ADULT CANCER: THE POSSIBLE IMPACT AND EXPLANATION FOR DIFFERENT CLINICAL OUTCOME

Jan Styczynski[1] and Lidia Gil[2]*

[1]Department of Pediatric Hematology and Oncology, Collegium Medicum, Nicolaus Copernicus University, Bydgoszcz, Poland; [2]Department of Hematology, University of Medical Sciences, Poznan, Poland

ABSTRACT

Age has an important prognostic impact in therapy of cancer. Adults usually have a worse prognosis compared to children with the same type of cancer. This may be due to: (1) different, unfavourable cancer biology, (2) poor treatment tolerance, (3) cellular drug resistance, (4) higher expression of drug resistance related proteins, (5) development of other mechanisms of resistance. Regarding possible mechanisms of resistance, an almost endless number can be envisaged along the signal transduction pathways triggered by anticancer drugs. The difference in current cure rate between adult and childhood cancer may be caused by differences in regulation of drug resistance, both primary and acquired. The aim of this study was the systematic review of the literature on the role and impact of Multidrug Resistance-Associated Protein's (MRP's) expression in various types of childhood and adult cancer. This paper describes an update in differences of research on the biology of MRP's of various types of childhood and adult cancer with stress on differences in protein expression and clinical outcome. A panel of proliferative disorders is reviewed, including hematological malignancies, with emphasis on acute leukemias, both at diagnosis and at relapse; as well as brain tumors, bone tumors, soft tissue

---

* Address for correspondence: Jan Styczynski, MD, PhD, Department of Pediatric Hematology and Oncology, Collegium Medicum, Nicolaus Copernicus University, ul. Curie-Sklodowskiej 9, 85-094 Bydgoszcz, Poland, E-mail: jstyczynski@cm.umk.pl

sarcomas, rhabdomyosarcomas, neuroblastomas and liver tumors. A large variety and discrepancy of results is presented in performed studies. MRP's are physiologically present in various tissues. MRP's are also markers of immature cells, thus are shown to be more often present in acute myeloid leukemia in adults, however recent data suggest the possible relevance of MRP's family in childhood acute lymphoblastic leukemia. In general, their overexpression is more often observed in solid tumors, which occur more frequently in adults. MRP seems to be disease specific, so overall distribution of cancer determine the occurrence and clinical prognostic impact in malignancies in adults. It may correlate and contribute to worse clinical outcome of cancer in adults. The impact of MRP's and association with resistant disease in childhood and adult cancer is analysed in this review, with emphasis on results of multivariate analyses, variety of diseases and possible geographical influence. Possible strategies of modulation or circumvention of resistance caused by MRP's are reviewed. In summary, it seems that the greater the age, the higher the drug resistance. Age itself, more than drug resistance profile, reflects factors with more direct effect on chemotherapy response in adult cancer. This might contribute to the difference in outcome between children and adults with malignancies. Induction of drug resistance proteins during chemotherapy and co-existence of various mechanisms are common phenomena in adult cancer. Differences in resistance to different drugs might contribute to the impact of age on cancer outcome. The underlying mechanisms for these differences are still largely unknown; however, knowledge about drug resistance mechanisms can lead to the development of new therapeutic options.

INTRODUCTION

The results of anticancer therapy in most types of cancer both in children and adults are still unsatisfactory. Age has important prognostic impact in therapy of cancer. Adults have usually a worse prognosis compared to children with the same type of cancer. This may be due to: different, unfavourable biology of cancer in adults, poor treatment tolerance by adults, development of cellular drug resistance, or higher expression of drug resistance related proteins.

The difference in current cure rate between adult and childhood cancer may be caused by differences in regulation of drug resistance phenomenon, both primary and acquired. One of (possible reason) major problems in therapy is the development of cellular drug resistance. Regarding possible mechanisms of resistance, an almost endless number can be envisaged along the signal transduction pathways triggered by anticancer drugs. One of the most important remains family of multidrug resistance proteins. The family of multidrug resistance-associated proteins (MRPs) belongs to the ATP-binding cassette superfamily of transporters, which have the ability to function as outward pumps for chemotherapeutic drugs. Their structure, function, and substrate specificity have been studied intensively, but still little is known about their clinical relevance in malignant diseases [1].

Drug resistance remains one of the primary causes of suboptimal outcomes in cancer therapy. ATP-binding cassette (adenosine triphosphate-binding-cassette, i.e. ABC transporters, which have the ability to function as outward pumps for chemotherapeutic drugs and therefore might be involved in drug resistance) transporters are a family of transporter proteins that contribute to drug resistance via ATP-dependent drug efflux pumps. ABC transporters might have an important role in clinical practice. The best known proteins of this family are P-glycoprotein (PGP), family of multidrug-resistance-associated protein (MRP) and breast cancer related protein (BCRP). MRP family transporters are involved in normal physiologic functions. It also confers resistance to certain chemotherapeutic agents. The expressions of MRP family members and ABCG2 have not been well worked out in cancer. MRP1 is overexpressed at baseline in chemotherapy-resistant tumors, such as solid tumors, and is upregulated after disease progression following chemotherapy in malignancies such as leukemia and ovarian cancer. Further optimism is warranted with the advent of potent, nontoxic inhibitors and new treatment strategies, including the combination of new targeted therapies with therapies aimed at the prevention of drug resistance [2].

Since the recognition of the multidrug resistance-associated protein (MRP) gene [3], many studies on the expression, function and prognostic role of MRP was performed in human cancers. MRP mRNA appeared to be ubiquitously expressed at low levels in all normal tissues, including peripheral blood, the endocrine glands (adrenal and thyroid), striated muscle, the lymphoreticular system (spleen and tonsil), the digestive tract (salivary gland, esophagus, liver, gall bladder, pancreas, and colon), the respiratory tract (lung), and the urogenital tract (kidney, bladder, testis, and ovary) [4]. Nooter et al [4] divided the human cancers into three groups with regard to MRP expression. Group 1 consists of tumors that often exhibit high to very high MRP mRNA levels (e.g., chronic lymphocytic leukemia). Group 2 comprises the tumors that often exhibit low, but occasionally exhibit high MRP mRNA expression (e.g., esophagus squamous cell carcinoma, non-small cell lung cancer, and acute myelocytic leukemia). Group 3 comprises the tumors with predominantly low levels of MRP mRNA, comparable to the levels found in normal tissues (e.g., other hematological malignancies, soft tissue sarcomas, melanoma, and cancers of the prostate, breast, kidney, bladder, testis, ovary, and colon).

Another major problem in the treatment of cancer might be drug resistance. There are many ways for cancer cells to develop resistance or defense mechanisms against cytotoxic drugs, so the response to treatment can be related both to pharmacokinetics and chemosensitivity in particular age groups. The aim of this study is the systematic review of the literature in order to define differences in multidrug-resistance related proteins profiles in various types of adult and childhood cancer.

METHODS OF DATA COLLECTION

References were retrieved using the online data base of the National Library of Medicine (PubMed; http://www.ncbi.nlm.nih.gov/PubMed), as well as Embase and Medline 1966 to March 2006. Terms used included: MRP, multidrug-resistance related protein, multidrug resistance-associated protein, child*, adult*, drug resistance, chemoresistance, chemosensitivity, acute lymphoblastic leukemia, acute myeloid leukemia, brain tumors, bone tumors, soft tissue sarcomas, rhabdomyosarcomas, neuroblastomas and liver tumors. The retrieved references were supplemented by references from the author's own data base and results.

RESULTS

Epidemiology of Cancer in Children and Adults

Only 1% of all cases of malignancy occur in childhood. Distribution of cancer in children is based mainly on histological picture. The most frequent types of childhood malignancy are acute leukemias, lymphomas (Hodgkin and non-hodgkin), brain tumors, neuroblastoma, nephroblastoma, bone tumors, soft tissue sarcomas (including rhabdomyosarcoma). There is little prevalence of cancer incidence in boys.

In adults, epidemiology is different from children, and it is also different between males and females. Classification in adults is based on organ localization. Females suffer from malignant tumors localized mainly in: breast, uterus, lungs, ovarium, colon, and stomach. Males suffer from tumors localized mainly in: lungs, stomach, bladder, prostate, and colon.

Table 1: Examples of possible clinical significance of MRP's family in cancer

	Children	Adults
MRP1	ALL [9] Neuroblastoma [10]	AML [11] ALL [9]
MRP2 (cMOAT)	No impact in ALL [12] ALL [9]	ALL [9]
MRP3	ALL [9, 12]	Pancreatic carcinoma [6] CML [13] AML [14] ALL [9]
MRP4 (MOAT-B)	Marker for immature stem cells [12]	CML [13] Gliomas [15]
MRP5 (ABCC5)	No impact in ALL [12] ALL [9]	Pancreatic carcinoma [6] CML [13] AML [14] Gliomas [15] Lung cancer [16] ALL [9]
MRP6	ALL [9]	AML [17] Low levels in CML [13] Glial cells [18] Liver and kidneys [19] Renal cell carcinoma [20] ALL [9]
MRP7 (ABCC10)		Small cell lung cancer [8] Testes, intestine, and kidney [7]
MRP8 (ABCC11)		Breast cancer [5]
MRP9 (ABCC12)		Pancreatic carcinoma [6], Breast cancer [21]

According to the study of Nooter et al [4] who divided the human cancers into three groups with regard to MRP expression, the expression, function and role of this protein might by higher in adults, since chronic lymphocytic leukemia, esophagus squamous cell carcinoma, non-small cell lung cancer occur exclusively in adults, and acute myeloid leukemia has its prevalence mainly in adults.

Clinical Features of MRP's Family: From MRP1 to MRP9

The multidrug resistance-associated proteins (MRP's) are ATP-dependent transporters that export a variety of conjugated and unconjugated compounds out of cells. So far, nine members of MRP family transporters has been identified in humans, and numbered from 1 to 9 (Table 1). Some of them were studied both in children and adults, however there are no data regarding expression of MRP7-MRP9 in children, while presence of these proteins was already documented in solid tumors in adults [5-8]. Most studies in children are related to acute leukemias.

A large number of studies was performed in acute leukemias. As these are the most frequent childhood cancer, it is relatively possible to compare the roleof MRP's family in children and adults. Expression of MRP's in various types of cancer, with possible impact as prognostic factor on therapy results is reviewed in leukemias and solid tumors with respect to patient age.

Acute Lymphoblastic Leukemia: Variability of Results and Significance

In acute lymphoblastic leukemia (ALL), MRP1 expression in general at diagnosis is not associated with response and long-term survival in the few studies on this aspect which have been reviewed previously [22]. Several new reports are available, however results show discrepancies, not only in age groups, but also in with respect to method of MRP's detection, or even with differences with respect to geographical region. Latest reports of Dutch and German groups [1, 9, 12, 23] indicate possible, however differentiated role of MRP1-6 in ALL, both in children and adults. These MRPs probably have strongly overlapping functional activities. Important role of MRP1 was found in adult T-cell leukemia in Japan, both in newly diagnosed and in refractory and relapsed patients [24] (Table 2). The frequency of MRP expression at initial diagnosis is similar in Ad-ALL and Ch-ALL and varies largely in different studies [22, 25-30]. The expression of MRP mRNA did not differ between initial (iALL) and relapsed (rALL) both in adults [26] and in children, however the MRP protein level was higher in multiple relapse samples [22, 25].

Children: Possible Role of all MRP's

Analysis based on data shown in Table 2, suggests higher expression and impact on inferior therapy outcome in adults. Recent reports indicate possible adverse prognostic role of expression of MRP's family also in childhood ALL [9, 12, 23].

Table 2. Significance of MRP in acute lymphoblastic leukemia

	Children	**Adults**
Prognostic significance	Adverse effect of MRP-3 in childhood ALL, in male patients and T-ALL [12] Lower CR in MRP-positive patients [31] MRP 1-6, except MRP4 [9]. MRP2 and MRP3 [1]	In ATL [24] In relapsed / refractory [32] MRP 1-6, except MRP4 [9].
Increased expression	In pre-B ALL [33]	In ALL with hyperleukocytosis [34] In GSTπ and GSTμ positive [30] Higher expression [35] In ALL de novo [36] In ATL [25]
No significance	No impact of MRP1, MRP2, MRP3 [23] In ALL de novo and at relapse [37, 38] In My+ALL [39], at relapse [40] No impact [41, 42]	No impact of MRP1, MRP2, MRP3 [23] No impact [29, 43]

In the study of Plasschaert et al [9] leukemic blasts of 105 de novo ALL patients (adults, n=49; children, n=56) including 70% B-lineage and 30% T-lineage ALL patients, the mRNA expression levels of MRP1 to MRP6 were analyzed by quantitative real-time PCR. Adults showed a higher expressions of MRP1, MRP2, and MRP3 than children. Relapsed patients showed a higher expression of all MRP genes, except MRP4. For the total group of ALL patients, the expressions of MRP1, MRP2, MRP3, MRP5, and MRP6 predicted relapse. High expression of all MRP genes, except MRP4, was associated with a reduced relapse-free survival both in children and adults. This study shows that a subset of ALL patients with high MRP expression has an unfavorable prognosis independently of age [9]. Thus expression of multidrug resistance-associated proteins predicts prognosis in childhood and adult acute lymphoblastic leukemia.

In another report of that group, it has been shown that MRP functional activity determined by flow cytometry did not correlate with the mRNA expression of MRP1, MRP2 and MRP3 determined with RT-PCR [23].

Steinbach et al [12] studied the MRP2, MRP3, MRP4, MRP5, and SMRP genes using TaqMan real-time polymerase chain reaction (PCR) in 103 children with previously untreated ALL (precursor B-cell ALL, n = 71; T-cell ALL, n = 32). All 5 genes were expressed with a great variability, however only MRP3 expression was associated with a significantly worse prognosis. The median expression of MRP3 was 10-fold higher in T-ALL than in precursor B-ALL and 4-fold higher in male patients than in female patients. The prognostic impact of MRP3 was independent of immunophenotype or sex. Higher levels of MRP3 were found in patients with a poor in vivo response to prednisone, but this could not be confirmed in an independent case-control study (40 patients) for prednisone response. In healthy donors, the median expression of MRP4 was 4-fold higher in bone marrow and 8-fold higher in CD34+ stem cells compared with peripheral blood. These results suggest that MRP3 is involved in drug resistance in childhood ALL. High levels of MRP3 could possibly be the reason for the poorer prognosis of male patients or patients who have T-cell immunophenotype of ALL [12].

Most of other studies shows however lack of correlation between expression of MRP1 and its clinical significance. In the study of Sauerbrey et al [38], expression of both MRP and LRP was tested by semiquantitative RT-PCR, normalized for beta-microglobulin expression, in 86 children (58 initial ALL and 28 children with relapsed disease). Expression of both transcripts was found to be significantly correlated. Both resistance mechanisms had no prognostic significance in that retrospective study, however, patients who showed high LRP expression exhibited a lower tendency of remaining in continuous first remission [38].

No differences in MRP or PGP, but the expression of LRP was found in Ph+ALL group of pediatric and adult patients. Both childhood and adult Ph+ precursor B-cell ALL samples display a heterogeneous in vitro resistance profile, with relatively sensitive and resistant cases. The adult Ph+ samples, however, are generally more resistant compared to matched Ph- controls, reaching significance for prednisolone. There is a correlation of prednisolone resistance with age within the Ph+ cases which might, at least partially, explain the poorer prognosis of adult Ph+ALL [44]. Overexpression of MRP1 and LRP was found in children with pre-B ALL compared with T-cell ALL and AML tested [33].

In Japaneese study, expression of the MDR1, MRP and LRP genes did not contribute to risk factors in newly diagnosed 40 childhood acute lymphoblastic leukemia. No positive correlations between expression of these genes and age or leukocyte count were found [37].

Den Boer et al [40] showed that MRP1 does not contribute to drug resistance in childhood ALL. PGP, MRP, and LRP expression did not differ between 112 initial and 29 unrelated relapsed ALL samples nor between paired initial and relapse samples from 9 patients. No significant correlations were found between PGP or MRP expression and in vitro drug resistance. Samples with a marked expression of two or three resistance proteins did not show increased resistance to the tested drugs compared with the remaining samples. The expression of PGP, MRP, and LRP was not higher in initial ALL patients with prognostically unfavorable immunophenotype, white blood cell count, or age. The expression of PGP and MRP in 20 initial AML samples did not differ or was even lower compared with 112 initial ALL samples [40]. Expression of LRP, but not of PGP and MRP, significantly correlated with daunorubicin resistance in childhood ALL [45]. Expression of GSTπ, but not of GSTα or GSTμ, weakly correlated with the expression of MRP but not with PGP in ALL. However, a high expression of both GSTπ and MRP was not associated with in vitro resistance to ifosfamide, daunorubicin or prednisolone [39]. Drug resistance in myeloid-positive My+ALL was not related to increased expression of PGP, MRP or LRP compared with My-ALL [39].

In the study of the expression of LRP and MRP in 38 children with acute leukemia measured with reverse transcription-polymerase chain reaction (RT-PCR), MRP was overexpressed in 21 of the 38 patients; CR rate was significantly lower in MRP-positive patients than in MRP-negative patients. The positive rate of LRP was significantly lower in ALL than in AML. The positive rate of MRP was 59.3% in ALL, and 45.5% in AML. The positive rate of MRP was 28.6% in LRP-positive patients, and 29.4% in LRP-negative patients; there was no correlation between LRP and MRP. Authors concluded that childhood acute leukemia patients with overexpression of LRP and MRP suffer severe disease and achieve low remission rate lower remission rate of childhood AML patients may relate to LRP expression [31].

No effect of overexpression of MRP1, PGP and LRP functional drug efflux pumps at diagnosis of 295 newly diagnosed pediatric ALL did not contribute to treatment failure in pediatric ALL in the study of the Children's Oncology Group. A small number of patients (2%, 6/295) also overexpressed both PGP and MRP1 [42].

In the groups of 30 children with a diagnosis of acute lymphoblastic leukemia studied, only the increased expression of LRP was related to worsened event-free survival. The presence of the common ALL antigen was correlated with increased LRP expression and increased risk of relapse or death. The relative risk of relapse or death was six times higher among children with high LRP expression upon diagnosis, as confirmed by multivariate analysis of the three genes studied [46].

Adults: MRP1 Overexpression in ALL is Rare

In the study of Gurbuxani et al [34] in Indian 167 ALL patients (adults+children), higher MRP1 and glutathione transpherases expression in patients with WBC counts >100x10(9)/l was observed. However, relapse or shorter event free survival was independent of mRNA expression levels of its gene, in terms of either achieving a complete remission or predilection to early relapse [34]. In view of some recent studies that envisage MRP as an energy-dependent pump involved in the efflux of GSH conjugates, the simultaneous up-regulation of transcription of all these genes might well be part of an integrated detoxification response that has been switched on after exposure to an environmental stress [30].

Study of Beck et al [35] suggested that a multifactorial MDR including MRP appears particularly in recurrent relapses of ALL, which often do not respond to chemotherapy. Low MRP expression levels were detected in acute lymphocytic leukemia (n=14), by DNA analysis by Southern blotting [29].

Damiani et al [43] in 95 previously untreated cases of adult acute lymphoblastic leukaemia (ALL), showed that 45 out of 95 (47%) patients were PGP positive (+), 12/66 (18%) were LRP+ and 11/66 (17%) were MRP+. They concluded that PGP overexpression associated with a defect in daunorubicin accumulation is a frequent feature in adult ALL at onset and seems to be related to poorer therapy outcome and, consequently, a shorter disease-free survival. On the other hand, LRP and MRP overexpression seems to be a rare event and no conclusion can be drawn on its prognostic role [43].

Adult T-lymphocyte ALL: MRP1 Is a Strong Adverse Prognostic Factor in ATL

Adult T-lymphocyte ALL (T-ALL) is a subtype of leukemia with bad prognosis. Adult T-cell leukemia (ATL) is a T-cell malignancy caused by human T-cell-leukemia-virus-I (HTLV-I) infection. ATL comprises 4 clinical forms: acute, chronic, smoldering and lymphoma types. The response of ATL to chemotherapy is poor, and a major obstacle to successful treatment is intrinsic or acquired drug resistance. ATL is usually resistant to conventional chemotherapy and has a relatively poor prognosis; however, not all resistance mechanisms remain undetermined. Two studies show that MRP1 has in important adverse influence on therapy results in ATL. In the study of Ohno et al [24] of MRP1 mRNA in leukemia cells from 48 ATL patients membrane vesicles prepared from ATL cells with high expression of MRP1 mRNA showed a higher ATP-dependent leukotriene C4 uptake than did those with low expression of MRP1 mRNA. This uptake was almost completely inhibited by LTD4 antagonists ONO-1078 and MK571. In acute- and lymphoma-type ATL, high expression of MRP1 mRNA at diagnosis correlated with shorter survival, and Cox regression analysis revealed that MRP1 expression was an independent prognostic factor. These findings suggest that functionally active MRP1 is expressed in some ATL cells and that it is involved in drug resistance and has a possible causal relationship with poor prognosis in ATL. Multidrug resistance-reversing agents, such as ONO-1078 and MK571, that directly interact and inhibit the transporting activity of MRP1 may be useful for treating ATL patients [24].

In the second study, performed by Ikeda et al [25] peripheral blood mononuclear cells (PBMC) from ATL patients expressed similar or higher levels of MRP, LRP and MRP2 (canalicular multispecific organic anion transporter, cMOAT) mRNAs, as compared with normal PBMC. In normal controls and ATL patients, MDR1 mRNA expression was undetectable in this study. PBMC from acute and chronic ATL patients expressed significantly higher levels of MRP and LRP mRNA than did normal PBMC. In chronic ATL, positive correlations were apparent between levels of MRP and LRP mRNA expression, and between each mRNA level and the absolute number of abnormal lymphocytes in peripheral blood. Probenecid, an inhibitor of the MRP pump, significantly increased the accumulation of calcein in PBMC from 3 chronic ATL patients. These findings suggest that the MRP and LRP genes in ATL are often activated by HTLV-I infection and may confer MDR of ATL cells in vivo. Combined chemotherapy with inhibitors of these MDR genes may be promising in the treatment of ATL [25].

Aplastic Anemia: Expression of Multidrug Resistance Proteins Might be Decreased in Acquired Aplastic Anaemia

Although acquired aplastic anaemia (AA) is not a malignant disorder, however due to the clinical picture, methods of therapy and possible transformation to acute leukemia, this disease is often analyzed together with hematological malignancies. To address a possible impairment of multidrug resistance mechanisms in acquired aplastic anemia (AA), the functions of PGP and multidrug resistance-associated protein (MRP) were respectively assessed by rhodamine 123 (Rh123) and daunorubicin (DNR) efflux in peripheral blood lymphocytes from AA patients. The proportion of Rh123-effluxing T cells was significantly decreased in AA, relative to controls. Interestingly, these changes were also present in patients with AA in remission. Conversely, Rh123 efflux in B and natural killer (NK) cells and DNR efflux in peripheral blood lymphocytes were unchanged. These data indicated that activity of multidrug resistance proteins might be decreased in AA not only during the development of the disease, but also after remission, introducing a new concept on the pathophysiology of AA by suggesting that it may contribute to drug-induced injury to haemopoietic cells in some cases of AA, by increasing the proportion of susceptible cells [47].

Acute Myeloid Leukemia: Possible Significance, in spite of Variability of Results

More than 80% of all cases of acute myeloid leukemia (AML) occur in adults, while it is not often disease in childhood and accounts for 15% of pediatric acute leukemias. Thus, most of data related to the role of MRP in AML is based on studies performed in adults. General rule that in AML, MRP1 expression at diagnosis is not correlated with clinical response and survival in most studies [22], was faced with the results of several reports published lately and showing possible prognostic role of MRP in adult AML (Table 3).

Table 3. Significance of multidrug resistance-associated proteins in acute myeloid leukemia

	Children	Adults
Prognostic significance	MRP3 and MRP2 [1]	Coexpression of PGP, MRP3, or BCRP [48] Poor CR rate [49] MRK (MRP) expression is an adverse prognostic factor [11] MRP associated with inferior overall survival [50]
No significance	In de novo and relapsed paired samples [51]	MRP activity in 26/44 cases [52] Low incidence [49, 53] PGP and MRP are not upregulated in relapsed AML [54] No significance of MRP1 and MRP2 in any phase of AML [55] No significance [56, 57] In relapsed AML [58]

Children: MRP3 and MRP2, but not MRP1 Might Contribute to Resistance in Pediatric AML

The data reflecting the role of MRP in childhood AML are scanty. In the study of Steinbach et al [1], the expression of the MRP2, MRP3, MRP4, MRP5, and SMRP genes was measured using TaqMan real-time PCR in 53 children with de novo and 9 with relapsed acute myeloid leukemia. MRP3 gene expression was higher in patients who did not achieve remission. Expression of MRP2 or MRP3 was associated with a lower rate of survival, and patients who expressed high levels of both genes had a particularly poor prognosis. No significant association was found for overall survival or remission rate and the expression of MRP4, MRP5, and SMRP. This study provides first data on the clinical relevance of five MRPs in acute myeloid leukemia patients. The results strongly suggest that MRP3 and possibly also MRP2 are involved in drug resistance in this disease. Those two proteins therefore represent interesting markers for risk-adapted therapy and possible targets for the development of specific drugs to overcome multidrug resistance [1].

In a previous study of 20 AML de novo children, the expression of PGP and MRP1 did not differ or was even lower compared with 112 initial ALL samples [40]. These studies showed that MRP1 does not contribute to drug resistance in childhood AML.

Adults: MRP3, BCRP and PGP Might Have Prognostic Impact in AML

To identify prognostic factors alternative or additional to drug-resistance and apoptosis proteins, the impact of the expression of heat-shock proteins (HSPs) and MRP was analyzed in 98 newly diagnosed AML. Cytogenetics, CD34 positive expression, MRP positive expression, and HSP110 positive expression remained as pejorative prognostic factors for OS in the multivariate analysis. When considering patients with intermediate risk cytogenetics, HSP110 and MRP positive expressions and CD33 negative expression were of poor outcome, while HSP27 and HSP60 positive expressions appeared of pejorative prognostic value in patients with unfavorable karyotypes [11]. The significant increases of MDR1, MRP, GST pi, and PKC (protein kinase C) theta gene expression was observed in relapsed AML in the study from primary (n=14) or relapsed (n=23) samples of AML [59].

Studies of ATP-binding cassette proteins MRP1, MRP2, MRP3, MRP5, PGP and BCRP, for their potential implication in chemoresistance performed by Benderra et al [48] in 85 AML patient samples showed that MRP3 function was higher in patients which had a high level of leukocytes, a M5 FAB subtype, and an intermediate or poor cytogenesis. BCRP activity was not correlated with clinical or biological variables, but high PGP activity was correlated with the following variables: CD34 expression, FAB subtype, intermediate or poor cytogenesis, and elderly patients. Second, PGP, MRP3, and BCRP activities were correlated with complete remission, disease-free survival, and overall survival in multivariate analysis. Important observation was that patient samples expressing one or none of these Pgp, MRP3, or BCRP functional proteins have a better prognosis than the patients expressing two or three of these functional proteins. Thus, BCRP and MRP3 may also be involved in chemoresistance in AML, especially MRP3 in patients with M5 FAB [48]

In another analysis of MRP1, MDR1, LRP/MVP and BCRP mRNA expression in 20 paired clinical AML samples from diagnosis and relapse or refractory disease, using quantitative Taqman analysis, MDR1 and MRP1 mRNA levels were not different at relapse as compared to diagnosis. These results suggested that BCRP, but not MDR1, MRP1 or LRP/MVP was associated with clinical resistant disease in AML [51].

No informative conclusion regarding MRP1 role could be drawn from the study 96 previously untreated cases of de novo AML, since only 8/96 (8%) patients were classified as MRP+, however 5/8 cases showed unfavourable karyotypic abnormalities, and 6/8 failed to achieve remission [49]. No role of MRP in 145 patients (109 initial and 36 relapsed or refractory AML) was found by Han et al [60], with the expression of the protein in 8.3% samples [60].

In the study of samples from 67 patients with AML examined for expression of LRP, MRP, and multidrug resistance (MDR1) mRNA using a semiquantitative reverse transcription polymerase chain reaction (RT-PCR) assay, levels of LRP, but not of MRP or MDR1 mRNA, were significantly higher in eight patients who failed to achieve complete remission (CR) compared with 25 patients who achieved CR. A positive correlation was demonstrated between LRP and MRP and between MRP and MDR1 mRNA levels in the 77 clinical samples analyzed. These data suggest that LRP, but not MRP1 gene overexpression may constitute a novel mechanism of multidrug resistance [53].

Patients with high GSTμ expression appeared to co-express MRP what support the theory that altered detoxification through the glutathione pathway contributes towards drug resistance in AML [61].

In AML M3, acute promyelocytic leukemia (APL), the high sensitivity to anthracyclines appears to be attributable to the low frequency of MDR proteins overexpression at onset even if 30% of patients still relapse and become resistant to therapy. However no changes were demonstrated in MRP1 and MRP2 expression in any phase of disease in 45 analyzed patients, while PGP and LRP overexpressing cases significantly grew up during disease progression and at second relapse were significantly higher than at onset. These data confirm the low expression at diagnosis of proteins related to development of drug resistance in APL. The evidence of a relative easy induction of PGP and LRP, but not of MRP, can be useful in choosing drugs to employ for consolidation or rescue therapy [55].

Also, in the study of Galimberti et al [62] in 35 AML patients, MRP was significantly co-expressed with topoisomerase II beta, GSTπ was co-expressed with LRP and MRP. Neither the expression nor the co-expression of the tested genes was significantly correlated with the response to the induction treatment and long-term outcome [62].

Gemtuzumab ozogamicin (GO) is a novel immunoconjugate therapy for AML. PGP, MRP1, and MRP2 expression were characterized in CD33+ cell lines and in CD33+ AML samples and analyzed the effect of the PGP inhibitor cyclosporine (CSA) and the MRP inhibitor MK-571 on GO-induced cytotoxicity. MRP1, but not MRP2, expression correlated with MRP activity. MK-571 enhanced GO-induced cytotoxicity in PGP-negative/MRP-positive NB4 and HL-60 cells. CSA, but not MK-571 alone, restored GO susceptibility in PGP-positive/MRP-positive TF1 cells; however, MK-571 enhanced cytotoxicity in the presence of CSA. All patient samples exhibited MRP activity, and 17 of 23 exhibited PGP activity. CSA increased GO-induced cytotoxicity in 12 PGP-positive samples, whereas MK-571 alone was effective in only one sample with minimal PGP activity. In 3 PGP-positive/MRP-positive samples, MK-571 enhanced GO-induced cytotoxicity in the presence of CSA. Thus, MRP1 may attenuate susceptibility to GO. This effect was comparatively less than that for PGP and required the inhibition of PGP for detection in cells that coexpressed both transporters. However, because MK-571 and CSA failed to affect cytotoxicity in a portion of PGP-positive/MRP-positive AML samples, this shows that additional resistance mechanisms are likely important [63].

Function of the ABC transporters, PGP, multidrug resistance protein and breast cancer resistance protein, in AML was tested with a fluorescent probe assay with substrate/ modulator: Syto16/PSC833 (PGP), calcein-AM/probenecid (MRP) and prazosin/Ko143 (BCRP); efflux profiles were directly compared with blasts at diagnosis and relapse from the same patient [52]. At diagnosis BCRP activity was undetectable in AML blasts from 23/26 cases, while PGP activity was present in 36/45 and MRP activity in 26/44 of the cases. Furthermore, no subpopulations of blasts with considerably higher drug efflux capacities were found. Overall, no consistent changes were observed at follow-up in forty-five patients, the mean activities (as percentages of values at diagnosis) were 97% (PGP), 103% (MRP) and 102% (BCRP). Thus, multidrug resistance protein probably have limited function in drug efflux-related resistance in AML [52].

Also, no association was observed between the multidrug resistance parameters and overall survival of de novo AML patients [56], and no significant changes in PGP, LRP or MRP1 expression are likely to occur at first relapse [58].

Laupeze et al [50] showed that high multidrug resistance associated proteins activity in acute myeloid leukaemias is associated with poor response to chemotherapy and reduced patient survival. Multidrug resistance protein (MRP) activity was investigated in 44 newly diagnosed acute myeloid leukaemia (AML) patients using a functional assay based on efflux of carboxy-2',7'-dichlorofluorescein, an anionic dye handled by both MRP1 and MRP2. Elevated MRP transport was detected in 29% of cases, but was not significantly correlated with sex, age, white blood cell count at diagnosis or karyotype. In contrast, it was associated with secondary AML, CD34 positivity and PGP activity. There was a lower rate of complete remission in MRP-positive patients versus MRP-negative patients; overall survival was also better for MRP-negative patients. These data indicate a probable role for MRP activity in the clinical outcome of AML [50].

Data compared prior to and after therapy start (paired samples) revealed that among AML patients who did not respond to therapy (NR) expressed increased levels of MDR1 mRNA, as well as MRP and Bcl-2 cDNA, when compared to patients achieving complete remission. The results indicate that high individual activity of the investigated genes might be associated with poor clinical outcome in treated acute leukemia [27].

In 127 AML patients, MRP expression was low, intermediate and high in 30%, 46% and 24% of the patients, respectively. MRP expression was independent of age and sex of the patients, white blood cell count, FAB subtype, serum lactate dehydrogenase levels and karyotype aberrations. MRP expression had no impact no response to induction chemotherapy. The complete remission rates were 75%, 70% and 64% for patients with low, intermediate and high expression, respectively. Patients with intermediate or high MRP expression showed a trend toward shorter overall survival as compared to patients with low MRP expression. MRP did not predict for response to induction chemotherapy but intermediate or high MRP expression possibly could be associated with shorter overall survival of the patients [64].

Role of MRP in AML with inv(16): the Sensitivity of AML M4Eo with inv(16) Might be Related to Loss of the Gene for MRP1

This gene of MRP1 maps to 16p13.13, centromeric to the primary short arm breakpoint, separated from MYH11 by a distance of approximately 150kb. Deletion of the MRP gene has been demonstrated by in situ hybridisation, gene dosage studies and by loss of heterozygosity of a flanking microsatellite marker (D16S405) [65]. Acute myeloid leukaemia associated with the inversion chromosome 16: inv(16)(p13q22) has a favourable prognosis and is known to be chemosensitive. The inversion chromosome is seen in a number of FAB subclasses but is most commonly associated with acute myelomonocytic leukaemia with abnormal eosinophils, M4Eo. It results in the creation of a fusion between the myosin heavy chain gene (MYH11) on the short arm and the gene for a transcription factor, core binding factor beta (CBFB) on the long arm. In a subset of these inv(16) AML patients, inversion also results in loss of the gene for the multidrug resistance-associated protein (MRP) at the short arm breakpoint. Kuss et al [66] have demonstrated deletion of MRP by in situ hybridisation, by gene dosage studies and by studying loss of heterogeneity of a flanking microsatellite marker. Among 13 AML patients with inv(16), MRP deletion was detected in 5 while 7 had no deletion. Deletion of MRP gene was associated with longer time from diagnosis until death or relapse from complete remission [66]. Twenty two patients with inv(16) leukaemia were analysed for deletion of the MRP gene. Deletion of the gene was detected in 7/22 AML M4Eo patients, fourteen patients showed retention of the gene and in one case the findings were indeterminate. Clinical data from 13 of these patients were analysed revealing deletion of the MRP gene to be significantly associated with longer time from diagnosis until failure in these patients. It appears likely that the deletion of an MRP allele, may favourably affect the biology of inv(16) AML and may have important prognostic implications [65].

On the pther hand, Van Der Kolk et al [17] showed in the group of inv(16) AML patients, that MRP1 mRNA was detected in patients with 1 or 2 MRP1 FISH signals, but not in patients with no MRP1 signals. MRP2 and MRP6 mRNA were expressed predominantly in AML samples with 1 MRP1 signal, whereas in normal bone marrow cells no MRP2 and MRP6 mRNA was observed. This study shows that MRP activity varies among inv(16) AML cases and does not differ from that in normal hematopoietic cells; this might be in part due to the up-regulation of other MRP genes [17].

MRP Is a Marker of Immature Cells

Members of the family of ABC transporters are regarded to be markers for immature stem cells [12]. In the study of van der Kolk et al [54], the mRNA expression and activity of PGP and the MRPs was determined with RT-PCR and flow cytometry, in conjunction with phenotype, as measured with the monoclonal antibodies CD34, CD38 and CD33, in 30 paired samples of de novo and relapsed AML. PGP and MRP activity varied strongly between the cases (rhodamine 123 efflux-blocking by PSC833, and carboxyfluorescein efflux-blocking by MK-571, n = 60). PGP and MRP activity were increased in 23% and 40% of the relapse samples, and decreased in 30% and 20% of the relapse samples, respectively (as defined by a difference of >2 x standard deviation of the assays). Up- or downregulation of mRNA expression was observed for MDR1 (40%), MRP1 (20%), MRP2 (15%), MRP3 (30%), and MRP5 (5%). Phenotyping demonstrated a more mature phenotype in 23% of the relapsed AML cases, and a more immature phenotype in 23% of the relapses, which was independent of the karyotypic changes that were observed in 50% of the studied cases. PGP and MRP activity correlated with the phenotypic changes, with higher PGP and MRP activities in less mature cells. This study shows that PGP and MRP activity are not consistently upregulated in relapsed AML. However, PGP and MRP activities were correlated with the maturation stage as defined by immune phenotype, which was observed to be different in 46% of the relapses. The activity of these proteins, might be upregulated at relapse as compared with de novo AML due to clonal selection [54]. Also MRP4 seems to be a marker for immature stem cells [12].

In the study of Suarez et al [67], bone marrow samples from 150 elderly patients (> 65 years) with de novo AML and 30 younger AML, quantitative expression of proteins associated with apoptosis (Bcl-2, bax, APO2.7) and MDR (PGP, MRP, LRP) in 3 blast cell subpopulations, defined according to their maturation stage was analyzed in a 4-color immunofluorescence technique. Although a homogeneous CD34+ blast cell population was more frequent in the elderly patients, no statistically significant differences were detected between the two age groups in the expression of either apoptosis- or MDR-associated proteins, except for slightly higher quantities of LRP protein in the more immature CD34+ blast cell subset in the elderly AML cases. Interestingly, when different blast cell populations were compared, immature (CD34+) blast cells were characterized by higher levels of Bcl-2 in both age groups and lower levels of APO2.7 in the elderly group. In addition, higher PGP levels were found in CD34+ blast cells than in CD34- ones in elderly AML patients. Reactivity for LRP was low in both elderly and younger patients. These results suggest that the higher resistance to chemotherapy observed in elderly AML patients could be related to a higher incidence of cases with a CD34+ homogeneous blast cell population, since these blast cells frequently display a more pronounced anti-apoptotic and MDR1 phenotype [67].

Elderly patients with AML the more immature blast cells are also more resistant to apoptotic processes, which could explain why the blast cells at relapse frequently display a more immature phenotype than that observed at diagnosis. Contradictory results in multidrug resistance profile support the hypothesis that failure to respond to chemotherapeutic drugs in AML is a multifactorial phenomenon [68].

AML and MDS: No Impact of MDR in Myelodysplastic Syndromes

In the study of CD34+ cells from acute myeloid leukemia, myelodysplastic syndromes, and normal bone marrow no significant differences were found in the expression of PGP, MRP, and LRP between low-risk myelodysplastic syndrome patients and normal BM, but decreased expression of MRP in AML and high-risk myelodysplastic syndromes and PGP in high-risk myelodysplastic syndromes were detected. The authors concluded that increased resistance to chemotherapy of CD34+ cells from both AML and high-risk myelodysplastic syndromes would be explained more appropriately in terms of an increased antiapoptotic phenotype rather than a MDR phenotype. In low-risk myelodysplastic syndromes abnormally high apoptotic rates would be restricted to the CD34- cell compartments [69].

In the study of bone marrow from 56 patients with MDS, including six with refractory anaemia (RA)/RA with ringed sideroblasts (RARS), 23 cases of RA with excess blasts/in transformation (RAEB/T), four patients with chronic myelomonocytic leukaemia (CMML) and 23 cases of MDS having progressed to acute myeloid leukaemia (MDS-AML), MRP1 expression was investigated by immunocytochemistry (ICC) and by flow cytometry using MRPm6 monoclonal antibody. The efflux test using calcein-AM (CAM) +/- probenecid to evaluate MRP1 activity was also performed. No correlation was observed between MRP1 expression and PGP, lung resistance-associated protein (LRP) or CD34 expression, although there was a trend for more frequent MRP1 expression in PGP-positive cases in MDS-AML. It seems that MRP1 expression was correlated with disease stage in MDS in that study. As for PGP, discordant expression/function of MRP1 could be found in some cases, suggesting the existence of non-functional transport proteins in MDS. MRP1 expression did not seem to be a prognostic factor in MDS [70].

Chronic Myeloid Leukemia: No Significance of MRP's

Carter et al [13] found that cells from chronic myelogenous leukaemia (CML) patients at presentation exhibit multidrug resistance not mediated by either MDR1 or MRP1. All cells from the CML patients transcribed high levels of MRP3, MRP4 and MRP5 compared with healthy donors. Low levels of MDR1, MRP1, MRP2, MRP6, LRP and anthracycline resistance-associated protein were equally transcribed in cells from healthy donors and CML patients. These results indicate that neither MDR1 nor MRP1 mediate the resistance in these cells. Our results shed light on a resistance mechanism operative in CML patients, which, together with the resistance to apoptosis, is responsible for the lack of response of CML patients to induction-type protocols used to treat acute myeloid leukaemia patients [13].

Chronic Lymphocytic Leukemia: Usually High Expression of MRP

Burger et al [29] determined the expression of the multidrug resistance-associated protein (MRP), in 60 patients with acute or chronic leukemia, using an RNase protection assay. MRP appeared to be ubiquitously expressed at low levels in all nonmalignant hemopoietic cell types, reflecting its basal constitutive expression. In chronic lymphocytic leukemia (CLL) (n=21), either treated (n=8) or untreated (n=13), a high percentage (15 of 21, ie. 71%) had relatively high expression levels of the MRP gene. In contrast, low MRP expression levels were detected in acute lymphocytic leukemia (n=14), and in chronic myelocytic leukemia (n = 9). In acute myelocytic leukemia (AML) (n=16), one of nine untreated patients and two of seven patients with prior chemotherapy showed significant hyperexpression of MRP. DNA analysis by Southern blotting did not reveal amplification of the MRP gene in the leukemia samples, including those with elevated MRP mRNA levels. Authors concluded that relatively high expression of MRP is occasionally observed in AML and at high frequency in CLL, irrespective of treatment, probably due to transcriptional activation and/or increased mRNA stability [29].

Juszczynski et al [71] reported that the level of constitutive MRP gene's expression in peripheral blood lymphocytes is higher in CLL patients than in healthy controls. They found increased MRP gene expression levels in patients with higher white blood cells and lymphocytes' counts as well as in more advanced disease stages according to Rai or Binet scale. Finally, MRP gene's expression was higher in patients with progressive CLL, especially in cases refractory to chemotherapy salvage. These results of the present study suggest that expression of MRP gene might be relevant in the pathogenesis of the MDR phenotype in CLL [71].

Consoli et al. [72] evaluated the presence of PGP, MRP, LRP and Bcl-2 in CD19-positive cells from 100 cases of chronic lymphocytic leukaemia (CLL). PGP was found in 73% of the CLL cases with no significant difference regarding stage or previous treatment. LRP protein was homogeneously distributed with no differences for stage or treatment. MRP protein was detected at a low level of expression in 49.4% of CLL patients with no differences for stage or treatment. Bcl-2 protein was expressed at a high level in all CLL patients and higher levels were found in the advanced stage. Authors concluded that PGP, MRP, LRP and Bcl-2 are frequently expressed in CLL, however PGP, MRP and LRP were not correlated to stage or previous treatment. Bcl-2 is higher in advanced-stage patients. The clinical and biological significance of these MDR mechanisms in CLL remains to be fully explained [72].

Lymphomas: No Role of MRP Gene

In the study of the lymph nodes of 23 untreated and 23 recurrent lymphoma (HD and NHL) patients, there was no difference in MRP gene expression level and positive rate between recurrent and untreated patients, while the expression levels and positive rates of MDR1 and PGP in recurrent patients were higher than those in untreated patients. The chemotherapy effective rates were lower in MDR1 gene and PGP positive expression patients (33% and 26%) than in negative expression patients (85% and 83%). Relevant analysis showed that there was a significant relevance in expression level between MDR1 gene and PGP, but there was no correlation between MDR1 and MRP or between MRP and PGP.

Authors concluded that MDR1 gene and PGP expression levels were dominant mechanisms of clinical drug resistance of lymphomas, whereas, MRP gene did no play a role. MDR1 gene and PGP expression levels were relevant to chemotherapy efficacy, however, MRP gene expression level seems to have no impact in lymphoma [73].

Brain Tumors: Overexpression of MRP's in Brain Tumors in Children and Adults Might Contribute to Worse Therapy Outcome

In molecular studies in pediatric medulloblastomas, the correlation coefficients between MRP and Bcl-2, as well as Bcl-2 and Bax, p53 and p21, Ki67 and PCNA were positive and significant, indicating their possible coregulated expression. The relationship between these markers indicates their relative and cumulative effect on cellular drug resistance, apoptosis, and/or cell proliferation in pediatric medulloblastomas [74]. A high expression of MRP1 in medulloblastomas was detected also in another study [75].

Expression of multidrug resistance protein gene might increase in patients with glioma after chemotherapy. MRP expression was observed in 16 (70%) of 23 untreated patients, and the proportion of MRP-positive cells in the whole cell population ranged from 3 to 32% in the 16 MRP-positive patients. PGP-positive tumors were observed in 4 (18%) of 23 patients, and the proportional rates of PGP-positive cells in the whole cell population ranged from 4 to 23%. The proportional rate of MRP-positive or PGP-positive glioma cells increased after chemotherapy when compared with that before chemotherapy in all patients examined. There was no significant correlation between expression of MRP or PGP and tumor grade. These results suggest that MRP as well as PGP may be involved in acquired or intrinsic drug resistance in human glioma [76].

In the study of Vogelgesang et al [77] of expression of MRP, PGP and BCRP in dysembryoplastic neuroepithelial tumors (DNT) showed their overexpression with a different labeling pattern. MRP5 was detected primarily in endothelial cells, but notably also in neurons. PGP and BCRP were predominantly located in the endothelium of brain vessels. Examination of MDR1 gene polymorphisms revealed no correlation with PGP expression whereas the MRP2 exon 10 G1249A polymorphism was associated with different MRP2 labelling. These results show that multidrug transporters are overexpressed in DNT, thus these transport proteins may play an important role in the mechanisms of drug resistance in brain tissue [77].

Bone Tumors: Possible Role of MRP

In 45 osteosarcomas analysed by immunohistochemistry, the expression of MRP1 was observed in 32 (71%) specimens. More specimens expressed MRP1 in high-grade osteosarcomas (30/38, 79%) than in low-grade osteosarcomas (2/7, 28.6%). The correlation coefficient between expression of MRP1 and grade of pathology was 0.844. In a limited number of patients, the expression of MRP1 was not related to the the age and sex of the patients, Enneking surgical stage, osteosarcoma size, serum concentration of ALP and duration before diagnosis. No expression of MRP1 in 6 normal bone specimens was observed. Possibly, MRP1 is expressed in osteosarcoma and its expression is positively correlated with the malignancy of osteosarcoma [78].

Fifteen of 24 osteosarcoma samples (62.5%) showed significant expression of MRP. The level of MRP expression was significantly correlated with the percentage washout rate of (99m)Tc-MIBI, and the washout rate of (99m)Tc-MIBI was significantly faster in patients with high MRP expression than in those with a low MRP score. It has been suggested that the washout rate of (99m)Tc-MIBI is correlated with MRP expression. Both the washout rate of (99m)Tc-MIBI and MRP expression were correlated with therapy response. (99m)Tc-MIBI can be used as a general probe for functional imaging of both PGP and MRP; however, it is not capable of differentiating the functional status of either MDR-related glycoprotein [79].

The analysis of the expression of multidrug resistance-associated protein mRNA in ten samples of Ewing's sarcoma and malignant peripheral neuroectodermal tumor of bone showed that MRP mRNA expression was recognized in eight of the ten clinical specimen and the expression of multidrug resistance gene (MDR1) was demonstrated in three of the ten clinical samples and all three cell lines, what may contribute to elucidation of the mechanism of anti-cancer-drug resistance in this tumor [80].

Soft Tissue Sarcomas: MRP Possibly Play a Role in Most Types of STS

The biological behaviour of different histological types and grades of soft tissue sarcomas (STS) varies. This might result in a differing sensitivity to cytotoxic drugs. Cross-resistance to functionally and structurally distinct natural-product drugs, known as multidrug resistance (MDR), is associated with the overexpression of PGP, MRP1 and LRP. Study performed in 141 chemotherapy-naive STS patients, showed that expression of PGP and LRP was observed more frequently than the expression of MRP1 (P<0.0001). PGP expression was most pronounced in malignant fibrous histiocytoma (MFH), MRP1 was expressed in most malignant peripheral nerve sheath tumours (MPNST), while LRP was strongly expressed in MFH and unspecified sarcomas. MRP1 and LRP expression was significantly more common in grades 2 and 3 compared with grade 1 tumours. PGP expression was correlated with MRP1, especially in grade 3 STS. It seems that PGP, MRP1 and LRP are expressed in the majority of STS, but this expression varies according to the histological type. MRP1 and LRP, but not PGP expression, were found to be correlated to tumour grade. Thus, MDR proteins might contribute to the observed differences in clinical behaviour within the heterogeneous group of STS [81].

On the other hand, enhanced levels of MDR1 and MRP1 were rare events in 21 STS or malignant melanoma patients [82]. PGP, and to less extent MRP1, MRP2, and MRP3 expression is an important independent prognostic factor in synovial sarcoma in series of 54 cases, however it was not prognostic in multivariate Cox analysis [83].

In 86 cases soft tissue sarcomas analysed for MDR1, MRP1, MRP2 and MRP3 using a quantitative reverse transcriptase-PCR (RT-PCR) method, malignant peripheral nerve sheath tumor (MPNST) showed significantly high levels of MDR1 (p=0.01) and MRP3 (p=0.03) mRNA expression, compared to the other tumor types. PGP expression was significantly correlated with large tumor size (> or =5 cm, p=0.04) and high clinical stage (stages III and IV) (p=0.03). Furthermore, cases with nuclear expression of p53 revealed significantly higher levels of MDR1 mRNA expression, compared to those with negative immunoreaction for p53 (p=0.03). These results suggest that MDR1/PGP expression may have an important role to play in tumor progression in the cases of soft tissue sarcoma, with p53 being one of the active regulators of the MDR1 transcript. Also, the high levels of both MDR1 and MRP3 mRNA expression in MPNST might help to explain the poor response of this tumor to anticancer-drugs [84].

In the analysis of the mRNA expression of MRP and MDR1 in soft-tissue sarcomas with RT-PCR in 39 samples from 33 cases of soft-tissue sarcomas (11 liposarcomas, 9 malignant fibrous histiocytomas, 6 leiomyosarcomas, 4 malignant schwannomas, 3 fibrosarcomas, 3 synovial sarcomas, and 3 epithelioid sarcomas) and 7 benign soft-tissue tumors obtained prior to chemotherapy, an expression of MRP mRNA was noted in 56% of soft-tissue sarcoma specimens. The co-expression of MRP and MDR1 was recognized in 15 samples (38%) (5/11 liposarcomas, 5/9 malignant fibrous histiocytomas, 3/6 leiomyosarcomas, 2/3 fibrosarcomas) and significantly correlated with histological grade. A positive and significant correlation was found between MRP and MDR1 expression in soft-tissue sarcomas (P=0.0013). In benign soft-tissue tumors the expression of multidrug resistance proteins was low: 1 chemodectoma and 1 neurothekeoma showed low MRP expression; however, and no case showed co-expression of MRP and MDR1 [85].

Clinical outcome was evaluated in 29 patients with LMS and 26 patients with a primary malignant GIST for immunohistochemical detection of PGP, MRP1, LRP, and c-kit. PGP and MRP1 expression was more pronounced in GIST than in LMS, and the mean percentage MRP1 expressing cells was 13.3% in patients with LMS and 35.4% in patients with GIST. LRP expression did not differ between LMS and GIST. c-kit was expressed in 5% of the LMS patients and in 68% of the GIST patients. LMS patients have a better survival than GIST patients, and the metastatic pattern is different. This might be due to lower expression of MDR proteins in LMS than in GIST [86].

Low expression of drug resistance proteins was observed in leiomyosarcoma: MRP [86, 87], and PGP and LRP [81].

Rhabdomyosarcoma: MRP is an Important Factor in Children and Adults

Pediatric rhabdomyosarcomas (RMS) have a more advantageous prognosis after multimodality treatment compared with adult RMS, which might be related to a decreased sensitivity to chemotherapy in adults. There is only 1 study comparing expression of multidrug resistance proteins in pediatric and adult rhabdomyosarcomas [88]. The expression of PGP, MRP1, and LRP was assessed immunohistochemically in 45 specimens of untreated RMS: 29 pediatric and 16 obtained from adults. All children had an embryonal or botryoid RMS. Among the adults, there were 10 embryonal, 3 alveolar, and 3 pleomorphic RMS. Expression of PGP and MRP1 did not differ significantly between children and adults. Expression of LRP was more pronounced in embryonal and pleomorphic RMS in adults compared with RMS in children. In addition, LRP expression correlated with age at diagnosis. Alveolar RMS had remarkably low LRP expression. In this series, an increased LRP expression was observed in adults, which may explain their worse response to chemotherapy. In alveolar RMS, a low LRP expression was observed, suggesting that other mechanisms are responsible for the resistant phenotype in most of these tumors [88].

In 23 the embryonal and the alveolar subtypes of pediatric rhabdomyosarcoma samples analyzed for the expression of MDR1 and MRP genes using a semi-quantitative competitive RT-PCR assay, MRP gene expression was associated with a reduction in survival. The overall survival of patients with tumors positive or negative for MRP expression were 50% and 93%, respectively. In contrast, the expression of MDR-1 gene was not predictive of survival. These findings suggest that MRP expression could be a prognostic factor in patients with rhabdomyosarcoma [89].

Cocker et al [90] did not confirm the presence of MRP1 and PGP in a pediatric rhabdomyosarcoma cell line. Also, indomethacin (MRP1 modulator) did not affect the development of resistance in this model. These experiments strongly suggest that the development of MDR may be preventable using modulators of multidrug resistance [90].

In the study of samples of 13 pairs of primary untreated rhabdomyosarcomas and their residual, recurrent, or metastatic lesions after chemotherapy for expression of multidrug resistance proteins, MRP1 and PGP expression did not change significantly, but LRP expression increased significantly after chemotherapy. In both untreated and treated samples, LRP was expressed primarily in differentiated cells. The findings indicate that the in vivo expression of LRP, but not of PGP and MRP1, is induced by chemotherapeutic treatment in rhabdomyosarcomas. It suggests that rather LRP, than PGP and MRP1, plays a role in therapy-induced differentiation [91].

Neuroblastoma: MRP1 Has Potent Prognostic Significance

The expression of MRP by neuroblastoma cells correlates with N-myc oncogene amplification, a well-established prognostic indicator in patients with neuroblastoma. In analysis of MRP expression in specimens of primary tumors from 60 patients with neuroblastoma, levels of MRP gene expression were significantly higher in tumors with N-myc amplification than in tumors without such amplification. High levels of MRP expression were strongly associated with reductions in both survival and event-free survival in the overall study population and in subgroups of patients without N-myc amplification and patients with localized disease. For the overall study population, the five-year cumulative survival rates in the groups with high and low levels of MRP expression were 57 percent and 94 percent, respectively. In contrast, expression of the MDR1 multi-drug-resistance gene was not predictive of survival or event-free survival. After adjustment by multivariate analysis for the effects of N-myc amplification and other prognostic indicators, high levels of MRP expression retained significant prognostic value for poor survival and poor event-free survival, whereas N-myc amplification had no prognostic value. Thus, high levels of MRP gene expression in patients with neuroblastoma correlate strongly with poor outcome. The findings suggest that expression of this multidrug-resistance gene accounts for the association between N-myc amplification and reduced survival [10].

MYCN and MRP gene expression were highly correlated in 60 primary untreated tumours both with and without MYCN gene amplification. Like MRP, high MYCN gene expression was significantly associated with reduced survival, both in the overall study population and in older children without MYCN gene amplification. Inhibition of MYCN, through the introduction of MYCN antisense RNA constructs into human neuroblastoma cells in vitro, resulted in decreased MRP gene expression, determined both by RNA-PCR and

Western analysis. The data are consistent with MYCN influencing neuroblastoma outcome by regulating MRP gene expression [92]. These results are to be confirmed by gene profiling of high risk neuroblastoma [93].

In the study of the expression of multidrug resistance proteins in 70 cases of untreated primary neuroblastoma, the frequencies of the expression of PGP, MRP, and LRP were 61.4%, 38.6%, and 24.3%, respectively. A significant positive correlation was observed between PGP and MRP expression, as well as between LRP and MRP expression. The rates of expression of PGP and MRP were higher in tumors from patients aged greater than one year old than in tumors from patients aged less than 1 year old at time of diagnosis. MRP expression in tumors that had metastasized was significantly more frequent than in tumors that had not metastasized. The expression of all tested proteins showed a significant relationship with whether or not the tumor had differentiated. MRP expression was significantly associated with a reduction in both median survival time and 2-year cumulative survival. By contrast, PGP and MRP expression did not correlate with survival. According to Cox regression analysis, only the co-expression of PGP and MRP had significant prognostic value [94].

The prognostic value of MDR1 gene expression in primary untreated neuroblastoma was shown in subsets of 60 primary untreated neuroblastomas for which MYCN gene copy number and expression of the multidrug resistance-associated-protein [95]. In contrast to MRP gene expression, MDR1 expression was lower in tumours with MYCN gene amplification compared with those without amplification. Strong correlations between MDR1 and MRP gene expression, and between MDR1 and MYCN gene expression, were observed in tumours lacking MYCN gene amplification. In these single-copy tumours, very high MDR1 gene expression was significantly associated with poor outcome. Very high MDR1 expression was also strongly predictive of poor outcome in older children, but not in infants. These findings suggest a clinical role for the MDR1 gene in specific subgroups of primary neuroblastoma [95].

Liver Tumor: Possible Role of MRP

The reports related to expression of MRP in malignant liver tumor in children are very scanty. In 10 malignant liver tumors tested for the expressions of MRP and canalicular multispecific organic anion transporter (cMOAT, MRP2) by quantitative RNA-polymerase chain reaction (PCR), cMOAT was frequently expressed in the malignant liver tumors. The expression of MRP and cMOAT in the childhood liver tumors was more common and higher, especially in advanced cases with a poor outcome, than that observed in normal liver or in 9 hepatocellular carcinomas from adult patients. The enhanced expression of these genes might be characteristic of childhood malignant liver tumors and related to their clinical chemoresistance [96].

Wilms Tumor: Possible Role of MRP

The reports related to expression of MRP in malignant renal tumor in children are also very scanty. Tumor samples from a variety of Wilms tumors (WT) obtained from three patients were analyzed by cytogenetic and array-based comparative genomic hybridization (CGH) methods. Array-based CGH examinations revealed a 2.6-fold genomic amplification of the multidrug resistance-associated protein 1 (MRP1) gene in the metachronous WT, but no amplification in the primary tumor. Polymerase chain reaction showed a sixfold overexpression of the MRP1 gene in this metachronous WT relative to the primary tumor. Isolated amplification and overexpression of the MRP1 gene in the metachronous WT, however, suggest that this gene may be an important factor in the development and progression of metachronous tumors [97].

Breast Cancer: Possible Role of MRP

Specimens from 64 patients with primary breast cancer were analysed for their individual expression levels of several MDR-associated genes (MDR1, MRP, LRP, topoisomerase II alpha/IIbeta, cyclin A and the PKC isozyme genes (alpha, beta1, beta2, eta, theta, and mu) by a cDNA-PCR approach. Significantly enhanced mean values for MRP, LRP and PKC eta gene expression were found, but significantly decreased Topo II alpha and cyclin A gene expression levels in G2 tumours compared with G3. Remarkably, significant positive correlations between the MDR1, MRP or LRP gene expression levels and PKC eta were determined. These findings point to the occurrence of a multifactorial drug resistance in the clinics and to PKC eta as a possible key regulatory factor for up-regulation of a series of MDR-associated genes in different types of tumours [98].

MULTIVARIATE ANALYSES

The impact of prognostic factors of anticancer therapy is usually presented as multivariate analysis. The possible adverse prognostic role of MRP was analyzed in a number of studies, is shown in Table 4. In general, there is only one study showing that MRP is an independent prognostic factor of anticancer therapy in children. This study is related to neuroblastoma [10]. On the other hand, there are at least 10 studies performed on adults, showing that MRP is an independent adverse prognostic factor. With respect to specific disease, most analyses are related to acute myeloid leukemia and ovarian cancer, thus these diseases are presented separately in Table 4.

MODULATION OF ACTIVITY OF
MULTIDRUG RESISTANCE-ASSOCIATED PROTEIN

MRP is expressed in most human tissues and is overexpressed in several tumor types. In such cases, this protein represents an interesting target to overcome multidrug resistance, e.g. MRP3 in childhood ALL [12]. The list of possible MRP modulators is presented in Table 5.

Table 4. Results of multivariate analyses of prognostic factors including MRP expression

Diagnosis	Prognostic significance of MRP	No prognostic significance (other factors)
AML	*Adults* Coexpression of two or three of functional proteins MRP3, BCRP, and PGP [48] Cytogenetics, CD34 positive expression, MRK positive expression, and HSP110 expression [11] MRP1, age, cytogenetics and FLT3 mutational status [99] Coexpression of at least 2 of: PGP, MRP1, bcl-2, mutant p53, hsp27 [100, 101] PGP, MRP, low expression of Topo II, age over 55 in acute leukemias [102]	*Adults* PGP, age and cytogenetics [49] LRP, older age, unfavourable karyotype [57]
ALL	*Adults* Adult T-cell leukemia: high expression of MRP1 mRNA [24]	*Adults* LRP, PGP, CD18 and Ki-67 [103] PGP, CD34 expression [104] *Children* LRP [46]
Ovarian carcinoma	High mRNA levels [105] Residual tumors 2 cm or larger and MRP expression [106]	FIGO stage, PGP expression [107] Pre-operative expression of p53 [108] Lower proliferation [109] No MDR proteins [110, 111] Stage, residual tumor [112] LRP status [113]
Other solid tumors	*Adults* Invasive breast cancer: Only in stage 1 or stage 2 high-grade tumours [114] Bladder cancer MDR1, MRP1, MRP2 and MRP3 [115] *Children* Neuroblastoma [10]	*Adults* Breast cancer: glutathione-S-transferase P1 (GSTP1) [116] Urothelial bladder carcinoma: large tumors and high Ki-67 expression [117] Non-small cell lung cancer [118] Choroidal melanoma [119] Squamous cell carcinoma of the oesophagus, (high MRP expression in samples after chemotherapy had significance) [120] Oral and oropharyngeal carcinomas. G-CSF receptor, angiogenic factors (platelet-derived endothelial cell growth factor) [121]

Table 5: Modulators of multidrug resistance-associated protein

Modulator	Effect
NSAIDs (indomethacin, sulindac, tolmetin, acemetacin, zomepirac and mefenamic acid)	In cell lines, in which multidrug resistance is due to overexpression of MRP, a significant increase in cytotoxicity was observed in the presence of the active NSAIDs [122]
Valproic acid (a histone deacetylase inhibitor)	Induction of apoptosis in AML patient cells expressing PGP and/or MRP1 [123]
PSC 833 and 280-446 (PGP inhibitors)	The PGP-/MRP+ cells (HL60/130) responded to PSC 833 and 280-446 by increased accumulation of daunorubicin [124]
PK11195 (peripheral benzodiazepine receptor ligand	Broad inhibition of ABC transporters in hematologic cancer cell lines and primary leukemia-cell samples [125]
Arsenic trioxide (As_2O_3)	As_2O_3 could significantly decrease the expression of PGP and MRP, but not LRP [126]
Verapamil, PSC833, cremophor	In the two MRP-over expressing cell lines, these modifiers only partially blocked the function of MRP and combinations of these optimal concentrations acted antagonistically [127]
Cyclosporin A (PGP inhibitor)	Cyclosporin A modulates PGP, MRP-1, BCRP, and LRP, and this broad-spectrum activity may contribute to its clinical efficacy [128]
Probenecid (the inhibitor of a wide variety of anion transporters)	Weak effect [52, 129]

Valproic acid (VPA) (a histone deacetylase inhibitor) can inhibit the proliferation of both PGP- and MDR-associated protein 1 (MRP1)-positive and -negative cells. VPA also induced apoptosis of PGP-positive cells. VPA as an interesting drug that should be tested in clinical trials for overcoming the MDR phenotype in AML patients [123].

The novel resistance modifying agents PSC 833, 280-446, and LY 335979 are primarily targeted at inhibition of PGP, and their MRP inhibitory potential is largely unknown. Drug-resistant human leukemia cells with PGP+/MRP- (KG1a/200, K562/150) and PGP-/MRP+ (HL60/130) phenotypes were maintained in suspension cultures for experimental studies of drug accumulation and drug sensitization by PGP inhibitors. The PGP-/MRP+ cells responded to PSC 833 and 280-446 by increased accumulation of daunorubicin. PGP inhibitory agents have differential effects on MRP-derived drug resistance which could be exploited in treatment of multidrug resistance in cancer patients [124].

The peripheral benzodiazepine receptor (pBR) ligand, PK11195, promotes mitochondrial apoptosis and blocks PGP-mediated drug efflux to chemosensitize cancer cells at least as well or better than the PGP modulator, cyclosporine A (CSA). We now show that PK11195 broadly inhibits adenosine triphosphate (ATP)-binding cassette (ABC) transporters in hematologic cancer cell lines and primary leukemia-cell samples, including multidrug resistance protein (MRP), breast cancer resistance protein (BCRP), and/or Pgp. Because PK11195 promotes chemotherapy-induced apoptosis by a pBR-dependent mitochondrial mechanism and broadly blocks drug efflux by an apparently pBR-independent, ABC transporter-dependent mechanism, PK11195 may be a useful clinical chemosensitizer in cancer patients [125].

The Pgp modulator cyclosporin A has shown clinical efficacy in AML, whereas its analogue PSC-833 has not. Cyclosporin A is known to also modulate MRP1. Cyclosporin A enhanced retention of the substrate drug mitoxantrone in cells overexpressing PGP (HL60/VCR), MRP-1 (HL60/ADR), and BCRP (8226/MR20, HEK-293 482R) and increased cytotoxicity 6-, 4-, 4-, and 3-fold, respectively. Cyclosporin A modulates PGP, MRP-1, BCRP, and LRP, and this broad-spectrum activity may contribute to its clinical efficacy [128].

Multidrug resistance protein (MRP), another drug efflux pump, may be inhibited by probenecid, i.e, the inhibitor of a wide variety of anion transporters [129].

Study of the effect of arsenic trioxide (As_2O_3) on expression of drug transporting molecules in APL MR2 cell line. Showed that As_2O_3 could significantly decrease the expression of PGP and MRP, but not that of LRP. Thus, PGP and MRP, but not LRP, may be the sensitive targets of As_2O_3 to overcome drug-resistance. ATRA might be the substrates of PGP and MRP [126].

Aszalos et al [127] showed that combinations of PGP blockers, verapamil, PSC833, and cremophor act differently on the multidrug resistance associated protein (MRP) and on PGP. Clinically optimal plasma levels of verapamil, cremophor, and PSC833 have been shown to completely block the function of PGP in PGP-over expressing cells. However, in the two MRP-overexpressing cell lines, these modifiers only partially blocked the function of MRP and combinations of these optimal concentrations acted antagonistically. These results also suggest that the identification of the specific mechanism of drug resistance is important for the selection of chemotherapeutic strategies to block the efflux pump on the cancer cell [127].

A specific group of NSAIDs (indomethacin, sulindac, tolmetin, acemetacin, zomepirac and mefenamic acid) all at non-toxic levels, significantly increased the cytotoxicity of the anthracyclines (doxorubicin, daunorubicin and epirubicin), as well as teniposide, VP-16 and vincristine, but not the other vinca alkaloids vinblastine and vinorelbine in a variety of chemotherapeutic drugs was examined in the human lung cancer cell lines DLKP, A549, COR L23P and COR L23R and in a human leukaemia line HL60/ADR.

A substantial number of other anticancer drugs, including methotrexate, 5-fluorouracil, cytarabine, hydroxyurea, chlorambucil, cyclophosphamide, cisplatin, carboplatin, mitoxantrone, actinomycin D, bleomycin, paclitaxel and camptothecin, were also tested, but displayed no synergy in combination with the NSAIDs. The synergistic effect was concentration dependent. The effect appears to be independent of the cyclo-oxygenase inhibitory ability of the NSAIDs, as (i) the synergistic combination could not be reversed by the addition of prostaglandins D2 or E2; (ii) sulindac sulphone, a metabolite of sulindac that does not inhibit the cyclooxygenase enzyme, was positive in the combination assay: and (iii) many NSAIDs known to be cyclo-oxygenase inhibitors, e.g. meclofenamic acid, diclofenac, naproxen, fenoprofen, phenylbutazone, flufenamic acid, flurbiprofen, ibuprofen and ketoprofen, were inactive in the combination assay. The enhancement of cytotoxicity was observed in a range of drug sensitive tumour cell lines, but did not occur in P-170-overexpressing multidrug resistant cell lines. However, in the HL60/ADR and COR L23R cell lines, in which multidrug resistance is due to overexpression of the multidrug resistance-associated protein MRP, a significant increase in cytotoxicity was observed in the presence of the active NSAIDs. Subsequent Western blot analysis of the drug sensitive parental cell lines, DLKP and A549, revealed that they also expressed MRP and reverse-transcription-polymerase chain reaction studies demonstrated that mRNA for MRP was present in both cell lines. It was found that the positive NSAIDs were among the more potent inhibitors of [3H]-LTC4 transport into inside-out plasma membrane vesicles prepared from MRP-expressing cells, of doxorubicin efflux from preloaded cells and of glutathione-S-transferase activity. The NSAIDs did not enhance cellular sensitivity to radiation. The combination of specific NSAIDs with anticancer drugs reported here may have potential clinical applications, especially in the circumvention of MRP-mediated multidrug resistance [122].

GEOGRAPHICAL DIFFERENCES

A large variability of results of studies on MRP performed worldwide with respect to different diagnosis of malignant disease, groups of patients, age and method is an interesting database showing that some differences related to geographical area. This might be related to more frequent occurrence of specific diseases in specific region, such as adult T-leukemia in Japan. A number of Chineese studies on acute leukemias show high expression and prognostic role of MRP both in children and adults. Possible geographical differences in multidrug resistance proteins in ALL is analyzed in Table 6.

Table 6: Possible geographical differences in multidrug resistance proteins in ALL

	Children	Adults
Europe	No impact of MDR, MRP1 and LRP, with some exceptions for LRP [23, 40, 45] Possible role of MRP3 [1, 9, 12]	Higher expression [35] Rare overexpression [43]
USA	Higher expression [33] Rarely overexpression (rather in T-ALL) and no influence of MRP1 on pDFS [42]	
China	Often overexpression, often coexpression, related to worse CR rate [32, 36]	Often overexpression, often coexpression, related to worse CR rate [31, 32, 36]
India	Often overexpression, but no relation to DFS [30, 34]	Often overexpression, but no relation to DFS [30, 34]
Japan	No impact [37]	MRP1 is a prognostic factor in ATL [24] High expression [25]
Brasil	No impact [46]	

CONCLUSION

A large variety and discrepancy of results is presented in performed studies. MRP's are physiologically present in various tissues. MRP's are also markers of immature cells, thus are shown to be more often present in acute myeloid leukemia in adults, however recent data suggest the possible relevance of MRP's family also in childhood acute lymphoblastic leukemia. In general, their overexpression is more often observed in solid tumors, which occur more frequently in adults. MRP seems to be disease specific, so overall distribution of cancer determine the occurrence and clinical prognostic impact in malignancies in adults. It may correlate and contribute to worse clinical outcome of cancer in adults. The impact of MRP's and association with resistant disease in childhood and adult cancer was analysed in this review, with emphasis on results of multivariate analyses, variety of diseases and possible geographical influence. Possible strategies of modulation or circumvention of resistance caused by MRP's are reviewed. In summary, it seems that the greater the age, the higher the drug resistance. Age itself, more than drug resistance profile, reflects factors with more direct effect on chemotherapy response in adult cancer. This might contribute to the difference in outcome between children and adults with malignancies. Induction of drug resistance proteins during chemotherapy and co-existence of various mechanisms are common phenomena in adult cancer. Differences in resistance to different drugs might contribute to the impact of age on cancer outcome. The underlying mechanisms for these differences are still largely unknown; however, knowledge about drug resistance mechanisms can lead to the development of new therapeutic options.

REFERENCES

[1]   Steinbach, D; Lengemann, J; Voigt, A; Hermann, J; Zintl, F; Sauerbrey, A. Response to chemotherapy and expression of the genes encoding the multidrug resistance-associated proteins MRP2, MRP3, MRP4, MRP5, and SMRP in childhood acute myeloid leukemia. *Clinical Cancer Research* 2003;9:1083-1086.

[2]   Leonard, GD; Fojo, T; Bates, SE. The role of ABC transporters in clinical practice. *Oncologist* 2003;8:411-424.

[3]   Cole, SP; Bhardwaj, G; Gerlach, JH; Mackie, JE; Grant, CE; Almquist, KC; Stewart, AJ; Kurz, EU; Duncan, AM; Deeley, RG. Overexpression of a transporter gene in a multidrug-resistant human lung cancer cell line. *Science* 1992;258:1650-1654.

[4]   Nooter, K; Westerman, AM; Flens, MJ; Zaman, GJ; Scheper, RJ; van Wingerden, KE; Burger, H; Oostrum, R; Boersma, T; Sonneveld, P. Expression of the multidrug resistance-associated protein (MRP) gene in human cancers. *Clinical Cancer Research* 1995;1:1301-1310.

[5]   Bera, TK; Lee, S; Salvatore, G; Lee, B; Pastan, I. MRP8, a new member of ABC transporter superfamily, identified by EST database mining and gene prediction program, is highly expressed in breast cancer. *Molecular Medicine* 2001;7:509-516.

[6]   Konig, J; Hartel, M; Nies, AT; Martignoni, ME; Guo, J; Buchler, MW; Friess, H; Keppler, D. Expression and localization of human multidrug resistance protein (ABCC) family members in pancreatic carcinoma. *International Journal of Cancer* 2005;115:359-367.

[7]   Maher, JM; Cheng, X; Slitt, AL; Dieter, MZ; Klaassen, CD. Induction of the multidrug resistance-associated protein family of transporters by chemical activators of receptor-mediated pathways in mouse liver. *Drug Metabolism and Disposition* 2005;33:956-962.

[8]   Boonstra, R; Timmer-Bosscha, H; van Echten-Arends, J; van der Kolk, DM; van den
      Berg, A; de Jong, B; Tew, KD; Poppema, S; de Vries, EG. Mitoxantrone resistance in a
      small cell lung cancer cell line is associated with ABCA2 upregulation. *British Journal
      of Cancer* 2004;90:2411-2417.

[9]   Plasschaert, SL; de Bont, ES; Boezen, M; van der Kolk, DM; Daenen, SM; Faber, KN;
      Kamps, WA; de Vries, EG; Vellenga, E. Expression of multidrug resistance-associated
      proteins predicts prognosis in childhood and adult acute lymphoblastic leukemia.
      Clinical Cancer Research 2005;11:8661-8668.

[10] Norris, MD; Bordow, SB; Marshall, GM; Haber, PS; Cohn, SL; Haber, M. Expression
      of the gene for multidrug-resistance-associated protein and outcome in patients with
      neuroblastoma. *The New England Journal of Medicine* 1996;334:231-238.

[11] Thomas, X; Campos, L; Mounier, C; Cornillon, J; Flandrin, P; Le, QH; Piselli, S;
      Guyotat, D. Expression of heat-shock proteins is associated with major adverse
      prognostic factors in acute myeloid leukemia. *Leukemia Research* 2005;29:1049-1058.

[12] Steinbach, D; Wittig, S; Cario, G; Viehmann, S; Mueller, A; Gruhn, B; Haefer, R;
      Zintl, F; Sauerbrey, A. *The multidrug resistance-associated protein* 3 (MRP3) is
      associated with a poor outcome in childhood ALL and may account for the worse
      prognosis in male patients and T-cell immunophenotype. *Blood* 2003;102:4493-4498.

[13] Carter, A; Dann, EJ; Katz, T; Shechter, Y; Oliven, A; Regev, R; Eytan, E; Rowe, JM;
      Eytan, GD. Cells from chronic myelogenous leukaemia patients at presentation exhibit
      multidrug resistance not mediated by either MDR1 or MRP1. *British Journal of
      Haematology* 2001;114:581-590.

[14] Van der Kolk, DM; de Vries, EG; Muller, M; Vellenga, E. The role of drug efflux
      pumps in acute myeloid leukemia. *Leukemia and Lymphoma* 2002;43:685-701.

[15] Bronger, H; Konig, J; Kopplow, K; Steiner, HH; Ahmadi, R; Herold-Mende, C;
      Keppler, D; Nies, AT. ABCC drug efflux pumps and organic anion uptake transporters
      in human gliomas and the blood-tumor barrier. *Cancer Research* 2005;65:11419-11428.

[16] Yoshida, M; Suzuki, T; Komiya, T; Hatashita, E; Nishio, K; Kazuhiko, N; Fukuoka, M.
      Induction of MRP5 and SMRP mRNA by adriamycin exposure and its overexpression
      in human lung cancer cells resistant to adriamycin. *International Journal of Cancer*
      2001;94:432-437.

[17] Van der Kolk, DM; Vellenga, E; van Der Veen, AY; Noordhoek, L; Timmer-Bosscha,
      H; Ossenkoppele, GJ; Raymakers, RA; Muller, M; van Den Berg, E; de Vries, EG.
      Deletion of the multidrug resistance protein MRP1 gene in acute myeloid leukemia: the
      impact on MRP activity. *Blood* 2000;95:3514-3519.

[18] Berezowski, V; Landry, C; Dehouck, MP; Cecchelli, R; Fenart, L. Contribution of glial
      cells and pericytes to the mRNA profiles of P-glycoprotein and multidrug resistance-
      associated proteins in an in vitro model of the blood-brain barrier. *Brain Research*
      2004;1018:1-9.

[19] Chassaing, N; Martin, L; Mazereeuw, J; Barrie, L; Nizard, S; Bonafe, JL; Calvas, P;
      Hovnanian, A. Novel ABCC6 mutations in pseudoxanthoma elasticum. *Journal of
      Invesigative Dermatology* 2004;122:608-613.

[20] Nomura, M; Matsunami, T; Kobayashi, K; Uchibayashi, T; Koshida, K; Tanaka, M;
      Namiki, M; Mizuhara, Y; Akiba, T; Yokogawa, K; Moritani, S; Miyamoto, K.
      Involvement of ABC transporters in chemosensitivity of human renal cell carcinoma,

and regulation of MRP2 expression by conjugated bilirubin. *Anticancer Research* 2005;25:2729-2735.

[21] Bera, TK; Iavarone, C; Kumar, V; Lee, S; Lee, B; Pastan, I. MRP9, an unusual truncated member of the ABC transporter superfamily, is highly expressed in breast cancer. *Proceedings of National Academy of Sciences USA* 2002;99:6997-7002.

[22] Van den Heuvel-Eibrink, MM; Sonneveld, P; Pieters, R. The prognostic significance of membrane transport-associated multidrug resistance (MDR) proteins in leukemia. *International Journal of Clinical Pharmacology and Therapeutics* 2000;38:94-110.

[23] Plasschaert, SL; Vellenga, E; de Bont, ES; van der Kolk, DM; Veerman, AJ; Sluiter, WJ; Daenen, SM; de Vries, EG; Kamps, WA. High functional P-glycoprotein activity is more often present in T-cell acute lymphoblastic leukaemic cells in adults than in children. *Leukemia and Lymphoma* 2003;44:85-95.

[24] Ohno, N; Tani, A; Chen, ZS; Uozumi, K; Hanada, S; Akiba, S; Ren, XQ; Furukawa, T; Sumizawa, T; Arima, T; Akiyama, SI. Prognostic significance of multidrug resistance protein in adult T-cell leukemia. *Clinical Cancer Research* 2001;7:3120-3126.

[25] Ikeda, K; Oka, M; Yamada, Y; Soda, H; Fukuda, M; Kinoshita, A; Tsukamoto, K; Noguchi, Y; Isomoto, H; Takeshima, F; Murase, K; Kamihira, S; Tomonaga, M; Kohno, S. Adult T-cell leukemia cells over-express the multidrug-resistance-protein (MRP) and lung-resistance-protein (LRP) genes. *International Journal of Cancer* 1999;82:599-604.

[26] Hart, SM; Ganeshaguru, K; Hoffbrand, AV; Prentice, HG; Mehta, AB. Expression of the multidrug resistance-associated protein (MRP) in acute leukaemia. *Leukemia* 1994;8:2163-2168.

[27] Kohler, T; Leiblein, S; Borchert, S; Eller, J; Rost, AK; Lassner, D; Krahl, R; Helbig, W; Wagner, O; Remke, H. Absolute levels of MDR-1, MRP, and BCL-2 MRNA and tumor remission in acute leukemia. *Advances in Experimental Medicine and Biology* 1999;457:177-185.

[28] Pall, G; Spitaler, M; Hofmann, J; Thaler, J; Ludescher, C. Multidrug resistance in acute leukemia: a comparison of different diagnostic methods. *Leukemia* 1997;11:1067-1072.

[29] Burger, H; Nooter, K; Zaman, GJ; Sonneveld, P; van Wingerden, KE; Oostrum, RG; Stoter, G. Expression of the multidrug resistance-associated protein (MRP) in acute and chronic leukemias. *Leukemia* 1994;8:990-997.

[30] Gurbuxani, S; Zhou, D; Simonin, G; Raina, V; Arya, LS; Sazawal, S; Marie, JP; Bhargava, M. Expression of genes implicated in multidrug resistance in acute lymphoblastic leukemia in India. *Annals of Hematology* 1998;76:195-200.

[31] Zhang, JB; Sun, Y; Dong, J; Liu, LX; Ning, F. [Expression of lung resistance protein and multidrug resistance-associated protein in naive childhood acute leukemia and their clinical significance]. *Ai Zheng* 2005;24:1015-1017.

[32] Zhao, Y; Yu, L; Lou, F; Wang, Q; Pu, J; Zhou, Q. [The clinical significance of lung resistance-related protein gene (lrp), multidrug resistance-associated protein gene (mrp) and mdr-1/p170 expression in acute leukemia]. *Zhonghua Nei Ke Za Zhi* 1999;38:760-763.

[33] Ogretmen, B; Barredo, JC; Safa, AR. Increased expression of lung resistance-related protein and multidrug resistance-associated protein messenger RNA in childhood acute lymphoblastic leukemia. *Journal of Pediatric Hematology and Oncology* 2000;22:45-49.

[34] Gurbuxani, S; Singh Arya, L; Raina, V; Sazawal, S; Khattar, A; Magrath, I; Marie, J; Bhargava, M. Significance of MDR1, MRP1, GSTpi and GSTmu mRNA expression in acute lymphoblastic leukemia in Indian patients. *Cancer Letters* 2001;167:73-83.

[35] Beck, J; Handgretinger, R; Dopfer, R; Klingebiel, T; Niethammer, D; Gekeler, V. Expression of mdr1, mrp, topoisomerase II alpha/beta, and cyclin A in primary or relapsed states of acute lymphoblastic leukaemias. *British Journal of Haematology* 1995;89:356-363.

[36] Zhao, Y; Yu, L; Wang, Q; Lou, F; Pu, J. [The relationship between expression of lung resistance-related protein gene or multidrug resistance-associated protein gene and prognosis in newly diagnosed acute leukemia]. *Zhonghua Nei Ke Za Zhi* 2002;41:183-185.

[37] Kakihara, T; Tanaka, A; Watanabe, A; Yamamoto, K; Kanto, K; Kataoka, S; Ogawa, A; Asami, K; Uchiyama, M. Expression of multidrug resistance-related genes does not contribute to risk factors in newly diagnosed childhood acute lymphoblastic leukemia. *Pediatric International* 1999;41:641-647.

[38] Sauerbrey, A; Voigt, A; Wittig, S; Hafer, R; Zintl, F. Messenger RNA analysis of the multidrug resistance related protein (MRP1) and the lung resistance protein (LRP) in de novo and relapsed childhood acute lymphoblastic leukemia. *Leuk Lymphoma* 2002;43:875-879.

[39] Den Boer, ML; Pieters, R; Kazemier, KM; Janka-Schaub, GE; Henze, G; Creutzig, U; Kaspers, GJ; Kearns, PR; Hall, AG; Pearson, AD; Veerman, AJ. Different expression of glutathione S-transferase alpha, mu and pi in childhood acute lymphoblastic and myeloid leukaemia. *British Journal of Haematology* 1999;104:321-327.

[40] Den Boer, ML; Pieters, R; Kazemier, KM; Rottier, MM; Zwaan, CM; Kaspers, GJ; Janka-Schaub, G; Henze, G; Creutzig, U; Scheper, RJ; Veerman, AJ. Relationship between major vault protein/lung resistance protein, multidrug resistance-associated protein, P-glycoprotein expression, and drug resistance in childhood leukemia. *Blood* 1998;91:2092-2098.

[41] Holleman, A; Cheok, MH; den Boer, ML; Yang, W; Veerman, AJ; Kazemier, KM; Pei, D; Cheng, C; Pui, CH; Relling, MV; Janka-Schaub, GE; Pieters, R; Evans, WE. Gene-expression patterns in drug-resistant acute lymphoblastic leukemia cells and response to treatment. *The New England Journal of Medicine* 2004;351:533-542.

[42] Olson, DP; Taylor, BJ; La, M; Sather, H; Reaman, GH; Ivy, SP. The prognostic significance of P-glycoprotein, multidrug resistance-related protein 1 and lung resistance protein in pediatric acute lymphoblastic leukemia: a retrospective study of 295 newly diagnosed patients by the Children's Oncology Group. *Leukemia and Lymphoma* 2005;46:681-691.

[43] Damiani, D; Michelutti, A; Michieli, M; Masolini, P; Stocchi, R; Geromin, A; Ermacora, A; Russo, D; Fanin, R; Baccarani, M. P-glycoprotein, lung resistance-related protein and multidrug resistance-associated protein in de novo adult acute lymphoblastic leukaemia. *British Journal of Haematology* 2002;116:519-527.

[44] Ramakers-van Woerden, NL; Pieters, R; Hoelzer, D; Slater, RM; den Boer, ML; Loonen, AH; Harbott, J; Janka-Schaub, GE; Ludwig, WD; Ossenkoppele, GJ; van Wering, ER; Veerman, AJ. In vitro drug resistance profile of Philadelphia positive acute lymphoblastic leukemia is heterogeneous and related to age: a report of the Dutch

and German Leukemia Study Groups. *Medical and Pediatric Oncology* 2002;38:379-386.

[45]   Den Boer, ML; Pieters, R; Kazemier, KM; Janka-Schaub, GE; Henze, G; Veerman, AJ. Relationship between the intracellular daunorubicin concentration, expression of major vault protein/lung resistance protein and resistance to anthracyclines in childhood acute lymphoblastic leukemia. *Leukemia* 1999;13:2023-2030.

[46]   Valera, ET; Scrideli, CA; Queiroz, RG; Mori, BM; Tone, LG. Multiple drug resistance protein (MDR-1), multidrug resistance-related protein (MRP) and lung resistance protein (LRP) gene expression in childhood acute lymphoblastic leukemia. *Sao Paulo Medical Journal* 2004;122:166-171.

[47]   Calado, RT; Garcia, AB; Falcao, RP. Decreased activity of the multidrug resistance P-glycoprotein in acquired aplastic anaemia: possible pathophysiologic implications. *British Journal of Haematology* 1998;102:1157-1161.

[48]   Benderra, Z; Faussat, AM; Sayada, L; Perrot, JY; Tang, R; Chaoui, D; Morjani, H; Marzac, C; Marie, JP; Legrand, O. MRP3, BCRP, and P-glycoprotein activities are prognostic factors in adult acute myeloid leukemia. *Clinical Cancer Research* 2005;11:7764-7772.

[49]   Michieli, M; Damiani, D; Ermacora, A; Masolini, P; Raspadori, D; Visani, G; Scheper, RJ; Baccarani, M. P-glycoprotein, lung resistance-related protein and multidrug resistance associated protein in de novo acute non-lymphocytic leukaemias: biological and clinical implications. *British Journal of Haematology* 1999;104:328-335.

[50]   Laupeze, B; Amiot, L; Drenou, B; Bernard, M; Branger, B; Grosset, JM; Lamy, T; Fauchet, R; Fardel, O. High multidrug resistance protein activity in acute myeloid leukaemias is associated with poor response to chemotherapy and reduced patient survival. British Journal of Haematology 2002;116:834-838.

[51]   Van den Heuvel-Eibrink, MM; Wiemer, EA; Prins, A; Meijerink, JP; Vossebeld, PJ; van der Holt, B; Pieters, R; Sonneveld, P. Increased expression of the breast cancer resistance protein (BCRP) in relapsed or refractory acute myeloid leukemia (AML). Leukemia 2002;16:833-839.

[52]   Van der Pol, MA; Broxterman, HJ; Pater, JM; Feller, N; van der Maas, M; Weijers, GW; Scheffer, GL; Allen, JD; Scheper, RJ; van Loevezijn, A; Ossenkoppele, GJ; Schuurhuis, GJ. Function of the ABC transporters, P-glycoprotein, multidrug resistance protein and breast cancer resistance protein, in minimal residual disease in acute myeloid leukemia. *Haematologica* 2003;88:134-147.

[53]   Hart, SM; Ganeshaguru, K; Scheper, RJ; Prentice, HG; Hoffbrand, AV; Mehta, AB. Expression of the human major vault protein LRP in acute myeloid leukemia. *Experimental Hematology* 1997;25:1227-1232.

[54]   Van der Kolk, DM; de Vries, EG; Noordhoek, L; van den Berg, E; van der Pol, MA; Muller, M; Vellenga, E. Activity and expression of the multidrug resistance proteins P-glycoprotein, MRP1, MRP2, MRP3 and MRP5 in de novo and relapsed acute myeloid leukemia. *Leukemia* 2001;15:1544-1553.

[55]   Damiani, D; Michieli, M; Michelutti, A; Candoni, A; Stocchi, R; Masolini, P; Geromin, A; Michelutti, T; Raspadori, D; Ippoliti, M; Lauria, F; Fanin, R. Antibody binding capacity for evaluation of MDR-related proteins in acute promyelocytic leukemia: Onset versus relapse expression. Cytometry B. *Clinical Cytometry* 2004;59:40-45.

[56] Van der Kolk, DM; de Vries, EG; van Putten, WJ; Verdonck, LF; Ossenkoppele, GJ; Verhoef, GE; Vellenga, E. P-glycoprotein and multidrug resistance protein activities in relation to treatment outcome in acute myeloid leukemia. *Clinical Cancer Research* 2000;6:3205-3214.

[57] Borg, AG; Burgess, R; Green, LM; Scheper, RJ; Yin, JA. Overexpression of lung-resistance protein and increased P-glycoprotein function in acute myeloid leukaemia cells predict a poor response to chemotherapy and reduced patient survival. *British Journal of Haematology* 1998;103:1083-1091.

[58] Michieli, M; Damiani, D; Ermacora, A; Geromin, A; Michelutti, A; Masolini, P; Baccarani, M. P-glycoprotein (PGP), lung resistance-related protein (LRP) and multidrug resistance-associated protein (MRP) expression in acute promyelocytic leukaemia. *British Journal of Haematology* 2000;108:703-709.

[59] Beck, J; Niethammer, D; Gekeler, V. MDR1, MRP, topoisomerase IIalpha/beta, and cyclin A gene expression in acute and chronic leukemias. *Leukemia* 1996;10 Suppl 3:S39-S45.

[60] Han, K; Kahng, J; Kim, M; Lim, J; Kim, Y; Cho, B; Kim, HK; Min, WS; Kim, CC; Lee, KY; Kim, BK; Kang, CS. Expression of functional markers in acute nonlymphoblastic leukemia. *Acta Haematologica* 2000;104:174-180.

[61] Sargent, JM; Williamson, C; Hall, AG; Elgie, AW; Taylor, CG. Evidence for the involvement of the glutathione pathway in drug resistance in AML. *Advances in Experimental Medicine and Biology* 1999;457:205-209.

[62] Galimberti, S; Testi, R; Guerrini, F; Fazzi, R; Petrini, M. The clinical relevance of the expression of several multidrug-resistant-related genes in patients with primary acute myeloid leukemia. *Journal of Chemotherapy* 2003;15:374-379.

[63] Walter, RB; Raden, BW; Hong, TC; Flowers, DA; Bernstein, ID; Linenberger, ML. Multidrug resistance protein attenuates gemtuzumab ozogamicin-induced cytotoxicity in acute myeloid leukemia cells. *Blood* 2003;102:1466-1473.

[64] Filipits, M; Stranzl, T; Pohl, G; Suchomel, RW; Zochbauer, S; Brunner, R; Lechner, K; Pirker, R. MRP expression in acute myeloid leukemia. An update. *Advances in Experimental Medicine and Biology* 1999;457:141-150.

[65] Kuss, BJ; Deeley, RG; Cole, SP; Willman, CL; Kopecky, KJ; Wolman, SR; Eyre, HJ; Callen, DF. The biological significance of the multidrug resistance gene MRP in inversion 16 leukemias. *Leukemia and Lymphoma* 1996;20:357-364.

[66] Kuss, BJ; Deeley, RG; Cole, SP; Willman, CL; Kopecky, KJ; Wolman, SR; Eyre, HJ; Lane, SA; Nancarrow, JK; Whitmore, SA. Deletion of gene for multidrug resistance in acute myeloid leukaemia with inversion in chromosome 16: prognostic implications. *Lancet* 1994;343:1531-1534.

[67] Suarez, L; Vidriales, MB; Moreno, MJ; Lopez, A; Garcia-Larana, J; Perez-Lopez, C; Tormo, M; Lavilla, E; Lopez-Berges, MC; de Santiago, M; San Miguel, JF; Orfao, A. Differences in anti-apoptotic and multidrug resistance phenotypes in elderly and young acute myeloid leukemia patients are related to the maturation of blast cells. *Haematologica* 2005;90:54-59.

[68] Suarez, L; Vidriales, B; Garcia-Larana, J; Lopez, A; Martinez, R; Martin-Reina, V; Tormo, M; Gonzalez-San Miguel, JD; Lavilla, E; Garcia-Boyero, R; Orfao, A; San Miguel, JF. Multiparametric analysis of apoptotic and multi-drug resistance phenotypes

according to the blast cell maturation stage in elderly patients with acute myeloid leukemia. *Haematologica* 2001;86:1287-1295.

[69]   Suarez, L; Vidriales, MB; Garcia-Larana, J; Sanz, G; Moreno, MJ; Lopez, A; Barrena, S; Martinez, R; Tormo, M; Palomera, L; Lavilla, E; Lopez-Berges, MC; de Santiago, M; de Equiza, ME; Miguel, JF; Orfao, A. CD34+ cells from acute myeloid leukemia, myelodysplastic syndromes, and normal bone marrow display different apoptosis and drug resistance-associated phenotypes. *Clinical Cancer Research* 2004;10:7599-7606.

[70]   Poulain, S; Lepelley, P; Preudhomme, C; Cambier, N; Cornillon, J; Wattel, E; Cosson, A; Fenaux, P. Expression of the multidrug resistance-associated protein in myelodysplastic syndromes. *British Journal of Haematology* 2000;110:591-598.

[71]   Juszczynski, P; Niewiarowski, W; Krykowski, E; Robak, T; Warzocha, K. Expression of the multidrug resistance-associated protein (mrp) gene in chronic lymphocytic leukemia. *Leukemia and Lymphoma* 2002;43:153-158.

[72]   Consoli, U; Santonocito, A; Stagno, F; Fiumara, P; Privitera, A; Parisi, G; Giustolisi, GM; Pavone, B; Palumbo, GA; Di Raimondo, F; Milone, G; Guglielmo, P; Giustolisi, R. Multidrug resistance mechanisms in chronic lymphocytic leukaemia. *British Journal of Haematology* 2002;116:774-780.

[73]   Yang, X; Jia, L; Wei, L; Zuo, W; Song, S. [Correlation of expression levels of multidrug resistance gene 1 (mdr1) mRNA, multidrug resistance-associated protein (MRP), amd P-glycoprotein (P-gp) with chemotherapy efficacy in malignant lymphomas]. *Zhonghua Yi Xue Za Zhi* 2002;82:1177-1179.

[74]   Ramachandran, C; Khatib, Z; Escalon, E; Fonseca, HB; Jhabvala, P; Medina, LS; D'Souza, B; Ragheb, J; Morrison, G; Melnick, SJ. Molecular studies in pediatric medulloblastomas. *Brain Tumor Pathol* 2002;19:15-22.

[75]   Vassal, G; Merlin, JL; Terrier-Lacombe, MJ; Grill, J; Parker, F; Sainte-Rose, C; Aubert, G; Morizet, J; Sevenet, N; Poullain, MG; Lucas, C; Kalifa, C. In vivo antitumor activity of S16020, a topoisomerase II inhibitor, and doxorubicin against human brain tumor xenografts. *Cancer Chemotherapy and Pharmacology* 2003;51:385-394.

[76]   Abe, T; Mori, T; Wakabayashi, Y; Nakagawa, M; Cole, SP; Koike, K; Kuwano, M; Hori, S. Expression of multidrug resistance protein gene in patients with glioma after chemotherapy. *Journal of Neurooncology* 1998;40:11-18.

[77]   Vogelgesang, S; Kunert-Keil, C; Cascorbi, I; Mosyagin, I; Schroder, E; Runge, U; Jedlitschky, G; Kroemer, HK; Oertel, J; Gaab, MR; Pahnke, J; Walker, LC; Warzok, RW. Expression of multidrug transporters in dysembryoplastic neuroepithelial tumors causing intractable epilepsy. *Clinical Neuropathology* 2004;23:223-231.

[78]   Tu, C; Tian, Y; Pei, F. [Expression of multidrug resistance-associated protein 1 in osteosarcoma and its relationship with clinicopathologic characteristics]. *Sichuan Da Xue Xue Bao Yi Xue Ban* 2003;34:684-687.

[79]   Burak, Z; Moretti, JL; Ersoy, O; Sanli, U; Kantar, M; Tamgac, F; Basdemir, G. 99mTc-MIBI imaging as a predictor of therapy response in osteosarcoma compared with multidrug resistance-associated protein and P-glycoprotein expression. *Journal of Nuclear Medicine* 2003;44:1394-1401.

[80]   Oda, Y; Dockhorn-Dworniczak, B; Jurgens, H; Roessner, A. Expression of multidrug resistance-associated protein gene in Ewing's sarcoma and malignant peripheral neuroectodermal tumor of bone. *Journal of Cancer Research and Clinical Oncology* 1997;123:237-239.

[81] Komdeur, R; Plaat, BE; van der Graaf, WT; Hoekstra, HJ; Hollema, H; van den Berg, E; Zwart, N; Scheper, RJ; Molenaar, WM. Expression of multidrug resistance proteins, P-gp, MRP1 and LRP, in soft tissue sarcomas analysed according to their histological type and grade. *European Journal of Cancer* 2003;39:909-916.

[82] Stein, U; Jurchott, K; Schlafke, M; Hohenberger, P. Expression of multidrug resistance genes MVP, MDR1, and MRP1 determined sequentially before, during, and after hyperthermic isolated limb perfusion of soft tissue sarcoma and melanoma patients. *Journal of Clinical Oncology* 2002;20:3282-3292.

[83] Oda, Y; Ohishi, Y; Saito, T; Hinoshita, E; Uchiumi, T; Kinukawa, N; Iwamoto, Y; Kohno, K; Kuwano, M; Tsuneyoshi, M. Nuclear expression of Y-box-binding protein-1 correlates with P-glycoprotein and topoisomerase II alpha expression, and with poor prognosis in synovial sarcoma. *Journal of Pathology* 2003;199:251-258.

[84] Oda, Y; Saito, T; Tateishi, N; Ohishi, Y; Tamiya, S; Yamamoto, H; Yokoyama, R; Uchiumi, T; Iwamoto, Y; Kuwano, M; Tsuneyoshi, M. ATP-binding cassette superfamily transporter gene expression in human soft tissue sarcomas. *International Journal of Cancer* 2005;114:854-862.

[85] Oda, Y; Schneider-Stock, R; Rys, J; Gruchala, A; Niezabitowski, A; Roessner, A. Expression of multidrug-resistance-associated protein gene in human soft-tissue sarcomas. *Journal of Cancer Research and Clinical Oncology* 1996;122:161-165.

[86] Plaat, BE; Hollema, H; Molenaar, WM; Torn Broers, GH; Pijpe, J; Mastik, MF; Hoekstra, HJ; van den Berg, E; Scheper, RJ; van der Graaf, WT. Soft tissue leiomyosarcomas and malignant gastrointestinal stromal tumors: differences in clinical outcome and expression of multidrug resistance proteins. *Journal of Clinical Oncology* 2000;18:3211-3220.

[87] Gaumann, A; Tews, DS; Mentzel, T; Petrow, PK; Mayer, E; Otto, M; Kirkpatrick, CJ; Kriegsmann, J. Expression of drug resistance related proteins in sarcomas of the pulmonary artery and poorly differentiated leiomyosarcomas of other origin. *Virchows Archives* 2003;442:529-537.

[88] Komdeur, R; Klunder, J; van der Graaf, WT; van den Berg, E; de Bont, ES; Hoekstra, HJ; Molenaar, WM. Multidrug resistance proteins in rhabdomyosarcomas: comparison between children and adults. *Cancer* 2003;97:1999-2005.

[89] Gallego, S; Llort, A; Parareda, A; Sanchez De Toledo, J. Expression of multidrug resistance-1 and multidrug resistance-associated protein genes in pediatric rhabdomyosarcoma. *Oncology Reports* 2004;11:179-183.

[90] Cocker, HA; Tiffin, N; Pritchard-Jones, K; Pinkerton, CR; Kelland, LR. In vitro prevention of the emergence of multidrug resistance in a pediatric rhabdomyosarcoma cell line. *Clinical Cancer Research* 2001;7:3193-3198.

[91] Klunder, JW; Komdeur, R; Van Der Graaf, WT; De Bont, EJ; Hoekstra, HJ; Van Den Berg, E; Molenaar, WM. Expression of multidrug resistance-associated proteins in rhabdomyosarcomas before and after chemotherapy: the relationship between lung resistance-related protein (LRP) and differentiation. *Human Pathology* 2003;34:150-155.

[92] Norris, MD; Bordow, SB; Haber, PS; Marshall, GM; Kavallaris, M; Madafiglio, J; Cohn, SL; Salwen, H; Schmidt, ML; Hipfner, DR; Cole, SP; Deeley, RG; Haber, M. Evidence that the MYCN oncogene regulates MRP gene expression in neuroblastoma. *European Journal of Cancer* 1997;33:1911-1916.

[93] Vasudevan, SA; Nuchtern, JG. Gene profiling of high risk neuroblastoma. *World Journal of Surgery* 2005;29:317-324.

[94] Lu, QJ; Dong, F; Zhang, JH; Li, XH; Ma, Y; Jiang, WG. Expression of multidrug resistance-related markers in primary neuroblastoma. *Chineese Medical Journal* 2004;117:1358-1363.

[95] Haber, M; Bordow, SB; Haber, PS; Marshall, GM; Stewart, BW; Norris, MD. The prognostic value of MDR1 gene expression in primary untreated neuroblastoma. *European Journal of Cancer* 1997;33:2031-2036.

[96] Matsunaga, T; Shirasawa, H; Hishiki, T; Enomoto, H; Kouchi, K; Ohtsuka, Y; Iwai, J; Yoshida, H; Tanabe, M; Kobayashi, S; Asano, T; Etoh, T; Nishi, Y; Ohnuma, N. Expression of MRP and cMOAT in childhood neuroblastomas and malignant liver tumors and its relevance to clinical behavior. *Japanese Journal of Cancer Research* 1998;89:1276-1283.

[97] Goldstein, M; Rennert, H; Bar-Shira, A; Burstein, Y; Yaron, Y; Orr-Urtreger, A. Combined cytogenetic and array-based comparative genomic hybridization analyses of Wilms tumors: amplification and overexpression of the multidrug resistance associated protein 1 gene (MRP1) in a metachronous tumor. *Cancer Genetics and Cytogenetics* 2003;141:120-127.

[98] Beck, J; Bohnet, B; Brugger, D; Bader, P; Dietl, J; Scheper, RJ; Kandolf, R; Liu, C; Niethammer, D; Gekeler, V. Multiple gene expression analysis reveals distinct differences between G2 and G3 stage breast cancers, and correlations of PKC eta with MDR1, MRP and LRP gene expression. *British Journal of Cancer* 1998;77:87-91.

[99] Schaich, M; Soucek, S; Thiede, C; Ehninger, G; Illmer, T. MDR1 and MRP1 gene expression are independent predictors for treatment outcome in adult acute myeloid leukaemia. *British Journal of Haematology* 2005;128:324-332.

[100] Kasimir-Bauer, S; Beelen, D; Flasshove, M; Noppeney, R; Seeber, S; Scheulen, ME. Impact of the expression of P glycoprotein, the multidrug resistance-related protein, bcl-2, mutant p53, and heat shock protein 27 on response to induction therapy and long-term survival in patients with de novo acute myeloid leukemia. *Experimental Hematology* 2002;30:1302-1308.

[101] Kasimir-Bauer, S; Ottinger, H; Meusers, P; Beelen, DW; Brittinger, G; Seeber, S; Scheulen, ME. In acute myeloid leukemia, coexpression of at least two proteins, including P-glycoprotein, the multidrug resistance-related protein, bcl-2, mutant p53, and heat-shock protein 27, is predictive of the response to induction chemotherapy. *Experimental Hematology* 1998;26:1111-1117.

[102] Shanghai Cooperative Leukemia Group. [Expressions of P-gp, mdr1, MRP and Topo II in acute leukemia patients and their correlation with prognosis]. *Zhonghua Xue Ye Xue Za Zhi* 2001;22:90-93.

[103] Oh, EJ; Kahng, J; Kim, Y; Kim, M; Lim, J; Kang, CS; Min, WS; Cho, B; Lee, A; Lee, KY; Kim, WI; Shim, SI; Han, K. Expression of functional markers in acute lymphoblastic leukemia. *Leukemia Research* 2003;27:903-908.

[104] Tafuri, A; Gregorj, C; Petrucci, MT; Ricciardi, MR; Mancini, M; Cimino, G; Mecucci, C; Tedeschi, A; Fioritoni, G; Ferrara, F; Di Raimondo, F; Gallo, E; Liso, V; Fabbiano, F; Cascavilla, N; Pizzolo, G; Camera, A; Pane, F; Lanza, F; Cilloni, D; Annino, L; Vitale, A; Vegna, ML; Vignetti, M; Foa, R; Mandelli, F. MDR1 protein expression is

an independent predictor of complete remission in newly diagnosed adult acute lymphoblastic leukemia. *Blood* 2002;100:974-981.

[105] Ohishi, Y; Oda, Y; Uchiumi, T; Kobayashi, H; Hirakawa, T; Miyamoto, S; Kinukawa, N; Nakano, H; Kuwano, M; Tsuneyoshi, M. ATP-binding cassette superfamily transporter gene expression in human primary ovarian carcinoma. *Clinical Cancer Research* 2002;8:3767-3775.

[106] Yokoyama, Y; Sato, S; Fukushi, Y; Sakamoto, T; Futagami, M; Saito, Y. Significance of multi-drug-resistant proteins in predicting chemotherapy response and prognosis in epithelial ovarian cancer. *Journal of Obstetrics and Gynaecology Research* 1999;25:387-394.

[107] Yakirevich, E; Sabo, E; Naroditsky, I; Sova, Y; Lavie, O; Resnick, MB. Multidrug resistance-related phenotype and apoptosis-related protein expression in ovarian serous carcinomas. *Gynecological Oncology 2006*;100:152-159.

[108] Eltabbakh, GH; Mount, SL; Beatty, B; Simmons-Arnold, L; Cooper, K; Morgan, A. Factors associated with cytoreducibility among women with ovarian carcinoma. *Gynecological Oncology* 2004;95:377-383.

[109] Itamochi, H; Kigawa, J; Sugiyama, T; Kikuchi, Y; Suzuki, M; Terakawa, N. Low proliferation activity may be associated with chemoresistance in clear cell carcinoma of the ovary. *Obstetrics and Gynecology* 2002;100:281-287.

[110] Katsaros, D; Fracchioli, S; Arts, HJ; de Vries, EG; Danese, S; Richiardi, G; Arisio, R; Gordini, G; Van der Zee, AG; Suurmeijer, AJ; Massobrio, M. [Expression and prognostic value of the drug resistance markers P-gp, Mrp1, Mrp2, and Lrp in ovarian carcinoma]. *Minerva Ginecologica* 1999;51:463-470.

[111] Brinkhuis, M; Izquierdo, MA; Baak, JP; van Diest, PJ; Kenemans, P; Scheffer, GL; Scheper, RJ. Expression of multidrug resistance-associated markers, their relation to quantitative pathologic tumour characteristics and prognosis in advanced ovarian cancer. *Analytical Cellular Pathology* 2002;24:17-23.

[112] Arts, HJ; Katsaros, D; de Vries, EG; Massobrio, M; Genta, F; Danese, S; Arisio, R; Scheper, RJ; Kool, M; Scheffer, GL; Willemse, PH; van der Zee, AG; Suurmeijer, AJ. Drug resistance-associated markers P-glycoprotein, multidrug resistance-associated protein 1, multidrug resistance-associated protein 2, and lung resistance protein as prognostic factors in ovarian carcinoma. *Clinical Cancer Research* 1999;5:2798-2805.

[113] Izquierdo, MA; van der Zee, AG; Vermorken, JB; van der Valk, P; Belien, JA; Giaccone, G; Scheffer, GL; Flens, MJ; Pinedo, HM; Kenemans, P. Drug resistance-associated marker Lrp for prediction of response to chemotherapy and prognoses in advanced ovarian carcinoma. *Journal of National Cancer Institute* 1995;87:1230-1237.

[114] Larkin, A; O'Driscoll, L; Kennedy, S; Purcell, R; Moran, E; Crown, J; Parkinson, M; Clynes, M. Investigation of MRP-1 protein and MDR-1 P-glycoprotein expression in invasive breast cancer: a prognostic study. *International Journal of Cancer* 2004;112:286-294.

[115] Tada, Y; Wada, M; Migita, T; Nagayama, J; Hinoshita, E; Mochida, Y; Maehara, Y; Tsuneyoshi, M; Kuwano, M; Naito, S. Increased expression of multidrug resistance-associated proteins in bladder cancer during clinical course and drug resistance to doxorubicin. *International Journal of Cancer* 2002;98:630-635.

[116] Moureau-Zabotto, L; Ricci, S; Lefranc, JP; Coulet, F; Genestie, C; Antoine, M; Uzan, S; Lotz, JP; Touboul, E; Lacave, R. Prognostic impact of multidrug resistance gene

expression on the management of breast cancer in the context of adjuvant therapy based on a series of 171 patients. *British Journal of Cancer* 2006, Jan 24 [Epub ahead of print]

[117] Su, JS; Arima, K; Hasegawa, M; Franco, OE; Yanagawa, M; Sugimura, Y; Kawamura, J. Proliferative status is a risk index for recurrence in primary superficial (pTa/T1) low-grade urothelial bladder carcinoma. *Hinyokika Kiyo* 2003;49:649-658.

[118] Yoh, K; Ishii, G; Yokose, T; Minegishi, Y; Tsuta, K; Goto, K; Nishiwaki, Y; Kodama, T; Suga, M; Ochiai, A. Breast cancer resistance protein impacts clinical outcome in platinum-based chemotherapy for advanced non-small cell lung cancer. Clinical Cancer Research 2004;10:1691-1697.

[119] Satherley, K; de Souza, L; Neale, MH; Alexander, RA; Myatt, N; Foss, AJ; Hungerford, JL; Hickson, ID; Cree, IA. Relationship between expression of topoisomerase II isoforms and chemosensitivity in choroidal melanoma. *Journal of Pathology* 2000;192:174-181.

[120] Nooter, K; Kok, T; Bosman, FT; van Wingerden, KE; Stoter, G. Expression of the multidrug resistance protein (MRP) in squamous cell carcinoma of the oesophagus and response to pre-operative chemotherapy. *European Journal of Cancer* 1998;34:81-86.

[121] Tsuzuki, H; Sunaga, H; Ito, T; Narita, N; Sugimoto, C; Fujieda, S. Reliability of platelet-derived endothelial cell growth factor as a prognostic factor for oral and oropharyngeal carcinomas. Archives of Otolaryngology *Head and Neck Surgery* 2005;131:1071-1078.

[122] Duffy, CP; Elliott, CJ; O'Connor, RA; Heenan, MM; Coyle, S; Cleary, IM; Kavanagh, K; Verhaegen, S; O'Loughlin, CM; NicAmhlaoibh, R; Clynes, M. Enhancement of chemotherapeutic drug toxicity to human tumour cells in vitro by a subset of non-steroidal anti-inflammatory drugs (NSAIDs). *European Journal of Cancer* 1998;34:1250-1259.

[123] Tang, R; Faussat, AM; Majdak, P; Perrot, JY; Chaoui, D; Legrand, O; Marie, JP. Valproic acid inhibits proliferation and induces apoptosis in acute myeloid leukemia cells expressing P-gp and MRP1. *Leukemia* 2004;18:1246-1251.

[124] Lehne, G; Morkrid, L; den Boer, M; Rugstad, HE. Diverse effects of P-glycoprotein inhibitory agents on human leukemia cells expressing the multidrug resistance protein (MRP). *International Journal of Clinical Pharmacology and Therapeutics* 2000;38:187-195.

[125] Walter, RB; Pirga, JL; Cronk, MR; Mayer, S; Appelbaum, FR; Banker, DE. PK11195, a peripheral benzodiazepine receptor (pBR) ligand, broadly blocks drug efflux to chemosensitize leukemia and myeloma cells by a pBR-independent, direct transporter-modulating mechanism. *Blood* 2005;106:3584-3593.

[126] Qian, XP; Liu, BR; Yin, HT; Wang, LF; Zou, ZY; Du, J. [Effect of arsenic trioxide on drug transporting molecules in acute promyelocytic leukemia cell line]. *Zhonghua Zhong Liu Za Zhi* 2004;26:601-605.

[127] Aszalos, A; Thompson, K; Yin, JJ; Ross, DD. Combinations of P-glycoprotein blockers, verapamil, PSC833, and cremophor act differently on the multidrug resistance associated protein (MRP) and on P-glycoprotein (Pgp). *Anticancer Research* 1999;19:1053-1064.

[128] Qadir, M; O'Loughlin, KL; Fricke, SM; Williamson, NA; Greco, WR; Minderman, H;, Baer, MR. Cyclosporin A is a broad-spectrum multidrug resistance modulator. *Clinical Cancer Research* 2005;11:2320-2326.

[129] Orlicky, J; Sulova, Z; Dovinova, I; Fiala, R; Zahradnikova, A; Breier, A. Functional fluo-3/AM assay on P-glycoprotein transport activity in L1210/VCR cells by confocal microscopy. *General Physiology and Biophysysics* 2004;23:357-366.

In: Multidrug Resistance-Associated Proteins
Editor: Christopher V. Aiello, pp. 119-136
ISBN 1-60021-298-0

Chapter 5

THE ROLE OF MULTIDRUG RESISTANCE-ASSOCIATED PROTEINS IN NEURODEGENERATIVE DISEASES

Silke Vogelgesang[1,], Lary C. Walker[2],*
Heyo K. Kroemer[3] and Rolf W. Warzok[1]

[1]Department of Neuropathology, [3]Department of Pharmacology,
University of Greifswald, Germany
[2]Yerkes National Primate Research Center and Department of Neurology,
Emory University, Atlanta, GA, USA

ABSTRACT

The blood-brain barrier (BBB) efficiently protects the brain against xenobiotics and plays an important part in the development of drug resistance in a wide range of neurological disorders such as brain cancer, epilepsy and infectious diseases. In this regard, the function of the members of the ABC transporter family, such as P-glycoprotein (P-gp) and multidrug resistance-associated proteins (MRP), in the integrity of the BBB recently has been the subject of intensive research. In particular, the importance of brain-to-blood transport across the BBB has garnered increasing attention as a potential mechanism in the pathogenesis of neurodegenerative disorders. According to the concept of "proteopathies", many neurodegenerative disorders such as Alzheimer's disease (AD), Creutzfeldt-Jakob-Disease (CJD), Parkinson's Disease (PD) and Huntington's Disease (HD) are the result of the aberrant polymerization and accumulation of misfolded proteins within the brain. In addition to their role in protecting the brain from exogenous toxins, there is now evidence that cellular transport proteins help to regulate the levels of some pathogenic proteins in the brain. In this review, we discuss the

* *Corresponding author:* Silke Vogelgesang, M.D. Department of Neuropathology, University of Greifswald, F.-Loeffler-Str. 23 e, D-17487 Greifswald, Germany, Email: sivogelg@uni-greifswald.de; Phone: +49-3834-865716 ; Fax: +49-3834-865704

possible role of drug efflux transporters, especially P-gp, in neurodegeneration, and consider how a fuller understanding of this process might promote the development of more efficacious treatment strategies.

INTRODUCTION

The ATP-binding cassette (ABC) superfamily of transporters mediate the transcellular trafficking of diverse endogenous and exogenous substances [Ambudkar et al. 2005]. Members of this superfamily include P-glycoprotein (P-gp; ABCB1) and multidrug resistance-associated proteins (MRPs), which act as efflux pumps at the blood-brain-barrier (BBB), thus playing an important role in the protection of the brain from potentially toxic xenobiotics [Schinkel 1997, Fromm 2000, Schinkel and Jonker 2003]. In cancer cells, overexpression of these transport proteins leads to drug resistance, a clinically problematic phenomenon that has been intensively investigated now for several decades [Juliano and Ling 1976, Bart et al. 2000, Leonard et al. 2003]. In recent years, a possible role of multidrug resistance proteins, especially P-gp (the protein product of the MDR1 gene), in the pathogenesis of neurodegenerative diseases has come to light. Whereas the drug-eliminating effects of ABC transporters in tumors are undesirable, the normal biological activity of the transporters could act to maintain organ homeostasis, and thereby mitigate the effects of aging and the probability of neurodegenerative disease.

Virtually all age-related neurodegenerative disorders are associated with the buildup of misfolded, aberrant proteins [Walker and Levine 2000]. A hallmark of these cerebral proteopathies is the transformation of normally soluble peptides or proteins into β-sheet-rich oligomers and insoluble fibrils that accumulate in the brain tissue. The pathogenic similarities among these disparate maladies suggest the possibility of congruent therapeutic strategies, including (1) lessening the production of the aggregation-prone proteins, (2) preventing their self-assembly and toxicity, or (3) promoting their degradation and removal [Walker and Levine 2002, Aguzzi and Haass 2003]. Below, we review the possible role of multidrug transporters in the pathogenesis of neurodegenerative diseases, and the implications of this involvement for developing disease-modifying therapies for these incurable disorders.

P-GP AND ALZHEIMER'S DISEASE

Alzheimer's disease (AD) is an age-associated neurodegenerative disorder that is characterized morphologically by the accumulation of the β-amyloid peptide (Aβ) as intraparenchymal Aβ plaques and cerebrovascular β-amyloid angiopathy (CAA) [Hardy and Selkoe 2002], as well as the formation of neurofibrillary tangles consisting of intracellular, hyperphosphorylated tau protein [Wood et al. 1986, Mandelkow and Mandelkow 1998]. Aβ is generated by the enzymatic cleavage of the amyloid precurser protein (APP) by β-secretase (β-amyloid cleaving enzyme, or BACE) and γ-secretase [Selkoe 1999, Li et al. 2006]. For unknown reasons, Aβ can assume a structure rich in β-sheet content that renders the peptide liable to self-aggregation. Although tauopathy is important for the behavioral manifestations of AD, genetic evidence strongly supports the concept that abnormalities of Aβ are upstream of tauopathy in the pathogenic cascade [Hardy and Selkoe 2002]. Hence, most therapeutic approaches to AD currently focus on reducing Aβ burden in the brain. It is hypothesized that Aβ accumulates because of an overproduction of the peptide, diminished enzymatic degradation, and/or impaired clearance from brain to blood or to cerebrospinal fluid (CSF) [Shibata et al. 2000, Walker and Levine 2000, Zlokovic and Frangione 2003, Tanzi et al. 2004]. Since the majority of AD cases are idiopathic in nature, and do not show constitutively increased Aβ production or elevated APP expression, it is conceivable that the underlying cause of Aβ accrual in these instances is the reduced degradation or clearance of Aβ from the brain [Shibata et al. 2000, Deane et al. 2003, Zlokovic and Frangione 2003, Deane et al. 2004, Tanzi et al. 2004]. It has been proposed also that CAA in AD develops slowly due to a progressive Aβ-clearance disorder, rather than to its uncontrolled production from APP [Zlokovic et al. 2005]. This *failure to purge* could be due, at least in part, to disturbed transcellular transport mechanisms that control the export of Aβ from the brain.

In 2001, Lam and collegues showed that P-gp, in the presence of ATP, can transport Aβ40 and Aβ42 across the plasma membranes of P-gp-enriched vesicles in cultured cells. Furthermore, using labeled vesicles enriched with hamster P-gp, the addition of synthetic human Aβ40 or Aβ42 revealed saturable quenching [Lam et al. 2001]. Since P-gp is highly expressed at the luminal surface of cerebrovascular endothelial cells and epithelial cells of the choroid plexus, it was hypothesized that P-gp could reduce intracerebral Aβ burden by promoting its removal into the blood or the CSF, respectively.

This hypothesis was supported by our immunohistochemical study of the relationship between P-gp expression and Aβ load in autopsied brains from 243 nondemented, elderly humans [Vogelgesang et al. 2002]. Since the objective of this analysis was to investigate the early stages of Aβ accumulation and to avoid ceiling effects associated with the pathologies of end-stage AD, cases with overt dementia were excluded from the analysis. The study revealed a significant inverse correlation between cerebrovascular P-gp expression and the deposition of Aβ, i.e., the risk of exhibiting Aβ plaques was significantly lower in cases with moderate or strong P-gp expression compared with individuals showing low P-gp expression. Homozygotes for apolipoprotein Eε4 (*apoEε4*), which is a well-recognised risk factor for the development of AD, manifested the highest Aβ plaque levels, as well as the lowest P-gp expression [Vogelgesang et al. 2002].

Regarding CAA, there was no colocalisation of endothelial P-gp and vascular Aβ, i.e. vessels with high P-gp expression showed no CAA, and vice versa. Aβ deposition appeared first in small- and medium-sized arterioles in which P-gp expression was low, and as the degree of CAA increased, P-gp-immunoreactivity disappeared completely. Interestingly, at early, mild stages of Aβ deposition, P-gp was *up*regulated in most capillaries, suggesting a compensatory attempt to enhance Aβ clearance from the brain. Capillaries were usually affected by Aβ only at more advanced stages of CAA, at which point P-gp was not detectable even in these vessels [Vogelgesang et al. 2004a].

Unexpectedly, analysis of all cases combined revealed no significant effect of age on P-gp expression. However, if the cases with CAA that showed an upregulation of capillary P-gp expression in the early stages of Aβ proteopathy were excluded from the analysis, there was a significant decrease of P-gp expression with age. This finding is supported by preliminary observations in four squirrel monkeys (*Saimiri* spp) one young (8 years) and three aged (22-23 years) animals. With increasing age, squirrel monkeys spontanously develop cerebral Aβ deposits, particularly CAA [Walker et al. 1990, Mackic et al. 2002]. In this small sample, the aged monkeys exhibited mild to moderate CAA and Aβ-plaques, but no P-gp immunoreactivity, whereas in the young animal, P-gp immunoreactivity was strongly evident in the absence of Aβ-lesions (Figure 1). This finding supports the view that P-gp declines with age, and indicates that the transporter may play an important role in Aβ clearance in nonhuman primate species as well.

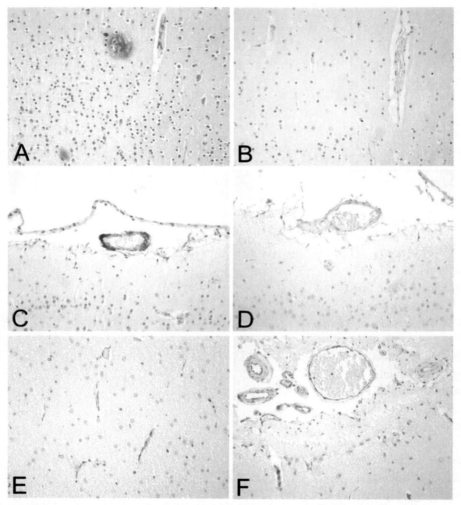

Figure 1: Brain tissue sections from squirrel monkeys (*Saimiri sciureus*) showing the inverse relationship between P-gp expression and Aβ deposition (Immunohistochemical demonstration of P-gp [JSB-1, Alexis, Gruenberg, Germany] and Aβ [DAKO, Hamburg, Germany]). Vascular P-gp expression is strong in the young animal and weak or absent in older animals with incipient Aβ accumulation. (Original magnification x 200).
A and B (case No. 85-55, 23 years old): A. Aβ plaques in neocortex; B. Adjacent histological section with absence of vascular P-gp expression.
C and D (case No. 86-3, 23 years old): C. Leptomeningeal vessel with strong CAA; D. Adjacent histological section with absence of P-gp staining.
E and F (case No. 86-6, 8 years old): Strong intraparenchymal (E) and leptomeningeal (F) endothelial P-gp expression in a young control (No Aβ deposits were seen in the young animal).

In a recent series of elegant experiments in genetically modified mice, Cirrito et al. (2005) provided further evidence for the involvement of P-gp in the accumulation of Aβ. Microinjection of radiolabeled Aβ40 or Aβ42 into the brains of P-gp-knockout mice revealed significantly higher Aβ retention within the brain than was seen in P-gp-competent, wild-type mice. Acute pharmacologic inhibition of P-gp activity in Tg2576 transgenic mice, which overexpress disease-mutant APP$_{Swe}$ and develop Aβ plaques and CAA with age, led to a significant increase of Aβ levels within the brain interstitial fluid. Furthermore, when Tg2576 mice were cross-bred with P-gpKO mice, brain Aβ load was significantly augmented compared with the P-gp-competent, Tg2576 littermates [Cirrito et al. 2005].

Taken together, the available data support the hypothesis that P-gp is involved in the clearance of Aβ from the brain via the BBB, and thus might modulate the pathogenic cascade of AD. The age-related decrease of cerebrovascular P-gp could be, at least in part, responsible for an imbalance between the production and clearance of Aβ that increases the levels of the peptide in brain tissue, and thereby promotes its multimerization into toxic oligomers and amyloid fibrils.

In addition to the brain-derived production of Aβ, it has been proposed that circulating Aβ arising from systemic organs could enter the brain, and that an increased influx of Aβ into the CNS across the BBB could lead to an accumulation of soluble and/or insoluble Aβ. There is support for this scenario from experimental studies showing that radiolabeled Aβ can enter the brain from the blood and bind to pre-existing amyloid deposits [Ghilardi et al. 1996, Mackic et al. 2002]. In this regard, under pathologic conditions, the receptor for advanced glycation end products (RAGE), a receptor of the immunglobulin superfamily, was shown to be involved in these processes [Deane et al. 2003]. P-gp, by acting to pump Aβ from the brain into blood, could also serve to protect the brain against peripherally circulating Aβ.

It is well-recognised that the activity of P-gp can be modulated pharmacologically by a range of frequently used drugs [Johne et al. 1999, Westphal et al. 2000, Izzo 2005, Rautio et al. 2006]. The selective up-regulation of cerebral P-gp therefore could be a new therapeutic strategy for reducing the buildup of Aβ. With regard to the drug-resistance of tumor cells, several inhibitors of P-gp have been investigated [Pan et al. 2005, Breedveld et al. 2006, Xu et al. 2006], but to date, little is known about the potential effects of P-gp modulators in AD. Recently, it was reported that three-month treatment with the antibiotic rifampin, one of the most recognised and potent inducers of P-gp, showed a positive influence on cognitive function in patients with mild-to-moderate dementia [Loeb et al. 2004]. The mechanism of this effect is unknown, but it is worth investigating the possibility that it is mediated by increased P-gp expression and enhanced Aβ export. If this can be demonstrated to be the case, the effects of such agents on blood levels of Aβ might be a convenient biomarker of efficacy. A potential advantage of the development of P-gp-inducers for AD is that the drugs may not need to cross the BBB because of the expression of P-gp on the luminal surface of the endothelial cells.

The 3-hydroxy-3-methylglutaryl-coenzyme A reductase inhibitors ("statins"), such as simvastatin and lovastatin, are known to reduce Aβ levels *in vitro* and *in vivo* [Fassbender et al. 2001]. There is evidence that the incidence of dementia is reduced in populations that were treated with statins to reduce blood lipid levels [Jick et al. 2000, Wolozin 2004], but there is still no definitive mechanistic explanation for this phenomenon. Since the statins are substrates for P-gp and can augment P-gp activity [Hooiveld et al. 1999, Bogman et al. 2001, Chen et al. 2005], it is conceivable that they might promote Aβ clearance. On the other hand, there are reports that some statins exhibit inhibitory effects on P-gp function [Wang et al. 2001]. The possible influence of statins on P-gp function and Aβ accumulation in the brain remains unclear, and further studies should shed more light on this issue. In this regard, it is important to note that P-gp itself appears to be involved in cholesterol metabolism [Santini et al. 2003, Troost 2004].

Finally, the expression of P-gp can be modulated by genetic polymorphisms of the MDR1 gene [Cascorbi et al. 2001]. More than 50 single nucleotide polymorphisms (SNPs) in the MDR1 gene have been detected to date [Loscher and Potschka 2005]. The strongest hints of an alteration in P-gp transport function were observed for the silent mutation in exon 26. In the intestine, the C-allele of this C3435T SNP was associated with increased P-gp levels [Hoffmeyer et al. 2000, Eichelbaum et al. 2004]. Other candidates are SNPs on exon 21 G2677T/A or exon 2G-1A, which were related to altered P-gp expression in human placenta [Tanabe et al. 2001, Eichelbaum et al. 2004]. To date, no significant relationship between these polymorphisms and Aβ burden or P-gp expression has been found in brain [Vogelgesang et al. 2002, Vogelgesang et al. 2004b]. However, it cannot be excluded that other polymorphisms in the MDR1 gene are associated with an increase or decrease of Aβ clearance, and thus might be related to an inherited increase in risk for the development of AD. Further genetic analysis of P-gp polymorphisms in relation to AD are needed to evaluate this hypothesis.

P-GP AND PARKINSONISM

Parkinson's disease is the second most common age-associated neurodegenerative disorder after AD. The characteristic neuropathological features of PD are a progressive loss of neurons in the substantia nigra with diminished dopaminergic innervation of the neostriatum, and the widespread occurrence of intraneuronal inclusions known as Lewy bodies [Jellinger and Mizuno 2003]. The resulting clinical presentation includes tremor, rigidity, postural instability and bradykinesia. Rare forms of genetically determined PD are the result of mutations in several genes, such as those for Parkin or α-synuclein [Kitada et al. 1998, Kruger et al. 1998, Mizuno et al. 2001]. In the more common idiopathic forms of PD, genetic and environmental factors (or both) may play a causative role [Payami et al. 2002]. For example, some pesticides have been shown to be neurotoxic and cause a Parkinsonian syndrome [Gorell et al. 2004, Bove et al. 2005]. In cases of unknown etiology, the term *Parkinsonism* is sometimes used to reflect the possible heterogeneity of cause(s) and underlying pathology. Since several pesticides are substrates for P-gp, variations in P-gp expression or function might be responsible for interindividual susceptibility to the effects of such environmental agents [Schinkel et al. 1994, Smit et al. 1999].

Based on the observation that the C3435T SNP on exon 26 of the MDR1 gene is related to modulated expression and function of P-gp [Hoffmeyer et al. 2000, Eichelbaum et al. 2004], the distribution of MDR1 polymorphisms in patients with and without Parkinsonism was investigated. A case-control study of the relationship between MDR1 polymorphisms and the risk of Parkinsonism revealed that the frequency of the 3435 TT genotype was highest in the early-onset Parkinsonian group, second highest in the late-onset group, and lowest in controls [Furuno et al. 2002]. The authors suggest that differences in the uptake and retention of neurotoxic agents due to differential P-gp expression at the BBB could influence interindividual vulnerability to Parkinsonism. A possible effect of P-gp on α-synuclein buildup was not mentioned; thus the differentiation between PD and Parkinsonism in this study is not clear. Additionally, the C3435T SNP in MDR1 has been reported to augment the damaging effect of pesticides leading to Parkinsonism [Drozdzik et al. 2003]. Similar results have been reported by others [Le Couteur et al. 2001, Lee et al. 2004, Tan et al. 2005]. A recent PET study found significantly elevated uptake of [^{11}C]verapamil (a P-gp substrate) in the midbrain of PD patients, suggesting that a dysfunction of P-gp at the BBB could be involved in the pathogenesis of PD [Kortekaas et al. 2005].

P-GP AND CREUTZFELDT-JAKOB-DISEASE

Creutzfeldt-Jakob-Disease (CJD) is a rare neurodegenerative disorder belonging to the transmissible spongiform encephalopathies, or prion diseases, and is characterized by the accumulation of misconformed prion protein (PrPScrapie, or PrP^{sc}). The principal histopathological features of CJD are the classical triad of spongiform change, neuronal loss, and gliosis, as well as immunohistochemically detectable PrP^{sc} deposits in certain brain regions [DeArmond and Prusiner 1995, Budka 2003a; Johnson 2005]. Although human prionosis can occur in uncommon hereditary and transmitted forms, most prion diseases are idiopathic, and generally affect older patients [Budka et al. 2003b]. Despite many clinicopathologic differences between CJD, PD and AD, these diseases share a critical pathogenic feature – the accumulation of aberrant, misfolded proteins [Walker and LeVine 2000, Aguzzi and Haass 2003; Tofaris and Spillantini 2005]. Since P-gp may play an important role in the pathogensis of AD and PD, the question arose as to whether P-gp might also be involved in the development of CJD. In a recent immunohistochemical study, we found significantly lower endothelial P-gp expression in the brains of patients who had died of sporadic CJD compared with controls [Vogelgesang et al. 2006]. Presently, there is no evidence that PrP is a substrate for P-gp, so it is not yet clear how a reduction in P-gp expression might contribute to the accumulation and toxicity of aberrant PrP, or whether the change in P-gp is a response to the disease. In some CJD cases, especially older patients, it is not uncommon to find both Aβ and PrP deposits in the brain [Budka 2003a]. In these instances, Aβ and PrP often colocalize in the same plaques, suggesting that either Aβ or PrP might act as a seeding factor, influencing the accumulation of one amyloidogenic protein onto a core composed of the other [Hainfellner et al. 1998, Kovacs and Budka 2002, Preusser et al. 2006, Vogelgesang et al. 2006]. Accordingly, the loss of P-gp might indirectly promote the misconformation and accumulation of PrP via the accrual of Aβ (see above).

A second potential point of interaction is that the accumulation of Aβ due to decreased P-gp expression could overwhelm the protein-degrading enzymes of the ubiquitin-proteasomal system (UPS), and thereby foster the cellular retention of other proteins, such as PrP. The UPS plays a major role in many basic cellular processes by degrading a broad range of proteins, including mutated and misfolded proteins [Ciechanover and Brundin 2003]. Disease-associated proteins that are degraded by this mechanism include α-synuclein [Petrucelli and Dawson 2004, Snyder and Wolozin, 2004], Aβ [Lopez Salon et al. 2003], tau [Oddo et al. 2004], and Huntingtin [Holmberg et al. 2004]. PrP also is believed to be degraded via the UPS [Yedida et al. 2001, Rane et al. 2004]. Downregulation of the UPS due to aging or drug treatment, or inundation of the UPS with other substrates such as Aβ, might bolster the intracellular levels of normal PrP^c, increasing the chances that the protein will convert to the pathogenic PrP^{sc} [Ma and Lindquist 2002]. Interestingly, recent data suggest that P-gp interacts actively with the proteasome complex [Begley et al. 2005]. Further studies are needed to clarify the relationship between PrP and P-gp. It cannot be excluded that, in neurodegenerative diseases such as CJD, there are additional mechanisms that impair the integrity of the BBB (e.g. the misfolded, toxic proteins themselves) and that secondarily reduce the expression of P-gp. Since P-gp acts as a critical detoxifying system in the brain [Terasaki and Ohtsuki 2005], we favour the hypothesis that the age-associated decline in P-gp function elevates the levels of potentially toxic proteins such as PrP in brain, thereby increasing the likelihood that they will misconform and accumulate to pathogenic levels.

NONSPECIFIC FUNCTIONS OF P-GP IN NEURODEGENERATION

Together with degrading and metabolizing enzymes, constitutive P-gp expression at the BBB is believed to protect the brain from injurious xenobiotics by forestalling their entry into the brain, as well as by exporting endogenous toxic compounds [Loscher and Potschka 2005]. Diminished P-gp expression could cause a pronounced influx of neurotoxic agents, leading to the impairment and loss of neurons. Differences in the uptake of neurotoxic substances, possibly due to genetic, pharmacologic or nutritive modulation of P-gp function, could influence interindividual susceptibility to neurological disorders. In particular, the age-related decrease of P-gp expression might diminish the protective mechanisms at the BBB, lowering the threshold for neurodegeneration in general.

Another possibility is that augmented P-gp could reduce neuronal damage by impeding the caspase-cascade. P-gp can inhibit apoptotic stimuli by suppressing the activation of caspases [Smyth et al. 1998, Tainton et al. 2004], an effect that has been investigated in tumor cells. Caspases are critical for apoptosis, and therefore are likely to mediate neuronal apoptosis in neurodegenerative diseases such as AD [Ivins et al. 1999, Nishimura et al. 2002] and CJD [Ferrer 2002, Sponne et al. 2004, Kristiansen et al. 2005]. In addition, caspases cleave specific proteins such as APP (resulting in elevated cerebral Aβ levels [Gervais et al. 1999, Wellington and Hayden 2000]), or huntingtin (generating toxic protein fragments [Qin and Gu 2004]). Thus, through inhibition of the caspase-cascade, increasing cerebral P-gp expression could have the dual benefits of impeding apoptotic cell loss and reducing the accumulation of abnormal proteins.

Alternatively, P-gp could reduce apoptosis through the removal of other cytotoxic, endogenously released compounds such as the excitatory (and excitotoxic) neurotransmitter glutamate, which is a substrate for P-gp [Liu and Liu 2001]. Interestingly, glutamate upregulates P-gp expression in rat brain microvessel endothelial cells [Zhu and Liu 2004], possibly as an adaptive mechanism that protects surviving brain cells from the devastating effects of toxic endogenous compounds [Loscher and Potschka 2005].

Finally, it is worth mentioning that, in addition to its presence in brain endothelial cells, P-gp also can be found (to a lesser extent) in astrocytes [Schlachetzky and Pardridge 2003] and microglia [Lee et al. 2001], and recently was shown to be induced by epileptic seizures in neurons [Volk et al. 2004, Volk et al. 2005]. Furthermore, in addition to the localization of P-gp in cell membranes, the transporter has been detected in intracellular compartments [Bendayan et al. 2002, Rajagopal and Simon 2003]. These findings suggest that the functions of P-gp in the brain could be more complex than previously realized.

OTHER ABC TRANSPORT PROTEINS

Compared to P-gp, only limited data are available for other members of the multidrug resistance family such as multidrug resistance-associated proteins (MRP, ABCC) or breast cancer-related protein (BCRP, ABCG2). Especially MRP1, MRP4, MRP5 and BCRP have been shown to be highly expressed in the brain [Eisenblatter and Galla 2002, Nies et al. 2004, Zhang et al. 2004].

MRP1 shares structural similarities and substantial pharmacological cross-reactivity with P-gp [Gottesmann et al. 2002]. The *in vitro* experiments of Lam and colleagues argue against the ability of MRP1 to transport Aβ as does P-gp [Lam et al. 2001]. *In vivo*, APPsw/P-gpKO mice showed increased MRP1 expression in hippocampal homogenates as compared with APPsw/P-gpWT littermates [Cirrito et al. 2005]. Whether MRP1 can transport Aβ *in vivo* has yet to be determined. Furthermore, in the brains of AD patients, 4-hydroxy-2-trans-nonenal (HNE) - a product of membrane lipid peroxidation during oxidative stress – was bound to glutathione S-transferase (GST) and MRP1 to a greater extent than in controls. MRP1 exports glutathione S-conjugates, and thus potentiates the GST-mediated protection against oxidative stress [Sultana and Butterfield 2004]. This observation suggests that MRP1 could play a protective role in the prevention of neuronal death through diminution of toxic endogenous compounds that are released during oxidative stress. Additionally, recent studies indicate that MRP1 could also protect cells from apoptosis [Gennuso et al. 2004].

The ATP-binding cassette transporter A1 (ABCA1), the cholesterol mobilizing-transporter, is another member of the ABC transport protein family [Borst and Elferink 2002, Jones and George 2004]. ABCA1 moves cholesterol from cells into high-density lipoproteins in plasma [Oram and Lawn 2001]. A lack of ABCA1 causes Tangier's disease, a rare hereditary disorder that is characterized by the absence of HDL cholesterol and an accumulation of cholesterol in macrophages, leading to severe coronary artery disease or peripheral neuropathy [Rust et al. 1999, Nofer and Remaley 2005]. In the brain, ABCA1 is localized within neurons and glial cells, and has been implicated in the pathogenesis of AD [Fukumoto et al. 2002, Katzov et al. 2004, Wahrle et al. 2004, Koldamova et al. 2005]. High cholesterol levels in the brain are associated with increased cleavage of APP, elevated Aβ-plaque burden, and a greater risk for AD [Shobab et al. 2005]. *In vivo* and *in vitro* studies found that intracellular cholesterol regulates the processing of APP, i.e., high levels increase Aβ formation and low levels decrease Aβ formation [Simons et al. 1998, Fassbender et al. 2001]. It is suggested that ABCA1 transfers lipids to other apolipoproteins abundant in brain, such as apoE, thus facilitating the elimination of (e.g.) injury-derived lipoidic membrane components from the brain. Induction of ABCA1 in central nervous system cells increases the secretion of Aβ [Fukumoto et al. 2002]. In ABCA1-KO mice, there was significantly decreased apoE in the cortex, plasma and cerebrospinal fluid, while there were no major differences in lipid levels (including cholesterol) as compared with controls. Since the *apoEε4* genotype represents a major risk factor for the accumulation of Aβ and the development of AD [Strittmatter et al. 1993, Warzok et al. 1998] it was proposed that ABCA1 might influence the apoE/Aβ interactions directly [Wahrle et al. 2004]. In a cross-breeding study of APP transgenic mice with ABCA1-KO mice, the animals lacking ABCA1 showed a strong decrease of apoE and an increase of Aβ deposition within the brain when compared to controls with intact ABCA1. Impaired clearance of Aβ in ABCA1-KO mice was also discussed [Koldamova et al. 2005]. Additionally, polymorphisms in the ABCA1 gene seem to influence intracerebral cholesterol levels, as well as the risk, or the age of onset, of AD [Wollmer et al. 2003, Katzov et al. 2004]. On the other hand, another study was unable to replicate this association [Li et al. 2004], and observations in our laboratory have failed to establish a correlation between the expression of ABCA1 and Aβ burden in the brains of nondemented elderly autopsy cases (unpublished data). However, ABCA1 could indirectly influence the pathogenesis of AD, an issue that needs further investigation.

CONCLUSION

In recent years, the involvement of ABC transporters in the pathogenesis of neurodegenerative disorders has garnered increasing interest. Within this superfamily of transporters, P-gp has been the subject of the most intense investigation. Evidence is accumulating that P-gp could play a role in the development of AD, possibly because the clearance of the amyloidogenic peptide Aβ (a substrate for P-gp) by the BBB is decreased in the aging brain. The deposition of aberrant proteins in other neurodegenerative diseases also may be linked to the reduced elimination of toxic proteins, such as PrP in prion diseases. In cases where the proteins are not known to be substrates for P-gp, such as PrP, other mechanisms might be involved, such as overburdening of the proteasomal degradation pathway by other proteins that normally are expelled by P-gp. Additionally, nonspecific effects of P-gp increase, such as protection of the brain from exogenous and endogenous neurotoxic compounds, or the inhibition of apoptosis, could positively influence the survival of brain cells and thus delay the development of neurodegenerative diseases. The age-related decline of endothelial P-gp expression in the brain correlates with the increased vulnerability to neurodegenerative disorders with advancing age. Knowledge of other members of the ABC transporter protein family in brain is still limited, but since a number of them are highly expressed within the brain, it is likely that these proteins could be involved in neurodegenerative processes as well. To overcome drug resistance in tumor cells, it is necessary to diminish the activity of P-gp, which transports the drugs from targeted neoplasms. In contrast, for neurodegenerative disorders the goal is to enhance cerebral P-gp expression, a strategy that could open new therapeutic pathways for the treatment or prevention of diseases involving the abnormal accumulation of proteins in brain. Further studies are needed to determine the feasibility and utility of this challenging, yet promising, objective.

REFERENCES

Aguzzi, A. and Haass, C. (2003). Games played by rogue proteins in prion disorders and Alzheimer's disease. *Science*, 302, 814-8.

Ambudkar, S.V.; Kim, I. W.; Sauna, Z. E. (2005). The power of the pump: Mechanisms of action of P-glycoprotein (ABCB1). *Eur J Pharm Sci*, 580, 1049-55.

Bart, J.; Groen, H. J.; Hendrikse, N. H.; van der Graaf, W. T.; Vaalburg, W.; de Vries, E. G. (2000). The blood-brain barrier and oncology: new insights into function and modulation. *Cancer Treat Rev*, 26, 449-62.

Begley, G. S.; Horvath, A. R.; Taylor, J. C.; Higgins, C. F. (2005). Cytoplasmic domains of the transporter associated with antigen processing and P-glycoprotein interact with subunits of the proteasome. *Mol Immunol*, 42, 137-41.

Bendayan, R.; Lee, G.; Bendayan, M. (2002). Functional expression and localization of P-glycoprotein at the blood brain barrier. *Microsc Res Tech*, 57, 365-80.

Bogman, K.; Peyer, A. K.; Torok, M.; Kusters, E.; Drewe, J. (2001). HMG-CoA reductase inhibitors and P-glycoprotein modulation. *Br J Pharmacol*, 132, 1183-92.

Borst, P. and Elferink, R.O. (2002). Mammalian ABC transporters in health and disease. *Annu Rev Biochem*, 71, 537-92.

Bove, J.; Prou, D.; Perier, C.; Przedborski, S. (2005). Toxin-induced models of Parkinson's disease. *NeuroRx*, 2, 484-94.

Breedveld, P.; Beijnen, J. H.; Schellens, J. H. (2006). Use of P-glycoprotein and BCRP inhibitors to improve oral bioavailability and CNS penetration of anticancer drugs. *Trends Pharmacol Sci*, 27, 17-24.

Budka, H. (2003a). Neuropathology of prion diseases. *Br Med Bull*, 66, 121-30.

Budka, H.; Head, M. W.; Ironside, J. W.; Gambetti, P.; Parchi, P.; Zeidler, M.; Tagliavini, F. (2003b). Sporadic Creutzfeldt-Jakob-Disease. In D.W. Dickson (Ed.), *Neurodegeneration: The molecular pathology of dementia and movement disorders* (pp. 287-297). Basel: ISN Neuropath Press.

Cascorbi, I.; Gerloff, T.; Johne, A.; Meisel, C.; Hoffmeyer, S.; Schwab, M.; Schaeffeler, E.; Eichelbaum, M.; Brinkmann, U.; Roots, I. (2001). Frequency of single nucleotide polymorphisms in the P-glycoprotein drug transporter *MDR1* gene in white subjects. *Clin Pharmacol Ther*, 69, 169-174.

Chen, C.; Mireles, R. J.; Campbell, S. D.; Lin, J.; Mills, J. B.; Xu, J. J.; Smolarek, T. A. (2005). Differential interaction of 3-hydroxy-3-methylglutaryl-coa reductase inhibitors with ABCB1, ABCC2, and OATP1B1. *Drug Metab Dispos*, 33, 537-46.

Ciechanover, A. and Brundin, P. (2003) The ubiquitin proteasome system in neurodegenerative diseases: sometimes the chicken, sometimes the egg. *Neuron* 40, 427-46.

Cirrito, J. R.; Deane, R.; Fagan, A. M.; Spinner, M. L.; Parsadanian, M.; Finn, M. B.; Jiang, H., Prior, J. L.; Sagare, A.; Bales, K. R.; Paul, S. M.; Zlokovic, B. V.; Piwnica-Worms, D.; Holtzman, D. M. (2005). P-glycoprotein deficiency at the blood-brain barrier increases amyloid-beta deposition in an Alzheimer disease mouse model. *J Clin Invest*, 115, 3285-90.

Deane, R.; Du Yan, S.; Submamaryan, R. K.; LaRue, B.; Jovanovic, S.; Hogg, E.; Welch, D.; Manness, L.; Lin, C.; Yu, J.; Zhu, H.; Ghiso, J.; Frangione, B.; Stern, A.; Schmidt, A.M.;

Armstrong, D. L.; Arnold, B.; Liliensiek, B.; Nawroth, P.; Hofman, F.; Kindy, M.; Stern, D.; Zlokovic, B. (2003). RAGE mediates amyloid-beta peptide transport across the blood-brain barrier and accumulation in brain. *Nat Med,* 9, 907-13.

Deane, R.; Wu, Z.; Zlokovic, B. V. (2004). RAGE (yin) versus LRP (yang) balance regulates alzheimer amyloid beta-peptide clearance through transport across the blood-brain barrier. *Stroke,* 35(11 Suppl 1), 2628-31.

DeArmond, S. J. and Prusiner, S.B. (1995) Etiology and pathogenesis of prion diseases. *Am J Pathol,* 146, 785-811.

Drozdzik, M.; Bialecka, M.; Mysliwiec, K.; Honczarenko, K.; Stankiewicz, J.; Sych, Z. (2003). Polymorphism in the P-glycoprotein drug transporter MDR1 gene: a possible link between environmental and genetic factors in Parkinson's disease. *Pharmacogenetics,* 13, 259-63.

Eichelbaum, M.; Fromm, M. F.; Schwab, M. (2004). Clinical aspects of the MDR1 (ABCB1) gene polymorphism. *Ther Drug Monit,* 26, 180-5.

Eisenblatter, T. and Galla, H. J. (2002). A new multidrug resistance protein at the blood-brain barrier. *Biochem Biophys Res Commun,* 293, 1273-8.

Fassbender, K.; Simons, M.; Bergmann, C.; Stroick, M.; Lutjohann, D.; Keller, P.; Runz, H.; Kuhl, S.; Bertsch, T.; von Bergmann, K.; Hennerici, M.; Beyreuther, K.; Hartmann, T. (2001). Simvastatin strongly reduces levels of Alzheimer's disease beta -amyloid peptides Abeta 42 and Abeta 40 in vitro and in vivo. *Proc Natl Acad Sci* U S A, 98, 5856-61.

Ferrer, I. (2002). Synaptic pathology and cell death in the cerebellum in Creutzfeldt-Jakob disease. *Cerebellum,* 1, 213-22.

Fromm, M.F. (2000). P-glycoprotein: a defense mechanism limiting oral bioavailability and CNS accumulation of drugs. *Int J Clin Pharmacol Ther,* 38, 69-74.

Fukumoto, H.; Deng, A.; Irizarry, M. C.; Fitzgerald, M. L.; Rebeck, G. W. (2002). Induction of the cholesterol transporter ABCA1 in central nervous system cells by liver X receptor agonists increases secreted Abeta levels. *J Biol Chem,* 277, 48508-13.

Furuno, T.; Landi, M. T.; Ceroni, M.; Caporaso, N.; Bernucci, I.; Nappi, G.; Martignoni, E.; Schaeffeler, E.; Eichelbaum, M.; Schwab, M.; Zanger, U. M. (2002). Expression polymorphism of the blood-brain barrier component P-glycoprotein (MDR1) in relation to Parkinson's disease. *Pharmacogenetics,* 12, 529-34.

Gennuso, F.; Fernetti, C.; Tirolo, C.; Testa, N.; L'Episcopo, F.; Caniglia, S.; Morale, M. C.; Ostrow, J.D.; Pascolo, L.; Tiribelli, C.; Marchetti, B. (2004). Bilirubin protects astrocytes from its own toxicity by inducing up-regulation and translocation of multidrug resistance-associated protein 1 (Mrp1). *Proc Natl Acad Sci* U S A, 101, 2470-5.

Gervais, F. G.; Xu, D.; Robertson, G. S.; Vaillancourt, J.P.; Zhu, Y.; Huang, J.; LeBlanc, A.; Smith, D.; Rigby, M.; Shearman, M. S.; Clarke, E. E.; Zheng, H.; Van Der Ploeg, L. H.; Ruffolo, S. C.; Thornberry, N. A.; Xanthoudakis, S.; Zamboni, R. J.; Roy, S.; Nicholson, D. W. (1999) Involvement of caspases in proteolytic cleavage of Alzheimer's amyloid-beta precursor protein and amyloidogenic A beta peptide formation. *Cell,* 97, 395-406.

Ghilardi, J. R.; Catton, M.; Stimson, E. R.; Rogers, S.; Walker, L. C.; Maggio, J. E.; Mantyh, P. W. (1996). Intra-arterial infusion of [125I]A beta 1-40 labels amyloid deposits in the aged primate brain in vivo. *Neuroreport,* 7, 2607-11.

Gorell, J. M.; Peterson, E. L.; Rybicki, B. A.; Johnson, C. C. (2004). Multiple risk factors for Parkinson's disease. *J Neurol Sci,* 217, 169-74.

Gottesman, M. M.; Fojo, T.; Bates, S. E. (2002). Multidrug resistance in cancer: role of ATP-dependent transporters. *Nat Rev Cancer,* 2, 48-58.

Hainfellner, J. A.; Wanschitz, J.; Jellinger, K.; Liberski, P.P.; Gullotta, F.; Budka, H. (1998). Coexistence of Alzheimer-type neuropathology in Creutzfeldt-Jakob disease. Acta Neuropathol, 96, 116-22.

Hardy, J. and Selkoe, D.J. (2002). The amyloid hypothesis of Alzheimer's disease: progress and problems on the road to therapeutics. *Science,* 297, 353-6.

Hoffmeyer, S.; Burk, O.; von Richter, O.; Arnold, H. P.; Brockmöller, J.; Johne, A.; Cascorbi, I.; Gerloff, T.; Roots, I.; Eichelbaum, M.; Brinkmann, U. (2000). Functional polymorphisms of the human multidrug resistance gene: multiple sequence variations and correlation with P-glycoprotein expression and activity in vivo. *Proc Natl Acad Sci,* 97, 3473-3478.

Holmberg, C. I.; Staniszewski, K. E.; Mensah, K. N.; Matouschek, A.; Morimoto, R. I. (2004). Inefficient degradation of truncated polyglutamine proteins by the proteasome. *EMBO J,* 23, 4307-18.

Hooiveld, G. J.; Vos, T. A.; Scheffer, G. L.; Van Goor, H.; Koning, H.; Bloks, V.; Loot, A. E.; Meijer, D. K.; Jansen, P. L.; Kuipers, F.; Muller, M. (1999). 3-Hydroxy-3-methylglutaryl-coenzyme A reductase inhibitors (statins) induce hepatic expression of the phospholipid translocase mdr2 in rats. *Gastroenterology,* 117, 678-87.

Ivins, K. J.; Thornton, P. L.; Rohn, T. T.; Cotman, C. W. (1999). Neuronal apoptosis induced by beta-amyloid is mediated by caspase-8. *Neurobiol Dis,* 6, 440-9.

Izzo, A. A. (2005). Herb-drug interactions: an overview of the clinical evidence. Fundam Clin Pharmacol, 19, 1-16.

Jellinger, K. A. and Mizuno, Y. (2003). Parkinson's disease. In D.W. Dickson (Ed.), *Neurodegeneration: The molecular pathology of dementia and movement disorders* (pp. 159-187). Basel: ISN Neuropath Press.

Jick, H.; Zornberg, G. L.; Jick, S. S.; Seshadri, S.; Drachman, D. A. (2000). *Statins and the risk of dementia. Lancet,* 356, 1627-31.

Johne, A.; Brockmoeller, J.; Bauer, S.; Maurer, A.; Langheinrich, M.; Roots, I. (1999). Pharmacokinetic interaction of digoxin with an herbal extract from St John's wort (Hypericum perforatum). *Clin Pharmacol Ther,* 66, 338-345.

Johnson, R.T. (2005). Prion diseases. Lancet Neurol, 4, 635-42.

Jones, P. M. and George, A. M. (2004). The ABC transporter structure and mechanism: perspectives on recent research. *Cell Mol Life Sci,* 61, 682-99.

Juliano, R. L. and Ling, V. (1976). A surface glycoprotein modulating drug permeability in Chinese hamster ovary cell mutants. *Biochim Biophys Acta,* 455, 152-162.

Katzov, H.; Chalmers, K.; Palmgren, J.; Andreasen, N.; Johansson, B.; Cairns, N.J.; Gatz, M.; Wilcock, G. K.; Love, S.; Pedersen, N. L.; Brookes, A. J.; Blennow, K.; Kehoe, P. G.; Prince, J. A. (2004). Genetic variants of ABCA1 modify Alzheimer disease risk and quantitative traits related to beta-amyloid metabolism. *Hum Mutat,* 23, 358-67.

Kitada, T.; Asakawa, S.; Hattori, N.; Matsumine, H.; Yamamura, Y.; Minoshima, S.; Yokochi, M.; Mizuno, Y.; Shimizu, N. (1998). Mutations in the parkin gene cause autosomal recessive juvenile parkinsonism. *Nature,* 392, 605-8.

Koldamova, R.; Staufenbiel, M.; Lefterov, I. (2005). Lack of ABCA1 considerably decreases brain ApoE level and increases amyloid deposition in APP23 mice. *J Biol Chem,* 280, 43224-35.

Kortekaas, R.; Leenders, K. L.; van Oostrom, J. C.; Vaalburg, W.; Bart, J.; Willemsen, A. T.; Hendrikse, N. H. (2005). Blood-brain barrier dysfunction in parkinsonian midbrain in vivo. *Ann Neurol,* 57, 176-9.

Kovacs, G. G. and Budka, H. (2002) Aging, the brain and human prion disease. *Exp Gerontol,* 37, 603-5.

Kristiansen, M.; Messenger, M. J.; Klohn, P. C.; Brandner, S.; Wadsworth, J. D.; Collinge, J.; Tabrizi, S.J. (2005). Disease-related prion protein forms aggresomes in neuronal cells leading to caspase activation and apoptosis. *J Biol Chem,* 280, 38851-61.

Kruger, R.; Kuhn, W.; Muller, T.; Woitalla, D.; Graeber, M.; Kosel, S.; Przuntek, H.; Epplen, J. T.; Schols, L.; Riess, O. (1998). Ala30Pro mutation in the gene encoding alpha-synuclein in Parkinson's disease. *Nat Genet,* 18, 106-8.

Lam, F. C.; Liu, R.; Lu, P.; Shapiro, A. B.; Renoir, J. M.; Sharom, F. J.; Reiner, P. B. (2001). beta-Amyloid efflux mediated by p-glycoprotein. *J Neurochem,* 76, 1121-8.

Le Couteur, D. G.; Davis, M. W.; Webb, M.; Board, P. G. (2001). P-glycoprotein, multidrug-resistance-associated protein and Parkinson's disease. *Eur Neurol,* 45, 289-90.

Lee, G.; Schlichter, L.; Bendayan, M.; Bendayan, R. (2001). Functional expression of P-glycoprotein in rat brain microglia. *J Pharmacol Exp Ther,* 299, 204-12.

Lee, C. G.; Tang, K.; Cheung, Y. B.; Wong, L. ; Tan, C.; Shen, H.; Zhao, Y.; Pavanni, R.; Lee, E. J.; Wong, M. C.; Chong, S. S.; Tan, E. K. (2004). MDR1, the blood-brain barrier transporter, is associated with Parkinson's disease in ethnic Chinese. *J Med Genet,* 41, e60.

Leonard, G. D.; Fojo, T.; Bates, S. E. (2003). The role of ABC transporters in clinical practice. *Oncologist,* 8, 411-24.

Li, Y.; Tacey, K.; Doil, L.; van Luchene, R.; Garcia, V.; Rowland, C.; Schrodi, S.; Leong, D.; Lau, K.; Catanese, J.; Sninsky, J.; Nowotny, P.; Holmans, P.; Hardy, J.; Powell, J.; Lovestone, S.; Thal, L.; Owen, M.; Williams, J.; Goate, A.; Grupe, A. (2004). Association of ABCA1 with late-onset Alzheimer's disease is not observed in a case-control study. *Neurosci Lett,* 366, 268-71.

Li, Y.; Zhou, W.; Tong, Y.; He, G.; Song, W. (2006). Control of APP processing and Abeta generation level by BACE1 enzymatic activity and transcription. *FASEB J,* 20, 285-92.

Liu, X. D. and Liu, G. Q. (2001). P glycoprotein regulated transport of glutamate at blood brain barrier. *Acta Pharmacol Sin,* 22, 111-6.

Loeb, M. B.; Molloy, D. W.; Smieja, M.; Standish, T.; Goldsmith, C. H.; Mahony, J.; Smith, S.; Borrie, M.; Decoteau, E.; Davidson, W.; McDougall, A.; Gnarpe, J.; O'DONNell, M.; Chernesky, M. (2004). A randomized, controlled trial of doxycycline and rifampin for patients with Alzheimer's disease. *J Am Geriatr Soc,* 52, 381-7.

Lopez Salon, M.; Pasquini, L.; Besio Moreno, M.; Pasquini, J. M.; Soto, E. (2003). Relationship between beta-amyloid degradation and the 26S proteasome in neural cells. *Exp Neurol,* 180, 131-43.

Loscher, W. and Potschka, H. (2005). Role of drug efflux transporters in the brain for drug disposition and treatment of brain diseases. *Prog Neurobiol,* 76, 22-76.

Ma, J. and Lindquist, S. (2002). Conversion of PrP to a self-perpetuating PrPSc-like conformation in the cytosol. *Science,* 298, 1785-8.

Mackic, J. B.; Bading, J.; Ghiso, J.; Walker, L.; Wisniewski, T.; Frangione, B.; Zlokovic, B. V. (2002). Circulating amyloid-beta peptide crosses the blood-brain barrier in aged monkeys and contributes to Alzheimer's disease lesions. *Vascul Pharmacol,* 38, 303-13.

Mandelkow, E. M. and Mandelkow, E. (1998). Tau in Alzheimer's disease. *Trends Cell Biol,* 8, 425-7.

Mizuno, Y.; Hattori, N.; Kitada, T.; Matsumine, H.; Mori, H.; Shimura, H.; Kubo, S.; Kobayashi, H.; Asakawa, S.; Minoshima, S.; Shimizu, N. (2001). Familial Parkinson's disease. Alpha-synuclein and parkin. *Adv Neurol,* 86, 13-21.

Nies, A. T.; Jedlitschky, G.; Konig, J.; Herold-Mende, C.; Steiner, H. H.; Schmitt, H. P.; Keppler, D. (2004). Expression and immunolocalization of the multidrug resistance proteins, MRP1-MRP6 (ABCC1-ABCC6), in human brain. *Neuroscience, 129,* 349-60.

Nishimura, I.; Uetsuki, T.; Kuwako, K.; Hara, T.; Kawakami, T.; Aimoto, S.; Yoshikawa, K. (2002) Cell death induced by a caspase-cleaved transmembrane fragment of the Alzheimer amyloid precursor protein. *Cell Death Differ,* 9, 199-208.

Nofer, J. R. and Remaley, A.T. (2005). Tangier disease: still more questions than answers. *Cell Mol Life Sci,* 62, 2150-60.

Oddo, S.; Billings, L.; Kesslak, J. P.; Cribbs, D. H.; LaFerla, F. M. (2004). Abeta immunotherapy leads to clearance of early, but not late, hyperphosphorylated tau aggregates via the proteasome. *Neuron,* 43, 321-32.

Oram, J. F. and Lawn, R. M. (2001). ABCA1. The gatekeeper for eliminating excess tissue cholesterol. J Lipid Res, 42, 1173-9.

Pan, Q.; Lu, Q.; Zhang, K.; Hu, X. (2005). Dibenzocyclooctadiene lingnans: a class of novel inhibitors of P-glycoprotein. *Cancer Chemother Pharmacol,* 18, 1-8.

Payami, H.; Zareparsi, S.; James, D.; Nutt, J. (2002). Familial aggregation of Parkinson disease: a comparative study of early-onset and late-onset disease. *Arch Neurol,* 59, 848-50.

Petrucelli, L. and Dawson, T. M. (2004). Mechanism of neurodegenerative disease: role of the ubiquitin proteasome system. *Ann Med,* 36, 315-20.

Preusser, M.; Strobel, T.; Gelpi, E.; Eiler, M.; Broessner, G.; Schmutzhard, E.; Budka, H. (2006). Alzheimer-type neuropathology in a 28 year old patient with iatrogenic Creutzfeldt-Jakob disease after dural grafting. *J Neurol Neurosurg Psychiatry,* 77, 413-6.

Qin, Z. H. and Gu, Z. L. (2004). Huntingtin processing in pathogenesis of Huntington disease. *Acta Pharmacol Sin,* 25, 1243-9.

Rajagopal, A. and Simon, S. M. (2003). Subcellular localization and activity of multidrug resistance proteins. *Mol Biol Cell,* 14, 3389-99.

Rane, N. S.; Yonkovich, J. L.; Hegde, R. S. (2004). Protection from cytosolic prion protein toxicity by modulation of protein translocation. *EMBO J,* 23, 4550-9.

Rautio, J.; Humphreys, J. E.; Webster, L. O.; Balakrishnan, A.; Keogh, J. P.; Kunta, J. R.; Serabjit-Singh, C. J.; Polli, J. W. (2006). In Vitro P-glycoprotein Inhibition Assays for Assessment of Clinical Drug Interaction Potential of New Drug Candidates: A Recommendation for Probe Substrates. *Drug Metab Dispos,* Feb 7, Epub ahead of print.

Rust, S.; Rosier, M.; Funke, H.; Real, J.; Amoura, Z.; Piette, J. C.; Deleuze, J. F.; Brewer, H. B.; Duverger, N.; Denefle, P.; Assmann, G. (1999). Tangier disease is caused by mutations in the gene encoding ATP-binding cassette transporter 1. *Nat Genet,* 22, 352-5.

Santini, M. T.; Napolitano, M.; Ferrante, A.; Rainaldi, G.; Arancia, G.; Bravo, E. (2003). Differential control of cholesterol and fatty acid biosynthesis in sensitive and multidrug-resistant LoVo tumor cells. *Anticancer Res,* 23, 4737-46.

Schinkel, A. H.; Smit, J. J.; van Tellingen, O.; Beijnen, J. H.; Wagenaar, E.; van Deemter, L.; Mol, C. A.; van der Valk, M. A.; Robanus-Maandag, E. C.; te Riele, H. P.; Berns, A. J.

M.; Borst, P. (1994). Disruption of the mouse mdr1a P-glycoprotein gene leads to a deficiency in the blood-brain barrier and to increased sensitivity to drugs. *Cell*, 77, 491-502.

Schinkel, A. H. (1997). The physiological function of drug transporting P-glycoproteins. *Semin Cancer Biol*, 8, 161-170.

Schinkel, A. H. and Jonker, J. W. (2003). Mammalian drug efflux transporters of the ATP binding cassette (ABC) family: an overview. *Adv Drug Deliv Rev*, 55, 3-29.

Schlachetzki, F. and Pardridge, W. M. (2003). P-glycoprotein and caveolin-1alpha in endothelium and astrocytes of primate brain. *Neuroreport*, 14, 2041-6.

Selkoe, D. J. (1999). Translating cell biology into therapeutic advances in Alzheimer's disease. *Nature*, 399, A23-A31.

Shibata, M.; Yamada, S.; Kumar, S. R.; Calero, M.; Bading, J.; Frangione, B.; Holtzman, D. M.; Miller, C. A.; Strickland, D. K.; Ghiso, J.; Zlokovic, B. V. (2000). Clearance of Alzheimer's amyloid-ß 1-40 peptide from brain by LDL receptor-related protein-1 at the blood-brain barrier. *J Clin Invest*, 106, 1489-1499.

Shobab, L. A.; Hsiung, G. Y.; Feldman, H. H. (2005). Cholesterol in Alzheimer's disease. *Lancet Neurol*, 4, 841-52.

Simons, M.; Keller, P.; De Strooper, B.; Beyreuther, K.; Dotti, C. G.; Simons, K. (1998). Cholesterol depletion inhibits the generation of beta-amyloid in hippocampal neurons. *Proc Natl Acad Sci* U S A, 95, 6460-4.

Smit, J. W.; Huisman, M. T., van Tellingen, O.; Wiltshire, H. R.; Schinkel, A. H. (1999). Absence or pharmacological blocking of placental P-glycoprotein profoundly increases fetal drug exposure. *J Clin Invest*, 104, 1441-7.

Smyth, M. J.; Krasovskis, E.; Sutton, V. R.; Johnstone, R. W. (1998). The drug efflux protein, P-glycoprotein, additionally protects drug-resistant tumor cells from multiple forms of caspase-dependent apoptosis. *Proc Natl Acad Sci* U S A, 95, 7024-9.

Snyder, H. and Wolozin, B. (2004). Pathological proteins in Parkinson's disease: focus on the proteasome. *J Mol Neurosci*, 24, 425-42.

Sponne, I.; Fifre, A.; Koziel, V.; Kriem, B.; Oster, T.; Olivier, J. L.; Pillot, T. (2004). Oligodendrocytes are susceptible to apoptotic cell death induced by prion protein-derived peptides. *Glia*, 47, 1-8.

Strittmatter, W. J.; Saunders, A. M.; Schmechel, D.; Pericak-Vance, M.; Enghild, J.; Salvesen, G. S.; Roses, A. D. (1993). Apolipoprotein E: high-avidity binding to beta-amyloid and increased frequency of type 4 allele in late-onset familial Alzheimer disease. *Proc Natl Acad Sci* U S A, 90, 1977-81.

Sultana, R. and Butterfield, D. A. (2004). Oxidatively modified GST and MRP1 in Alzheimer's disease brain: implications for accumulation of reactive lipid peroxidation products. *Neurochem Res*, 29, 2215-20.

Tainton, K. M.; Smyth, M. J.; Jackson, J. T.; Tanner, J. E.; Cerruti, L.; Jane, S. M.; Darcy, P. K.; Johnstone, R. W. (2004) Mutational analysis of P-glycoprotein: suppression of caspase activation in the absence of ATP-dependent drug efflux. *Cell Death Differ*, 11, 1028-37.

Tan, E. K.; Chan, D. K.; Ng, P.W.; Woo, J.; Teo, Y. Y.; Tang, K.; Wong, L. P.; Chong, S. S.; Tan, C.; Shen, H.; Zhao, Y.; Lee, C. G. (2005). Effect of MDR1 haplotype on risk of Parkinson disease. *Arch Neurol*, 62, 460-4.

Tanabe, M.; Ieiri, I.; Nagata, N.; Inoue, K.; Ito, S.; Kanamori, Y.; Takahashi, M.; Kurata, Y.; Kigawa, J.; Higuchi, S.; Terakawa, N.; Otsubo, K. (2001). Expression of P-glycoprotein in human placenta: relation to genetic polymorphism of the multidrug resistance (MDR)-1 gene. *J Pharmacol Exp Ther*, 297, 1137-43.

Tanzi, R. E.; Moir, R. D.; Wagner, S. L. (2004). Clearance of Alzheimer's Abeta peptide: the many roads to perdition. *Neuron*, 43, 605-8.

Terasaki, T. and Ohtsuki, S. (2005) Brain-to-blood transporters for endogenous substrates and xenobiotics at the blood-brain barrier: an overview of biology and methodology. *NeuroRx*, 2, 63-72.

Tofaris, G. K. and Spillantini, M. G. (2005). Alpha-synuclein dysfunction in Lewy body diseases. *Mov Disord*, 20 (Suppl 12), S37-44.

Troost, J. (2004). Modulation of cellular cholesterol alters P-glycoprotein activity in multidrug-resistant cells. *Mol Pharmacol*, 66, 1332-9.

Vogelgesang, S.; Cascorbi, I.; Schroeder, E.; Pahnke, J.; Kroemer, H. K.; Siegmund, W.; Kunert-Keil, C.; Walker, L. C.; Warzok, R. W. (2002). Deposition of Alzheimer's beta-amyloid is inversely correlated with P-glycoprotein expression in the brains of elderly non-demented humans. *Pharmacogenetics*, 12, 535-41.

Vogelgesang, S.; Warzok, R. W.; Cascorbi, I.; Kunert-Keil, C.; Schroeder, E.; Kroemer, H. K.; Siegmund, W.; Walker, L. C.; Pahnke, J. (2004a). The role of P-glycoprotein in cerebral amyloid angiopathy; implications for the early pathogenesis of Alzheimer's disease. *Curr Alzheimer Res*, 1, 121-5.

Vogelgesang, S.; Kunert-Keil, C.; Cascorbi, I.; Mosyagin, I.; Schroder, E.; Runge, U.; Jedlitschky, G.; Kroemer, H. K.; Oertel, J.; Gaab, M. R.; Pahnke, J.; Walker, L. C.; Warzok, R. W. (2004b). Expression of multidrug transporters in dysembryoplastic neuroepithelial tumors causing intractable epilepsy. *Clin Neuropathol*, 23, 223-31.

Vogelgesang, S.; Glatzel, M.; Walker, L. C.; Kroemer, H. K.; Aguzzi, A.; Warzok, R. W. (2006) Cerebrovascular P-glycoprotein expression is decreased in Creutzfeldt-Jakob disease, *Acta Neuropathologica*, Mar 07, Epub ahead of print.

Volk, H. A.; Burkhardt, K.; Potschka, H.; Chen, J.; Becker, A.; Loscher, W. (2004). Neuronal expression of the drug efflux transporter P-glycoprotein in the rat hippocampus after limbic seizures. *Neuroscience*, 123, 751-9.

Volk, H.; Potschka, H.; Loscher, W. (2005). Immunohistochemical localization of P-glycoprotein in rat brain and detection of its increased expression by seizures are sensitive to fixation and staining variables. *J Histochem Cytochem*, 53, 517-31.

Wahrle, S. E.; Jiang, H.; Parsadanian, M.; Legleiter, J.; Han, X.; Fryer, J. D.; Kowalewski, T.; Holtzman, D. M. (2004). ABCA1 is required for normal central nervous system ApoE levels and for lipidation of astrocyte-secreted apoE. *J Biol Chem*, 279, 40987-93.

Walker, L. C.; Masters, C.; Beyreuther, K.; Price, D. L. (1990). Amyloid in the brains of aged squirrel monkeys. *Acta Neuropathol*, 80, 381-7.

Walker, L. C. and LeVine, H. (2000). The cerebral proteopathies: neurodegenerative disorders of protein conformation and assembly. *Mol Neurobiol*, 21, 83-95.

Walker, L. C. and LeVine, H. (2002). Proteopathy: the next therapeutic frontier? *Curr Opin Investig Drugs*, 3, 782-7.

Wang, E.; Casciano, C. N.; Clement, R. P.; Johnson, W. W. (2001). HMG-CoA reductase inhibitors (statins) characterized as direct inhibitors of P-glycoprotein. *Pharm Res*, 18, 800-6.

Warzok, R.; Kessler, C.; Apel, G.; Schwarz, A.; Egensperger, R.; Schreiber, D.; Herbst, E. W.; Wolf, E.; Walther, R.; Walker, L. C. (1998). Apolipoprotein E promotes incipient Alzheimer pathology in the elderly. *Alzheimer Dis Rel Dis,* 12, 33-39.

Wellington, C. L. and Hayden, M. R. (2000) Caspases and neurodegeneration: on the cutting edge of new therapeutic approaches. *Clin Genet,* 57, 1-10.

Westphal, K.; Weinbrenner, A.; Gießmann. T.; Stuhr, M.; Franke, G.; Zschiesche, M.; Oertel, R.; Terhaag, B.; Kroemer, H. K.; Siegmund, W. (2000). Oral bioavailability of digoxin is enhanced by talinolol: Evidence for involvement of intestinal P-glycoprotein. *Clin Pharmacol Ther,* 68, 6-12.

Wollmer, M. A.; Streffer, J. R.; Lutjohann, D.; Tsolaki, M.; Iakovidou, V.; Hegi, T.; Pasch, T.; Jung, H. H.; Bergmann, K.; Nitsch, R. M.; Hock, C.; Papassotiropoulos, A. (2003). ABCA1 modulates CSF cholesterol levels and influences the age at onset of Alzheimer's disease. *Neurobiol Aging,* 24, 421-6.

Wolozin, B. (2004). Cholesterol, statins and dementia. *Curr Opin Lipidol,* 15, 667-72.

Wood, J. G.; Mirra, S. S.; Pollock, N. J.; Binder, L. I. (1986). Neurofibrillary tangles of Alzheimer disease share antigenic determinants with the axonal microtubule-associated protein tau (tau). *Proc Natl Acad Sci* U S A, 83, 4040-3.

Xu, D., Lu, Q.; Hu, X. (2006). Down-regulation of P-glycoprotein expression in MDR breast cancer cell MCF-7/ADR by honokiol. *Cancer Lett,* Jan 7, Epub ahead of print.

Yedidia, Y.; Horonchik, L.; Tzaban, S.; Yanai, A.; Taraboulos, A. (2001). Proteasomes and ubiquitin are involved in the turnover of the wild-type prion protein. *EMBO J,* 20, 5383-91.

Zhang, Y.; Schuetz, J. D.; Elmquist, W. F.; Miller, D. W. (2004). Plasma membrane localization of multidrug resistance-associated protein homologs in brain capillary endothelial cells. *J Pharmacol Exp Ther,* 311, 449-55.

Zhu, H. J. and Liu, G. Q. (2004). Glutamate up-regulates P-glycoprotein expression in rat brain microvessel endothelial cells by an NMDA receptor-mediated mechanism. *Life Sci,* 75, 1313-22.

Zlokovic, B. V. and Frangione, B. (2003). Transportclearance hypothesis for Alzheimer's disease and potential therapeutic implications. In T. C. Saido (Ed.), *Aβ Metabolism in Alzheimer's disease* (pp. 114-122). Georgetown, TX: Landes Bioscience.

Zlokovic, B. V.; Deane, R.; Sallstrom, J.; Chow, N.; Miano, J. M. (2005). Neurovascular pathways and Alzheimer amyloid beta-peptide. *Brain Pathol,* 15, 78-83.

In: Multidrug Resistance-Associated Proteins
Editor: Christopher V. Aiello, pp. 137-157

ISBN 1-60021-298-0
© 2007 Nova Science Publishers, Inc.

Chapter 6

NEUROFILAMENTS AS THE CENTRAL CORE OF AXONAL DAMAGE IN MULTIPLE SCLEROSIS

Catherine Fressinaud [1,*] and Véronique Sazdovitch [2]
[1]Neurology Department, Angers Cedex, France
[2]Neuropathology Laboratory, University Hospital Pitié-Salpêtrière, Paris, France

ABSTRACT

Little is known about the proteins involved in axonal damage (AD) which associates with demyelination during multiple sclerosis (MS). Axon transections, amyloid precursor protein accumulation and abnormal expression of the non-phosphorylated form of neurofilaments (NF) have been described. Characterization of AD is a main concern for at least two purposes. First, AD is probably involved in central nervous system (CNS) atrophy, and in patients permanent disability. Second, its impact on remyelination is unknown. Indeed, although neurons are dispensable for oligodendrocytes (OL), the myelinating cells in the CNS, to synthesize myelin-like membranes, neurons enhance this process *in vitro*. Thus, it may be that AD inhibits, in turn, remyelination.

To get insight into these axonal cytoskeleton alterations, we have analyzed by immunohistochemistry 18 chronic plaques from autopsy samples, originating from 6 MS patients (1 progressive, 5 remitting-progressive forms; mean disease duration : 18.5 years). In comparison to the normal appearing white matter decreased number of axons immunostained for the 3 NF subunits, βtubulin, and GAP-43 were - with demyelination and loss of oligodendrocytes (OL) - the hallmarks of plaques, and were extremely severe in 2/3. AD intensity did not correlate with demyelination : although severe demyelination always associated with a 90% decrease in NF+ axons, such severe NF loss also occurred in some plaques despite a moderate demyelination, suggesting it depends too upon other factors. CNP+ and MBP+ OL decreased by the same extent within one plaque, indicating that most OL have reached their final maturation. Nevertheless, residual cells show a

* Correspondence to: Dr. Catherine Fressinaud, Neurology Department, UPRES EA 3143, University Hospital, 4 rue Larrey, F49933 Angers Cedex 9, France. E-mail : Catherine.fressinaud@univ-angers.fr; Phone : (33) 2 41 35 46 13; Fax : (33) 2 41 35 35 94

lower capability to remyelinate axons, since the ratio of MBP+ fibers per OL decreased also.

These results enlarge previous descriptions of cytoskeleton and NF abnormalities in MS, since the expression of the 3 subunits of NF are decreased, providing evidence that their intimate constituents are impaired. As previously described in animal models, this decrease could lead to axonal atrophy (and slowness of axon potential conduction). Moreover severe impairment of NF associates with decreased tubulin expression which could result in altered axoplasmic transport. Finally one can hypothesized that the expression or localization of NF associated proteins (which copurify with NF) could be altered too.

Thus, the body of these results suggests that NF abnormalities are the core of more severe AD than previously hypothesized in MS. Detailing these lesions will help our understanding of permanent disability in MS patients, as well as cues to prevent them. Whether AD might be involved in MS remyelination impairment - which is one of the actual major target of therapeutic hopes such as cell grafts – is under current investigation at the laboratory.

Keywords: Axon cytoskeleton; Axonal damage; GAP-43; Myelin Basic Protein; Neurofilament; Oligodendrocyte; Tubulin

ABBREVIATIONS

AD	axonal damage
CNP	2',3'-cyclic nucleotide 3'-phosphodiesterase
CSF	cerebrospinal fluid
GAP-43	growth associated protein 43
GFAP	glial fibrillary acidic protein
LPC	lysophosphatidyl choline
MBP	myelin basic protein
MS	multiple sclerosis
NF	neurofilament proteins
OL	oligodendrocyte
TUB	tubulin

INTRODUCTION

In the course of multiple sclerosis (MS) demyelination is often associated with axonal damage (AD) (Trapp et al., 1998). Nevertheless, the severity of these axonal lesions compared to demyelination, the proteins of the cytoskeleton which are involved, and their mechanisms (Silber and Sharief, 1999), are yet unresolved questions (review in Frohman et al., 2006).

AD is probably involved in central nervous system (CNS) atrophy during MS, and in patient permanent disability (Brück et al., 2002; Losseff et al., 1996), but its impact on remyelination is unknown. Although oligodendrocytes (OL), the myelinating cells in the CNS are able to synthesize and to repair myelin-like membranes *in vitro* even in the absence of neurons (Fressinaud et al., 1990 ; 1996), neurons enhance myelin protein mRNAs and myelin synthesis *in vitro* (Demerens et al., 1996; Macklin et al., 1986). Moreover, axotomy decreases the number of OL precursors in the optic nerve (Barres and Raff, 1993). Thus, it may be that AD in MS inhibits, in turn, remyelination. Therefore it is necessary to clarify the pattern of axonal cytoskeleton lesions, and whether they might impair remyelination since experimentally remyelination can be improved by techniques such as growth factor supply (e. g. Allamargot et al., 2001 ; Jean et al., 2003) or myelinating cell grafts. Indeed, it has been known for years that myelin has a profound beneficial effect on axonal integrity and that remyelination restores the saltatory conduction of action potentials (review in Zhao et al., 2005). So, in order to remyelinate denuded axons numerous techniques of cell grafts from various origin have been developed including : Schwann cells (e. g. Baron-Van Evercooren et al., 1991; Bachelin et al., 2005), central and olfactory glia (review in Franklin, 2002), adult OL progenitors (Crang et al., 2004), as well as glial precursors derived from embryonic stem cells (Brustle et al., 1999), human embryonic stem cells (Nistor et al., 2005), neural stem cells (review in Cao et al., 2002; Ben-Hur et al., 2003) and bone marrow stromal cells (Akiyama et al., 2002).

Nevertheless, few reports have characterized axonal lesions in MS. Numerous axon transections (Trapp et al., 1998), amyloid precursor protein (APP) accumulation (Ferguson et al., 1997) and abnormal axons expressing the non-phosphorylated form of neurofilaments (NF) (Chang et al., 2002) within active plaques from autopsies, as well as abnormal ubiquitination of axons in the normal appearing white matter (NAWM) (Giordana et al., 2002) have been described. Axonal proteins involved in myelination are also modified : paranodin (which localizes to paranodes when myelination begins) is repressed (Guennoc et al., 2001), and PSA-NCAM, which is believed to inhibit myelination, is reexpressed by some axons in plaques (Charles et al., 2002).

Early in the course of the disease, and even in the NAWM (De Stefano et al., 2001; Narayanan et al., 1997), AD also is suggested by decreased N-acetyl-aspartate peak observed by MRI-spectroscopy. Axonal loss noticed in the NAWM might result from wallerian degeneration of axons transected in the plaques (Evangelou et al., 2000). The increase in the main cytoskeleton proteins (NF L isoform (Lycke et al., 1998), actin and tubulin (Semra et al., 2002), as well as TAU protein (Kapaki et al., 2000)) in the cerebrospinal fluid (CSF) of MS patients, correlates to the severity of the disease. Therefore, AD appears to be precocious during MS, nevertheless, its mechanisms are presently unknown: either secondary to the demyelinated status of the axons, and/or due to cytokines released during inflammation (Silber and Sharief, 1999) : OL death and axonal lesions may result from full complement activation (Schwab and McGeer, 2002), and cytotoxic T lymphocytes are able to induce neurite transections *in vitro* (Medana et al., 2001). Bystander killing of neurons by cytotoxic T cells specific for a glial antigen has recently been confirmed in transgenic animals (McPherson et al., 2006).

On the other hand, OL progenitors (Chang et al., 2002; Scolding et al., 1998) and mature OL are either spared, or strongly decreased, depending on plaques even in the same patient, or among authors (e.g. Brück et al., 1994, 2002; Mews et al., 1998; Ozawa et al., 1994 ; Rodriguez et al., 1993). These conflicting results have not yet received convincing explanations. OL density does not correlate with inflammatory cell infiltration or axonal loss (Lucchinetti et al., 1999). Expression of the anti-apoptotic protein bcl-2 by OL is associated with remyelination, and may contribute to OL preservation in MS (Kuhlmann et al., 1999). Some authors have proposed there could be different histological forms of MS (e. g. Brück et al., 1994; Ozawa et al., 1994). In a large group of actively demyelinating lesions Lucchinetti et al. (2000) identified 4 patterns of demyelination and inflammation, two closely similar with experimental autoimmune encephalomyelitis (EAE), and two suggestive of a primary viral or toxic OL insult. More recently Chang et al. (2002) have observed a high number of OL at a premyelinating stage in some areas of chronic plaques. These cells spread processes contacting demyelinated axons with a dystrophic aspect, suggesting that axons were unsuitable for remyelination. Dystrophic axons have already been described in EAE (Raine and Cross, 1989) or in MS, as well as atrophy (revue in Prineas and McDonald, 1997), but their cytoskeleton has not been characterized, the expression of abnormal non-phosphorylated NF excepted (Chang et al., 2002).

Axonal lesions are better characterized in animal models : in experimental optic neuritis, NF and microtubule loss in some axons, occasional NF ovoid staining, and axonal atrophy are observed (Zhu et al., 1999). Moreover, we have demonstrated that lysophosphatidyl choline (LPC)-induced demyelination in the rat corpus callosum decreases by 50% the axons immunolabelled for the 3 subunits of NF (NFL, NFM, NFH) and βtubulin (TUB), and that platelet-derived growth factor (PDGF), - which improves remyelination (Allamargot et al., 2001) - , largely reverses these abnormalities (Jean et al., 2002). Since there is no prominent axon loss in this model, this might suggest that demyelination on its own induces AD, and that remyelination alleviates these lesions (Jean et al., 2002). Interestingly we have already observed a similar pattern of cytoskeleton protein alterations in chronic inflammatory demyelinating neuropathy (CIDP, Fressinaud and Jean, 2002), which also shows similarities with MS (Hartung et al., 1999). Therefore, we thought of studying in detail the axonal cytoskeleton proteins in MS too : a decrease in NF and TUB immunostaining will traduce axonal lesions with more accuracy than the simple counts of transections, whereas an increase in TUB and in GAP-43 will be indicative of a trend to regeneration, since these two proteins are upregulated during development and regeneration (Hoffman et al., 1987 ; Hoffman, 1989).

MATERIALS AND METHODS

Samples

Brain autopsy samples from 6 patients suffering histologically confirmed MS (Neuropathology Laboratory, Pr. J.J. Hauw, University Hospital Pitié-Salpêtrière, Paris, France) were analyzed. The samples originated from 3 women and 3 men (mean age : 54.5 ± 11.5 years), 5 were remitting-progressive (RP) forms and one was a primary progressive (PP) form. All patients had EDSS scores > 8.5, and died from infectious or pulmonary . complications. Disease duration was in mean 18.5 ± 6 years.

Histology and Immunocytochemistry

Paraffin blocks containing the plaques (3 blocks per brain) were cut in serial sections (7 μm thick) which were used for luxol-fast blue (LFB)-phloxin-hematein staining and immunohistochemistry. Chronic plaques were recognized by the absence of LFB-positive inclusions in macrophages (Giordana et al., 2002; Prineas and McDonald, 1997).

The cytoskeleton components were labelled with antibodies raised against each of the 3 neurofilament subunits (light, medium, and heavy chain : NFL, NFM, NFH, Sigma) and βtubulin (TUB, Sigma). The axons were also stained with anti-growth associated protein antibody (GAP-43, Biotrend, Köln, Germany). Antibodies raised against myelin basic protein (MBP, Dako, Trappes, France), myelin proteolipid (PLP, gift of Dr. E. Trifilieff (Trifilieff et al., 1986)), 2',3'-cyclic nucleotide 3'-phosphodiesterase (CNP, Sigma Immunochemicals, St Louis, MO), and glial fibrillary acidic protein (GFAP, Dako) were used to label myelin and oligodendrocytes (MBP, PLP, CNP), or astrocytes (GFAP), respectively. Biotinylated secondary antibodies (Amersham, Les Ulis, France) and avidin-biotin-horseradish peroxydase H complex (Vectastain ABC kit, Vector Laboratories, Burlingame, CA) were used for 3,3'-diaminobenzidine tetrahydrochloride (Sigma) staining. Sections were counterstained with hematein. Procedures were performed as previously described (Fressinaud et al., 2002, 2005; Jean et al., 2002).

Cell and Fiber Counting

Axonal transections (i. e. interruption of fiber continuity) in plaques were semi-quantitatively estimated on LFB-stained sections and, depending on the number of preserved fibers, expressed as mild (-25%), moderate (-50%) or severe (-100%, i.e. virtually all the axons were transected) compared to the adjacent normal appearing white matter (NAWM).

Immunolabelled cells (OL and astrocytes) and the entire cell population (defined by nucleus staining with hematein) were counted in the totality of standardized microscopic fields defined by an ocular morphometric grid using a X 100 objective. Similarly the number of immunolabelled fibers for myelin antibodies, and the number of axons stained for antibodies to the cytoskeleton, or to GAP-43, were counted per optic field. All these measurements were performed in 5 optic fields within each of the plaques, and in 5 optic fields in the adjacent NAWM. In this latter the fibers were so dense that it precluded a perfectly accurate counting of myelinated fibers and of axons labelled for cytoskeleton components, these values represent therefore rather a precise estimation and are slightly underevaluated (i.e. between 2 counts in the same field differences from 10 to less than 50 fibers were encountered for a total number of 400 to 10^3 fibers, depending on the antibody used, and on the anatomic localization). Results were first expressed as mean ± SD of counts per optic field within the plaque, or in the NAWM. To allow comparison between plaques counts were subsequently expressed as percentage of variation compared to the NAWM.

Comparison of mean counting between plaques and NAWM employed Mann and Whitney test.

RESULTS

Since MS is primary characterized by demyelination we first characterized plaques on the basis of myelin and OL loss.

Demyelination and Oligodendrocyte Loss

Demyelination (Figures 1A and 2A), loss of OL, and axonal lesions (transections as well as decreased immunostaining for cytoskeleton proteins) (Figures 2B, 3, and 4) were the hallmarks of plaques, excepted in one block (4*2) where OL number was modestly increased (non significant). Comparison of the number of CNP+ and MBP+ cells within one plaque gave similar results (Figure 2A), as well as that of PLP+ OL (not shown), indicating that most OL have reached their final maturation stage and were therefore susceptible to remyelinate axons (attempts to use anti-MOG antibody were unsuccessful). OL number (CNP+, PLP+, and MBP+ cells per optic field) was generally decreased compared to the NAWM ($\alpha < 1\%$, Mann and Whitney test).

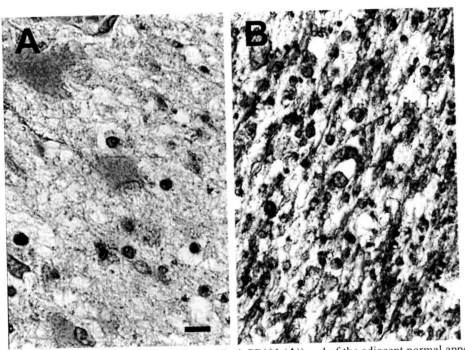

Figure 1. Immunohistochemistry of MS plaque (block PP6*1 (A)) and of the adjacent normal appearing white matter (B), with anti-MBP antibody (peroxydase, hematein counterstain). Despite preservation of quite numerous axons, note complete demyelination in (A) compared to (B), whereas some MBP+ oligodendrocytes are still present in the plaque. Bar = 10 µm.

Since the lack of remyelination could simply result from this decrease in mature (MBP+) OL, we also calculated the capability of theses cells to myelinate axons : i. e. the ratio of myelinated fibers per OL (MBP+ fibers / MBP+ OL). This demonstrated that residual cells showed a lower capability to myelinate axons, - or axons were unproper for remyelination - , since this ratio also decreased, by 37 to 100%, compared to the NAWM (Figures 1A and 2A). Moreover, it was also decreased in block 4*2, despite the increased number of MBP+ OL.

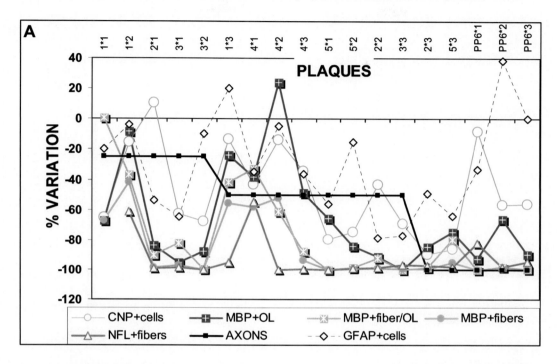

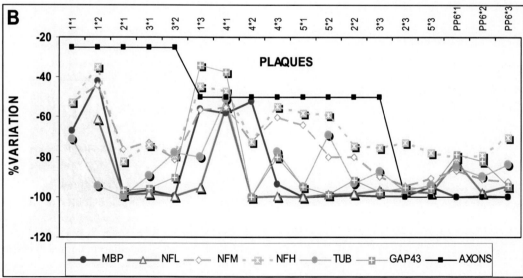

Figure 2. Continued.

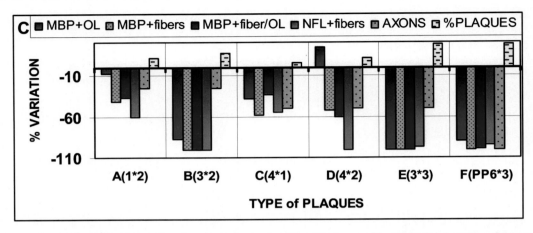

Figure 2. Results of immunohistochemistry for each of the 18 plaques (**A, B**) (patient number * block number, PP denotes the primary progressive form) presented by order of increasing axonal transections that were semi-quantitatively expressed as mild (-25%), moderate (-50%) or severe (-100%). (**A**) Labelled cells and/or fibers for antibodies directed against myelin (CNP, MBP, and the ratio of MBP+ fibers per MBP+ oligodendrocytes) are compared to astrocytes (GFAP+ cells), and to NFL. Results are expressed as percentage of variation compared to the adjacent normal appearing white matter (NAWM, mean of counts in 5 optic fields). (**B**) Results of axonal cytoskeleton immunohistochemistry compared to demyelination for each of the 18 plaques that have been analyzed (mean counts of 5 optic fields). (**C**) Classification of MS plaques in 6 types (A-F) by increasing severity of axonal transections, demyelination (MBP+ fibers), and NFL loss. Results are expressed as percentage of variation compared to the adjacent NAWM. One representative example of each type of plaque (number of patient * number of sample) is presented. The percentage of plaques of each type is given (yellow bars).

Astrocytic Gliosis

Astrocyte morphology was modified with a rigid aspect and an increase in the number of spine-like processes, suggestive of astrocytic gliosis (not shown). In most cases, however, the number of GFAP+ cells decreased (non significant) (Figure 2A) in the plaques compared to the NAWM. Rather an "astrocytic line" could be delineated at the edges of the plaques : rows of astrocytes were often delimiting the plaques (not shown).

Axonal Cytoskeleton Damage

Axonal lesions comprised axonal transections, which were constant (Figure 2B). Moreover, in 13/18 plaques (72%), they were semi-quantitatively quantified as moderate (50% axon loss) or severe (nearly 100% axon loss). Dystrophic axons were sometimes encountered (Figure 3C), but we did not observe ovoid.

Even in residual axons without transections the cytoskeleton was frequently affected : these axons (and the continuity of the axonal cylinder) were still observable with the hematein counterstain, but they were not labelled by the different antibodies (NFL, NFM, NFH, TUB, and GAP-43) used (Figures 3 and 4). It was striking that all the cytoskeleton proteins, as well as GAP-43, were strongly decreased (> 50%) compared to the NAWM ($\alpha < 1\%$, Mann and

Whitney test), although NFM and NFH were less severely affected than NFL, TUB and GAP-43 (Figure 2B). Indeed, TUB and GAP-43 were generally decreased by 80% (TUB) to 100% (GAP-43), in 2 lesions excepted (blocks 1*3 and 4*1), and correlated with NFL decrease, indicating that there was no trend to regeneration.

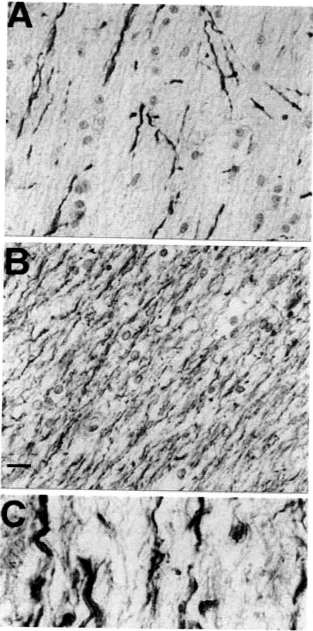

Figure 3. Immunohistochemistry of MS plaque (block 4*2) (**A** and **C**) and of the adjacent normal appearing white matter (**B**), with anti-NFH antibody (peroxydase, hematein counterstain). Despite preservation of some axons, note nearly complete loss of neurofilament immunostaining in (**A** and **C**) compared to (**B**), while still labelled axons appear tortuous and dystrophic in the plaque at higher magnification (**C**). Bar = 20 μm in **A** and **B**, 10 μm in **C**.

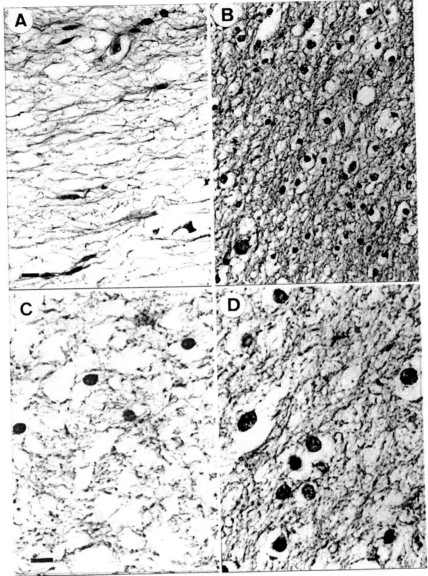

Figure 4. Immunohistochemistry of MS plaque (block 4*2) (**A** and **C**) and of the adjacent normal appearing white matter (**B** and **D**), with anti-β tubulin (**A**, **B**) and anti-GAP-43 (**C**, **D**) antibodies (peroxydase, hematein counterstain). Despite preservation of some axons, note nearly complete loss of axon immunostaining in (**A** and **C**) compared to (**B** and **D**) respectively. Bar = 20 μm in **A** and **B**, 10 μm in **C** and **D**.

Major axonal transections were, unsurprisingly, associated with severe defects in axonal cytoskeleton proteins immunolabelling (> 80%) (as observed in case PP6) (Figure 2B). Nevertheless, these defects also occurred in association with more moderate axonal transections. For example the number of fibers immunostained for NFL decreased by 98% in blocks 2*1, 3*1, and 3*2, whereas axon loss was only estimated by 25% in these 3 lesions. This indicated that axon loss did not account for the extent of decreased immunostaining in cytoskeletal proteins, and that additional AD was present in these cases.

Thus, the only PP form (case PP6) included in this study coincided with the most severe pattern of axonal transections, loss of staining for axonal cytoskeleton proteins, and complete demyelination. Nevertheless this pattern of complete destruction could also be observed in RP forms (blocks 5*3 and 2*3 for example, Figure 2B). So, in these latter several types of profiles could be delineated (Figure 2A, 2B): i) either moderate (block 4*1) or severe (block 5*3) destruction of myelin and axons that were correlated, ii) or, dissociation between severe demyelination and cytoskeleton lesions contrasting with moderate axonal loss (blocks 4*3, 5*1, and 5*2). Conversely, a strong decrease in NFL immunolabelling and pronounced axonal transections (block 1*3) could be observed, despite relative preservation of myelin. In some plaques (1*3, and 4*2) also moderate demyelination and axonal transections contrasted with nearly complete loss in NFL immunostaining. Finally, severe demyelination was always associated with major cytoskeleton abnormalities, but these latter could also accompanied more moderate demyelination.

Classification of Plaques

Depending on axonal transections, NFL loss and demyelination, we classified plaques in 6 representative types of lesions by increasing severity (Figure 2C) : i) mild axonal transections associated with either moderate demyelination and moderate NFL loss (2 lesions, 11.11%, type A), or with severe demyelination and severe NFL loss (3 lesions, 16.67%, type B); ii) moderate axonal transections associated with : either moderate demyelination and moderate NFL loss (1 lesion, 5.56%, type C), or moderate demyelination and severe NFL loss (2 lesions, 11.11%, type D), or severe demyelination and severe NFL loss (5 lesions, 27.78%, type E). This type E was therefore the most frequent encountered together with the last type (more than 55 % in all), i.e.: iii) severe axonal transections associated with severe demyelination and severe NFL loss (5 lesions, 27.78%, type F), this type corresponded to the 3 lesions of the PP form, and to 2 of RP forms.

Mean duration of disease was not significantly different between the PP form (20 years) and RP forms (18.2 ± 6.5 years). Nevertheless, it was striking that complete axonal transections and demyelination were observed in only 2/15 (13 %) of RP forms, versus 3/3 plaques of the PP form; moreover this type of lesion concerned only 1/3 plaques of these 2 RP forms. In all, 10/15 (67 %) plaques of RP forms comprised complete demyelination and NFL loss, 2 (13%) with major axonal transections (type F), 5 (33%) with moderate axonal transections (type E), and 3 (20%) with mild axonal transections (type B). Although there was a relative homogeneity of lesions for one given patient, i.e. at least 2/3 plaques of the same type were observed in 5/6 cases (83%), there was as many type of lesions as of patients.

In search for correlations with the classification of active plaques (Lassmann, 2002), we observed that most of these chronic plaques had sharp edges (types I, II and IV of Lassmann), and 10/18 (55 %), including the totality (3 blocks) of 3 cases were very well delimited (not shown). Only 5 plaques were centred by a vessel. Vessels were generally numerous within the plaques, with perivascular infiltration in one case (RP1*) only, and often distributed at random. In addition to the 5 plaques with at least one central vessel, 3 elongated plaques had venules centring their extremities. There was no correlation between these parameters and the intensity of myelin or axonal destruction.

DISCUSSION

Although the histology of MS has been described long ago, relatively few studies have analyzed in parallel the fate of myelin, OL and of axons. The severity of demyelination and of axonal cytoskeleton damage that we observed in these chronic lesions was striking since 72% showed complete demyelination and NFL loss. This appears a severe evolution for a disease duration that was in mean < 19 years in our cases, with a mean age of apparition of clinical signs of 32 years. Although our study is based on a small number of cases, it is important to note, despite a mean duration of disease similar to that of RP forms, that the more severe immunohistochemical pattern of axon destruction and demyelination (major axonal transections and complete MBP and NFL loss) corresponded mostly to the only PP form studied - since it was observed in 3/3 lesions analysed, a pattern which was never observed in the totality of the plaques for one case in RP forms - . Nevertheless, this PP form represented 16% of our cases, which is in the range of frequency (10-15%) of PP forms generally reported (e.g. Ingle et al., 2002; McDonnell and Hawkins, 2002). This in accordance with the literature pointing out the severity of MS PP forms (Bashir and Whitaker, 1999; Brück et al., 2002; McDonnell and Hawkins, 2002; Thompson et al., 1997). It has been reported that cerebrospinal fluid from patients with PP – but not those with RP forms – of MS induces neuron apoptosis *in vitro* (Øren et al., 2001). Such a neurotoxic factor could explain, at least partly, the severity of these forms, while primary OL degeneration, - which seems to be the hallmark of MS PP forms (Brück et al., 2002) - , might explain the failure of remyelination. The report of Wolswijk (2000) has already emphasized the decrease in mature and immature OL in chronic progressive MS, our results showing a 70-90% decrease in OL in case PP6 is in accordance with this observation.

Our results also strengthen the notion that axonal lesions (transections as well as decrease in cytoskeleton proteins expression) are a prominent feature of MS plaques, since they were constantly observed, and, most frequently (15/18, 83% with complete NFL loss), moderate or severe. AD therefore is not limited to acute lesions where it has been reported too (Bitsch et al., 2000). This is akin to the data of Mews et al. (1998) who found an average of 55-65% reduction in axon density. We have already observed very similar alterations of the cytoskeleton (without fiber transections) in experimental studies, where they appeared consecutive to demyelination itself, and improved during remyelination (Jean et al., 2002). In MS, nevertheless, and as shown here, they may occur even in the presence of moderate demyelination (5/18, 28%; and 5 out of 5 plaques with moderate demyelination). Given the early axonal degeneration observed for example in double mutant *plp-/-mag-/-* which lacks compact myelin (Uschkureit et al., 2000), this result is not surprising : sustained demyelination - even mild - in MS might be deleterious for axons. Nevertheless, the lack of congruence between the severity of demyelination and that of axonal impairment in our study could suggest that this latter depends also on other factors, such as cytotoxic cytokines, reactive oxygen and NO species, or glutamate (revue in Silber and Sharief, 1999). The fact that axonal injury is, at least in part, independent of demyelination has already been reported (Bitsch et al., 2000).

Profound decrease (around 100%) in immunolabelling for the axonal proteins studied (NF, TUB, and GAP-43) was observed in some of our cases even in the absence of severe axonal loss (-25%) indicating that : first, decreased number of immunostained axons is not only due to fiber loss, and , second, that additional AD appears more extended than previously reported. Similarly, we have previously demonstrated that LPC-induced demyelination induces decreased NF expression in rat corpus callosum despite the lack of significant fiber loss in this model (Allamargot et al., 2001), and that remyelination alleviates these lesions (Jean et al., 2002).

The precise nature of the axonal cytoskeleton lesions in MS also has not been described to our knowledge; most authors have used only the SMI-32 antibody (e.g. Chang et al., 2002; Trapp et al., 1998), which labels the abnormal non-phosphorylated forms of NF, or anti-amyloid antibody (Bitsch et al., 2000; Ferguson et al., 1997) and, for axonal transections excepted, only qualitative studies of axonal damage have been reported. It was remarkable that all the cytoskeleton proteins (the 3 NF subunits, and TUB) that we have studied were affected, although NFL and TUB were more severely decreased. Pronounced decrease in TUB and GAP-43 immunolabelling indicated that there was no trend to regeneration since these two proteins are upregulated during it (Hoffman et al., 1987; Hoffman, 1989). As TUB and GAP-43 decreased in parallel to NFL, this confirms that these proteins can be used as valuable markers of AD during MS, as previously reported by CSF studies (Lycke et al., 1998).

Since NF are major determinants of axonal caliber (Hoffmann et al., 1987; Eyer and Peterson, 1994), the strong decrease in NF we observed in plaques could have severe consequences on axonal architecture as well as metabolism, and might also account for axonal atrophy, which is a recognized feature of MS plaques (Prineas and McDonald, 1997). Decreased NF expression may arise from demyelination, as demonstrated in our LPC model (Jean et al., 2002). Indeed, during development axon ensheathment by OL processes induces local accumulation of NF, triggering thereby full axon radial growth (Sanchez et al., 1996; Windebank et al., 1985). Conversely, the lack of remyelination might be explained, at least in part, if axons do not reach the adequate caliber (Dyck et al., 1984; Hoffmann et al., 1987).

Nevertheless, other results from our group suggest that the lack of NF might not be per see the origin of the remyelination defect in MS. Indeed, we have observed in NFH-lacZ transgenic mice – which lack axonal NF (Eyer and Peterson, 1994) and show constitutive CNS (as well as PNS) axonal atrophy – that remyelination proceeds as well as in their wild-type littermates after LPC-induced demyelination of the corpus callosum (Jean and Fressinaud, 2003). This demonstrates that, at least, constitutive lack of axonal NF does not impair CNS remyelination. This model also confirmed that demyelination induces axonal atrophy in wild-type mice, a phenomenon known to slow down axon potential conduction (review in Sargent, 1992), and thus able to impair proper function of axons leading finally to disability.

Moreover, the profound decrease in TUB that we observed in MS also could result in altered axoplasmic transport along microtubules (review in Hammerschlag and Brady, 1989), which is likely to impair even more axon metabolism. Indeed, altered axoplasmic transport might affect too proteins involved in axon-glia interactions, and especially in myelination, providing thereby additional perturbations to the repair process. Such molecules comprise for example neuregulins which are expressed by axons and promote OL development and myelination (review in Falls, 2003) and which have been implicated in MS physiopathology (e. g. Cannella et al., 1999, Viehover et al., 2001).

In order to get insights into the putative impact of decreased NF expression observed in MS on the remyelination process, we have started another experimental approach to determine the effects of NF and/or their associated proteins on OL fate. Although these neurocytoskeletal elements are physiologically intracytoplasmic, they could either mediate a signal to OL through their binding to transmembrane proteins, or they could be present in the extracellular space following an axonal lesion and modulate remyelination. Indeed, during NF purification procedures (Fasani et al., 2004) numerous proteins copurify with NF (e. g. STOP proteins (Letournel et al., 2003)). Preliminary results reveal that *in vitro* adult rat brain NF enriched fractions, obtained by successive purification steps, significantly enhanced OL progenitor proliferation as well as their differentiation and maturation into OL (Fressinaud et al., 2006), compared to controls, in pure OL secondary cultures grown in chemically defined medium (Fressinaud et al., 1990; Fressinaud, 2005). Molecules responsible for these effects are currently under investigation at the laboratory, and their expression will be assessed in MS plaques in search for correlations with demyelination and AD.

Thus, the body of these results strengthen the hypothesis that severe impairment of axonal cytoskeleton, involving NF, TUB, (and/or their associated proteins) that we observed in MS plaques might have severe consequences on both axon metabolism, and remyelination, and finally create a vicious circle leading to patient permanent disability.

It is also important to draw comparisons between AD in MS and other pathological or experimental conditions. This pattern of decreased NF and TUB immunostaining in MS is similar to what we have observed in: i) toxic demyelination of the CNS in rodents - where there is no prominent fiber loss - (Jean et al., 2002); and ii) in cases of chronic inflammatory demyelinating neuropathy (CIDP) presenting with fiber loss (Fressinaud and Jean, 2002). On the contrary, in axonopathies of unknown aetiology, and in necrotizing vasculitis of the peripheral nervous system (Fressinaud et al., 2002, 2003, 2005), TUB increased and was inversely correlated with fiber density and NFL, which decreased. Thus, primary demyelination involving either the CNS (MS, LPC-induced demyelination) or the PNS (CIDP), whatever its mechanisms may be (probably autoimmune : MS and CIDP, or toxic : LPC-induced), could result in the same axonal cytoskeleton alterations, which are clearly distinct from those encountered in primary axonal pathologies. In a therapeutic perspective, it is important to note also that remyelination alleviates acute axonal damage in our toxic model (Jean et al., 2002).

In most of our MS cases OL were strongly decreased (over 50%) in the plaques, compared to the NAWM, in accordance with previous studies (Brück et al., 1994; Mews et al., 1998; Ozawa et al., 1994; Rodriguez et al., 1993). Recent *in vitro* studies using LPC toxicity have demonstrated that the repetition of attacks is deleterious for cells of the OL lineage (Fressinaud, 2005). Thus, it is likely that repeated relapses account – at least in part - for OL loss in RP MS plaques. Subsequently, this decrease in myelinating cells could represent one of the main factors limiting remyelination. From this point of view, our study in MS does not match with that of Chang et al. (2002), since we observed a number of MBP+ cells (as well as of PLP+ cells) that was generally equivalent to that of CNP+ cells in plaques. This demonstrates that nearly all surviving OL had reached their final maturation stage, and were therefore susceptible to remyelinate axons. Also, Chang et al. (2002) reported that "many" premyelinating OL extended processes contacting axons without myelination; in our cases we did not detect such type of cells. This apparent discrepancy could be due to the technique used by these authors (microwave pretreatment, thickness of sections > 30µm, and > 5 days incubation with primary antibody) that differs from ours.

Our data introduce a new notion concerning OL in MS plaques : we observed in addition that in all cases the capability of OL to remyelinate axons was decreased by 37 to 100%, even in the block where the number of OL was slightly increased. Indeed, fibers unlabelled for MBP (and counterstained by hematein), with a normal aspect (i.e. not dystrophic) and crossing the plaques could be observed in most cases, indicating that this lack of remyelination was unlikely due – at least in these cases - to axonal dystrophy or transections. Such disturbances of the myelinating function of OL have been reported (Rodriguez et al., 1993). To explain the failure of remyelination in MS this mechanism of OL dysfunction could represent an alternative to the hypothesis of a causal axonal impairment proposed by Chang et al. (2002), based on their observations of the association between OL processes and abnormal axons. Though, our results might in turn be compatible with the assumption that, despite their normal morphology, axons are unproper for remyelination, for example as a consequence of paranodin repression (Guennoc et al., 2001), or PSA-N CAM reexpression (Charles et al., 2002). Nevertheless, it cannot be concluded yet that these latters are sufficient to explain on their own the lack of remyelination. As demonstrated and discussed above, NF loss (resulting in axonal atrophy), decreased OL density, and impairment of OL capability to synthesize new membranes after several attacks, are also likely involved in the failure of myelin repair.

We were unable to match up the histology of these chronic lesions with the classification of active plaques (Lassmann, 2002), which could have explained the variabilty of histological damage depending on the situation of fibers compared to vessels. This could be due to the repetition of attacks in these chronic lesions, modifying the architecture of the plaques, for example by extension of the process to additional vessels.

As described previously (revue in Prineas and McDonald, 1997), astrocytic gliosis was not a prominent feature of MS plaques. Rather, as reported in EAE (Matsumoto et al., 1992), an "astrocytic limit" could be delineated at the edges of the plaques Although astrocytes are involved in the course of CNS repair (e.g. Matsumoto et al., 1992; Ridet et al., 1997; Westenbroek et al., 1998), and might protect newly generated OL by internalization (Wu and Raine, 1992), or terminal axonal sprouts by PSA-N CAM+ ensheathment (Dusart et al., 1999), there is little evidence from our results to draw conclusions about their role. At least it can be assumed that astrocyte density did not increase in the plaques in our cases. Nevertheless, the peculiar arrangement of their processes could be sufficient to modify significantly, even on the only architectural point of view, the environment of injured axons and damaged myelin sheathes.

CONCLUSION

Pronounced AD, involving all the major cytoskeleton components (NF and TUB) together with GAP-43, is now characterized in MS chronic plaques, and it occurs in nearly ¾ of the lesions, even in the absence of major axonal transactions or demyelination. This strengthens the hypothesis that axon injury also depends upon other components (probably involved in the inflammatory process). Comparative analyses reveal that NFL appears as a good marker of AD, since TUB and GAP-43 decrease to the same extent. Depending on the severity of axonal and myelin damage, we have identified several types of lesions, confirming the heterogeneity of pathological patterns among patients (Brück et al., 1994, 2002;

Lassmann, 2002; Ozawa et al., 1994), and the lack of correlation between demyelination and AD (Bitsch et al., 2000). In addition, this study emphasizes the facts that OL are decreased and that their capability to synthesize new myelin sheathes is impaired.

Although our study should be confirmed by analyses of a greater number of samples, its results bring arguments favouring the utilization, early in the course of MS, of efficient therapeutics that will take into account the axonal as well as the myelin components of plaques. From this point of view it is relevant to remember that, experimentally, growth factor supply alleviates, at least partly, both these demyelinating and axonal lesions (Jean et al., 2002).

ACKNOWLEDGMENTS

Supported by a grant (PHRC 21-01) from the University Hospital of Angers to CF. We thank the Neurologists from the Departments of Neurology from Pitié-Salpêtrière Hospital for their help in collecting clinical data, and Ms I. Viau and C. Dumez for skilful technical assistance.

REFERENCES

Akiyama Y, Radtke C, Kocsis JD. (2002). Remyelination of the rat spinal cord by transplantation of identified bone marrow stromal cells. *J Neurosci.* 22, 8823-8830.

Allamargot, C., Pouplard-Barthelaix, A., Fressinaud, C. (2001). A single intracerebral injection of platelet-derived growth factor (PDGF) accelerates the rate of remyelination in vivo. *Brain Res.* 918, 28-39.

Bachelin C, Lachapelle F, Girard C, Moissonnier P, Serguera-Lagache C et al., (2005). Efficient myelin repair in the macaque spinal cord by autologous grafts of Schwann cells. *Brain* 128, 540-549.

Baron-Van Evercooren, A., Gansmüller, A., Clerin, E., Gumpel, M. (1991). Visualization of Schwann cells transplanted in a demyelinated lesion of the adult mouse spinal cord. *Neurosci. Lett.* 131, 241-244.

Barres, B.A., Raff, M.C. (1993). Proliferation of oligodendrocyte precursor cells depends on electrical activity in axons. *Nature* 361, 258-260.

Bashir, K., Whitaker, J.N. (1999). Clinical and laboratory features of primary progressive and secondary progressive MS. *Neurology* 53, 765-771.

Ben-Hur T, Einstein O, Mizrachi-Kol R, Ben-Menachem O, Reinhartz E et al., (2003). Transplanted multipotential neural precursor cells migrate into the inflamed white matter in response to experimental autoimmune encephalomyelitis. *Glia* 41, 73-80.

Bitsch, A., Schuchardt, J., Bunkowski, S., Kuhlmann, T., Bruck, W. (2000). Acute axonal injury in multiple sclerosis. Correlation with demyelination and inflammation. *Brain* 123, 1174-1183.

Brück, W., Schmied, M., Suchanek, G., Brück, Y., Breitschopf, H., Poser, S., Piddlesden, S., Lassmann, H. (1994). Oligodendrocytes in the early course of multiple sclerosis. *Ann. Neurol.* 35, 65-73.

Brück, W., Lucchinetti, C., Lassmann, H. (2002). The pathology of primary progressive multiple sclerosis. *Mult. Scler.* 8, 93-97.

Brustle O, Jones KN, Learish RD, Karram K, Choudhary K et al., (1999). Embryonic stem cell-derived glial precursors : a source of myelinating transplants. *Science* 285, 650-651.

Cannella B, Pitt D, Marchionni M, Raine CS. (1999). Neuregulin and erbB receptor expression in normal and diseased human white matter. *J Neuroimmunol* 100, 233-242.

Cao Q, Benton RL, Whittemore SR. (2002). Stem cell repair of central nervous system injury. *J Neurosci Res* 68, 501-510.

Chang, A., Tourtelotte, W.W., Rudick, R., Trapp, B.D. (2002). Premyelinating oligodendrocytes in chronic lesions of multiple sclerosis. *N. Engl. J. Med.* 346, 165-173.

Charles, P., Reynolds, R., Seilhean, D., Rougon, G., Aigrot, M.S., Neizgoda, A., Zalc, B., Lubetzki, C. (2002). Re-expression of PSA-NCAM by demyelinated axons : an inhibitor of remyelination in multiple sclerosis ? *Brain* 125, 1972-1979.

Crang AJ, Gilson JM, Li WW, Blakemore WF. (2004). The remyelinating potential and in vitro differentiation of MOG-expressing oligodendrocyte precursors isolated from the adult rat CNS. *Eur J Neurosci* 20, 1445-1460.

Demerens, C., Stankoff, B., Anglade, P., Allinquant, B., Couraud, F., Zalc, B., Lubetzki, C. (1996). Induction of myelination in the central nervous system by electrical activity. *Proc. Natl. Acad. Sci. USA* 93, 9887-9892.

De Stefano, N., Narayanan, S., Francis, G.S., Arnaoutelis, R., Tartaglia, M.C., Antel, J.P., Matthews, P.M., Arnold, D.L. (2001). Evidence of axonal damage in the early stages of multiple sclerosis and its relevance to disability. *Arch. Neurol.* 58, 65-70.

Dusart, I., Morel, M.P., Wehrle, R., Sotelo, C. (1999). Late axonal sprouting of injured Purkinje cells and its temporal correlation with permissive changes in the glial scar. *J. Comp. Neurol.* 408, 399-418.

Dyck, P.J., Nukada, H., Lais, A.C., Karnes, J.L. (1984). Permanent axotomy: A model of chronic neuronal degeneration preceded by axonal atrophy, myelin remodeling and degeneration. In: Dyck PJ, Thomas PK, Lambert EH, Bunge R. (Eds), *Peripheral neuropathy, Saunders, Philadelphia*, pp. 666-690.

Evangelou, N., Konz, D., Esiri, M.M., Smith., S, Palace, J., Matthews, P.M. (2000). Regional axonal loss in the corpus callosum correlates with cerebral white matter lesion volume and distribution in multiple sclerosis. *Brain* 123, 1845-1849.

Eyer J, Peterson A. (1994). Neurofilament-deficient axons and perikaryal aggregates in viable transgenic mice expressing a neurofilament-b-galactosidase fusion protein. *Neuron* 12:389-405.

Falls DL. (2003). Neuregulins: functions, forms, and signalling strategies. *Exp Cell Res* 284, 14-30.

Fasani F, Bocquet A, Robert P, Peterson A, Eyer J. (2004). The amount of neurofilaments aggregated in the cell body is controlled by their increased sensitivity to trypsin-like proteases. *J Cell Sci* 117:861-869.

Ferguson, B., Matyszak, M.K., Esiri, M.M., Perry, V.H. (1997). Axonal damage in acute multiple sclerosis lesions. *Brain* 120, 393-399.

Franklin RJM, 2002). Remyelination of the demyelinated CNS: the case for and against transplantation of central, peripheral and olfactory glia. *Brain Res Bull* 57, 827-832.

Fressinaud, C., Vallat, J.M., Rigaud, M., Cassagne, C., Labourdette, G., Sarlièvre, L.L. (1990). Investigation of myelination in vitro: polar lipid content and fatty acid composition of myelinating oligodendrocytes in rat oligodendrocyte cultures. *Neurochem. Int.* 16, 27-39.

Fressinaud, C., Vallat, J.M., Pouplard-Barthelaix, A. (1996). Platelet-derived growth factor partly prevents chemically induced oligodendrocyte death and improves myelin-like membranes repair in vitro. *Glia* 16, 40-50.

Fressinaud, C., Jean, I. (2002). Polyradiculonévrites inflammatoires chroniques et cytosquelette axonal : données morphométriques et immunocytochimiques. *Rev. Neurol.* (Paris) 158, 713-718.

Fressinaud, C., Vigneron, I., Letournel, F., Nicolas, G., Jean, I., Dubas F. (2002). Cytoskeleton abnormalities in axonopathies of unknown aetiology: correlations with morphometry. *J. Neurol. Sci.* 196, 53-61.

Fressinaud, C., Jean, I., Dubas, F. (2003). Vascularites nécrosantes du système nerveux périphérique : comparaison des anomalies du cytosquelette axonal avec d'autres types de neuropathies. *Rev. Neurol.* (Paris) 159, 293-299.

Fressinaud, C. (2005). Repeated injuries dramatically affect cells of the oligodendrocyte lineage : effects of PDGF and NT-3 in vitro. *Glia* 49, 555-566.

Fressinaud, C., Jean, I., Dubas, F. (2005). Modifications des neurofilaments et des microtubules axonaux en fonction du mécanisme lésionnel : étude pathologique et expérimentale. *Rev. Neurol.* (Paris) 161, 55-60.

Fressinaud, C., Berges, R., Bocquet, A., Eyer, J. (2006). Neurofilament associated proteins specifically alter oligodendrocyte development in vitro : relevance for MS. *J. Neurochem.*, 2006, 96 (Suppl. 1), Abstract PTW08-2 p. 133.

Frohman EM, Racke MK, Raine CS. (2006). Multiple sclerosis – The plaque and its pathogenesis. *N Engl J Med* 354, 942-955.

Giordana, M.T., Richiardi, P., Trevisan, E., Boghi, A., Palmucci, L. (2002). Abnormal ubiquitination of axons in normally myelinated white matter in multiple sclerosis brain. *Neuropathol. Appl. Neurobiol.* 28, 35-41.

Guennoc, A.M., Stankoff, B., Barbin, G., Zalc, B., Lubetzki, C. (2001). Rôle de la paranodine dans la myélinisation du SNC. *Rev. Neurol.* (Paris) 157, suppl 3, 2S51 abstract F13.

Hammerschlag R, Brady ST. (1989). Axonal transport and the neuronal cytoskeleton. In: *Basic neurochemistry.* Siegel G, Agranoff B, Albert RW, Molinoff P (Eds), Raven Press, New York, pp. 457-478.

Hartung, H.P., Ritz, M.F., Steck, A.J. (1999). Eléments de neuro-immunologie. In: . Steck, A.J., coordinator, Bogousslavsky, J., Léger, J.M., Mas, J.L., (Eds), *Affections démyélinisantes. Neuroimmunologie et clinique. Traité de neurologie.* Doin, Rueil-Malmaison, pp. 35-60.

Hoffman, P.N., Cleveland, D.W., Griffin, J.W., Landes, P.N., Cowan, N.J., Price, D.L. (1987). *Neurofilament gene expression : a major determinant of axonal caliber.* Proc. Natl. Acad. Sci. USA 84, 3472-3476.

Hoffman, P.N. (1989). Expression of GAP-43, a rapidly transported growth-associated protein and class II beta tubulin, a slowly transported cytoskeletal protein, are coordinated in regenerating neurons. *J. Neurosci.* 9, 893-897.

Ingle, G.T., Thompson, A.J., Miller, D.H. (2002). Magnetic resonance imaging in primary progressive multiple sclerosis. *J. Rehabil. Res.* Dev. 39, 261-271.

Jean, I., Allamargot, C., Barthelaix-Pouplard, A., Fressinaud, C. (2002). Axonal lesions and PDGF-enhanced remyelination in the rat corpus callosum after lysolecithin demyelination. *Neuroreport* 13, 627-631.

Jean I, Fressinaud C. (2003). Spontaneous central nervous system remyelination is not altered in NFH-lacZ transgenic mice after chemical demyelination. *J Neurosci Res* 73:54-60.

Jean, I., Lavialle, C., Barthelaix-Pouplard, A., Fressinaud, C. (2003). Neurotrophin-3 specifically increases mature oligodendrocyte population and enhances remyelination after chemical demyelination of adult rat CNS. *Brain Res.* 972, 110-118.

Kapaki, E., Paraskevas, G.P., Michalopoulou, M., Kilidireas, K. (2000). Increased cerebrospinal fluid tau protein in multiple sclerosis. *Eur. Neurol.* 43, 228-232.

Kuhlmann, T., Lucchinetti, C., Zettl, U.K., Bitsch, A., Lassmann, H., Brück, W. (1999). Bcl-2 expressing oligodendrocytes in multiple sclerosis lesions. *Glia* 28, 34-39.

Lassmann, H., 2002. Mechanisms of demyelination and tissue destruction in multiple sclerosis. *Clin. Neurol. Neurosurg.* 104, 168-171.

Letournel F, Bocquet A, Dubas F, Barthelaix A, Eyer J. (2003). Stable tubule only polypeptides (STOP) proteins co-aggregate with spheroid neurofilaments in amyotrohic lateral sclerosis. *J Neuropathol Exp Neurol* 62:1211-1219.

Losseff, N.A., Webb, S.L., O'Riordan, J.I., Page, R., Wang, L., Barker, G.J., Tofts, P.S., McDonald, W.I., Miller, D.H., Thompson, A.J. (1996). Spinal cord atrophy and disability in multiple sclerosis. A new reproductible and sensitive MRI method with potential to monitor disease progression. *Brain* 119, 701-708.

Lucchinetti, C., Brück, W., Parisi, J., Scheithauer, B., Rodriguez, M., Lassmann, H. (1999). A quantitative analysis of oligodendrocytes in multiple sclerosis. A study of 113 cases. *Brain* 122, 2279-2295.

Lucchinetti, C., Brück, W., Parisi, J., Scheithauer, B., Rodriguez, M., Lassmann, H. (2000). Heterogeneity of multiple sclerosis lesions: implications for the pathogenesis of demyelination. *Ann. Neurol.* 47, 707-717.

Lycke, J.N., Karlsson, J.E., Andersen, O., Rosengren, L.E. (1998). Neurofilament protein in cerebrospinal fluid: a potential marker of activity in multiple scerosis. J. Neurol. Neurosurg. *Psychiatry* 64, 402-404.

Macklin, W.B., Weill, C.L., Deininger, P.L. (1986). Expression of myelin proteolipid and myelin basic protein mRNAs in culture cells. *J. Neurosci. Res.* 16, 203-217.

McDonnell, G.V., Hawkins, S.A. (2002). Primary progressive multiple sclerosis : increasing clarity but many unanswered questions. *J. Neurol. Sci.* 199, 1-15.

McPherson SW, Heuss ND, Roehrich H, Gregerson DS. (2006). Bystander killing of neurons by cytotoxic T cells specific for a glial antigen. Glia 53, 457-466.

Matsumoto, Y., Ohmori, K., Fujiwara, M. (1992). Microglial and astroglial reactions to inflammatory lesions of experimental autoimmune encephalomyelitis in the rat central nervous system. *J. Neuroimmunol.* 37, 23-33.

Medana, I., Martinic, M.A., Wekerle, H., Neumann, H. (2001). Tansection of major histocompatibility complex class I-induced neuritis by cytotoxic T lymphocytes. *Am. J. Pathol.* 159, 809-815.

Mews, I., Bergmann, M., Bunkowski, S., Gulotta, F., Brück, W. (1998). Oligodendrocyte and axon pathology in clinically silent multiple sclerosis lesions. *Mult. Scler.* 4, 55-62.

Narayanan, S., Fu, L., Pioro, E., De Stefano, N., Collins, D.L., Francis, G.S., Antel J.P., Matthews, P.M., Arnold, D.L. (1997). Imaging of axonal damage in multiple sclerosis: spatial distribution of magnetic resonance imaging lesions. *Ann. Neurol.* 41, 385-391.

Nistor GI, Totoiu MO, Haque N, Carpenter MK, Kierstead HS. (2005). Human embryonic stem cells differentiate into oligodendrocytes in high purity and myelinate after spinal cord transplantation. *Glia* 49, 385-396.

Øren, A., White, L.R., Aasly, J. (2001). Apoptosis in neurons exposed to cerebrospinal fluid from patients with multiple sclerosis or acute polyradiculoneuropathy. *J. Neurol. Sci.* 186, 31-36.

Ozawa, K., Suchanek, G., Breitschopf, H., Brück, W., Budka, H., Jellinger, K., Lassmann, H. (1994). Patterns of oligodendroglia pathology in multiple sclerosis. *Brain* 117, 1311-1322.

Prineas, J.W., McDonald, W.I. (1997). Demyelinating diseases. In: Graham DI, Lantos PL. (Eds), *Greenfield's neuropathology*, Arnold, London, pp. 813-896.

Raine, C.S., Cross ,A.H. (1989). Axonal dystrophy as a consequence of long-term demyelination. Lab. Invest. 60, 714-725.

Ridet, J.L., Malhotra, S.K., Privat, A., Gage, F.H., 1997). *Reactive astrocytes: cellular and molecular cues to biological function.* TINS 20, 570-577.

Rodriguez, M., Scheithauer, B.W., Forbes, G., Kelly, P. (1993). Oligodendrocyte injury is an early event in lesions of multiple sclerosis. *Mayo Clin. Proc.* 68, 627-636.

Sanchez, I., Hassinger, L., Paskevich, P.A., Shine, H.D., Nixon, R.A. (1996). Oligodendroglia regulate the regional expansion of axon caliber and local accumulation of neurofilaments during development independently of myelin formation. . *Neurosci.* 16, 5095-5105.

Sargent PB, 1992). Signalisation électrique. In : *Introduction à la neurobiologie moléculaire.* Hall ZW (Ed), Flammarion, Paris, pp. 33-80.

Schwab, C., McGeer, P.L. (2002). Complement activated C4d immunoreactive oligodendrocytes delineate small cortical plaques in multiple sclerosis. *Exp. Neurol.* 174, 81-88.

Scolding, N., Franklin, R., Stevens, S., Heldin, C.H., Compston, A., Newcombe, J. (1998). Oligodendrocyte progenitors are present in the normal adult human CNS and in the lesions of multiple sclerosis. *Brain* 121, 2221-2228.

Semra, Y.K., Seidi, O.A., Sharief, M.K. (2002). Heightened intrathecal release of axonal cytoskeletal proteins in multiple sclerosis is associated with progressive disease and clinical disability. *J. Neuroimmunol.* 122, 132-139.

Silber, E., Sharief, M.K. (1999). Axonal degeneration in the pathogenesis of multiple sclerosis. *J. Neurol. Sci.* 170, 11-18.

Thompson, A.J., Polman, C.H., Miller, D.H., McDonald, W.I., Brochet, B., Filippi, M., Montalban, X., De Sa, J. (1997). Primary progressive multiple sclerosis. *Brain* 120, 1085-1096.

Trapp, B.D., Peterson, J., Ransohof, R.M., Rudick, R., Mörk, S., Bö, L. (1998). Axonal transection in the lesions of multiple sclerosis. *N. Engl. J. Med.* 338, 278-285.

Trifilieff, E., Luu, B., Nussbaum, J.L., Roussel, G., Espinosa de los Monteros, A., Sabatier, J.M., Van Rietschoten, J. (1986). A specific immunological probe for the major myelin proteolipid. Confirmation of a deletion in DM 20. *FEBS Lett.* 198, 235-239.

Uschkureit, T., Spörkel, O., Stracke, J., Büssow, H., Stoffel, W. (2000). Early onset of axonal degeneration in double (plp-/-mag-/-) and hypomyelinosis in triple (plp-/-mbp-/-mag-/-) mutant mice. *J. Neurosci.* 20, 5225-5233.

Viehover A, Miller RH, Park SK, Fischbach G, Vartanian T. (2001). Neuregulin: an oligodendrocyte growth factor absent in active multiple sclerosis lesions. *Dev Neurosci* 23, 377-386.

Westenbroek, R.E., Bausch, S.B., Lin, R.C., Franck, J.E., Noebels, J.L., Catterall, W.A. (1998). Upregulation of L-type Ca2+ channels in reactive astrocytes after brain injury, hypomyelination, and ischemia. *J. Neurosci.* 18, 2321-2334.

Windebank, A.J., Wood, P., Bunge, R.P., Dyck, P.J. (1985). Myelination determines the caliber of dorsal root ganglion neurons in culture. *J. Neurosci.* 5, 1563-1569.

Wu, E., Raine, C.S. (1992). Multiple sclerosis, interactions between oligodendrocytes and hypertrophic astrocytes and their occurrence in other, nondemyelinating conditions. *Lab. Invest.* 67, 88-99.

Zhao C, Fancy SPJ, Magy L, Urwin JE, Franklin RJM. (2005. Stem cells, progenitors and myelin repair. *J Anat* 207, 251-258.

Zhu, B., Moore, G.R.W., Zwimpfer, T.J., Kastrukoff, L.F., Dyer, J.K., Steeves, J.D., Paty, D.W., Cynader, M.S. (1999). Axonal cytoskeleton changes in experimental optic neutitis. *Brain Res.* 824, 204-217.

In: Multidrug Resistance-Associated Proteins
Editor: Christopher V. Aiello, pp. 159-178

ISBN 1-60021-298-0
© 2007 Nova Science Publishers, Inc.

Chapter 7

MULTIDRUG RESISTANCE-ASSOCIATED PROTEINS AND EFFLUX OF ORGANIC ANIONS AT THE BLOOD-BRAIN AND BLOOD CEREBROSPINAL FLUID BARRIERS

Jan Wijnholds[*]

Department of Neuromedical Genetics, Netherlands Institute for Neuroscience,
and Division of Molecular Biology, The Netherlands Cancer Institute,
Amsterdam, the Netherlands

ABSRACT

Multidrug Resistance-associated Proteins (MRPs) are membrane proteins transporting organic anions. MRP1, MRP2, MRP4, and MRP5 (ABCC1, ABCC2, ABCC4, and ABCC5) and orphan organic anion efflux pump activities are detected in the brain. MRP1 is known to be a major basolateral transporter in epithelial cells, also expressed in the choroid plexus. MRP2 is a major apical canalicular multispecific organic anion transporter in the liver, also detected at brain blood capillaries. MRP4 and MRP5 are expressed in the choroid plexus and brain capillary endothelial cells. We discuss the putative roles of MRPs and orphan organic anion efflux pumps in the brain.

[*] Correspondence concerning this article should be addressed to Jan Wijnholds, Department of Neuromedical Genetics, Netherlands Institute for Neuroscience, Meibergdreef 47, 1105 BA, Amsterdam, The Netherlands, tel. +31-20-5664597, fax +31-20-5666121, e-mail j.wijnholds@nin.knaw.nl.

INTRODUCTION

The brain protects itself successfully against xenobiotics and metabolic waste products by an array of efflux pumps at the blood-brain barrier (BBB) and blood-cerebrospinal fluid barrier (BCSFB). The most well known of these pumps is P-glycoprotein (P-gp), the protein product of the Multidrug Resistance 1 gene (*MDR1* in human, *Mdr1a* and *Mdr1b* in rodents; *ABCB1*), which localizes at the apical or luminal plasma membrane of brain capillary endothelium and limits the delivery of drug substrates to their targets in the brain by actively transporting the substrates into the bloodstream. P-gp actively restricts the passage of many lipophilic compounds from the blood into the brain and can contribute to the efflux of substrates from the brain into the blood (Schinkel et al., 1996; Schinkel and Jonker, 2003). Similar to its function in the apical plasma membranes of intestinal epithelia, P-gp in brain endothelium regulates the availability of many non-charged or weakly basic substrates (e.g., lipophilic drugs).

Subsequent to the discovery of P-gp as one of the main efflux transporters at the BBB (Schinkel et al., 1994), the role of other ATP-binding cassette (ABC) proteins at the BBB or BCSFB has been investigated (reviewed in Ghersi-Egea and Strazielle, 2002; Hagenbuch et al., 2002). Several members of the Multidrug Resistance-associated Protein (MRP) family, MRP1, MRP2, MRP4, MRP5 (ABCC1, ABCC2, ABCC4, ABCC5) have been detected in the endothelium of brain capillaries and/or epithelium of the choroid plexus suggesting possible functions for these pumps at the BBB or BCSFB. However, whereas there are clear roles for P-gp in the BBB, the biochemical and physiological role(s) of the 9 MRP family members (MRP1-9; ABCC1-6 and ABCC10-12) need to be further clarified.

MRPs are multi-specific organic anion transporters that can transport negatively charged acidic anionic drugs, including several pyrimidine and purine based nucleotide analogs, and drugs or natural compounds conjugated to glutathione, sulfate or glucuronate (reviewed by Borst et al., 2000; Hipfner et al., 1999; Jedlitschky and Keppler, 2002; Kruh et al., 2001). Neutral drugs can also be transported by several of the MRPs (MRP1, MRP2, MRP4, MRP5) if co-transported with glutathione. MRP1, MRP2, MRP4 and MRP5 are prominently present in the brain (Kool et al., 1997; Lee et al., 2004; Miller et al., 2000; Rao et al., 1999; Wijnholds et al., 2000, 2002), whereas expression of MRP3 and MRP6 is low (Lee et al., 2004). Levels of MRP1 protein in brain capillaries are low (Cisternino et al., 2003; Wijnholds et al., 2000) thus excluding a main role for MRP1 in the BBB, however MRP2, MRP4, and MRP5 protein has been demonstrated in the endothelium of brain capillaries and other blood vessels (Leggas et al., 2004; Miller et al., 2000; Mitani et al., 2003; Nies et al., 2002; Zhang et al., 2000, 2004). Levels of MRP1 protein in the basal plasma membrane of the choroid plexus epithelium are high and MRP1 has been shown to contribute to the blood-CSF drug permeability barrier (Rao et al., 1999; Wijnholds et al., 2000). MRP4 and MRP5 are highly expressed in the epithelium of the choroid plexus as well (Lee et al., 2004; Leggas et al., 2004).

This chapter will focus on MRP1, MRP2, MRP4, and MRP5 and organic anion efflux pump activities readily detected in the brain. Various organic anion efflux transporter activities have been discovered at the BBB and BCSFB that have not yet been ascribed to a specific transporter and the potential involvement of MRP family members will be examined.

MRP1 AND MRP2

Human multidrug resistance-associated protein 1 (MRP1), also designated ABCC1 and 1531 amino acids in length, was discovered in 1992 and demonstrated to be involved in drug resistance against a broad variety of neutral and negatively charged drugs (Cole et al., 1992). Not long after the discovery of MRP1, a second member of the family comprising 1545 amino acids was identified as the liver canalicular multispecific organic anion transporter, cMOAT, ABCC2, or MRP2 (Paulusma et al., 1996). Subsequent database searches revealed the existence of 9 MRP or ABCC family members that show different tissue and subcellular plasma membrane distributions (Table 1) and substrate specificities (Borst et al., 2000; Kruh et al., 2001; Jedlitschky and Keppler, 2002). The 9 MRP family members share a predicted core structure and membrane topology with P-gp; two nucleotide-binding domains (ATP-binding cassettes) and two arrays of 6 transmembrane domains. MRP1-3 and MRP6-7 have a short extra amino-terminal intracellular domain, called the L0 domain, and an extra transmembrane domain consisting of 5 membrane-spanning regions for MRP1. MRP4-5 and MRP8-9 only have a short extra amino-terminal intracellular domain.

The tissue distribution and substrate specificities of MRP1 and other MRP family members are summarized in Table 1. MRP1 provides substantial resistance to multidrug resistance (MDR) drugs such as anthracyclins, *Vinca* alkaloids, and podophyllotoxins, as well as to various other xenobiotics (Borst et al., 2000; Kruh et al., 2001; Jedlitschky and Keppler, 2002). Transport studies demonstrate that MRP1 preferentially transports glutathione and glucuronide conjugates. Some substrates are transported unmodified in the presence of glutathione. This co-transport activity is shared by at least 3 other members of the MRP1 family, MRP2, MRP4, and MRP5, but not MRP3 which is the closest relative of MRP1 in the MRP family. MRP1 protein has a broad tissue distribution but is mainly detected on the basolateral surface of polarized cells including choroid plexus, kidney, and lung epithelium, and Sertoli cells. High protein levels are also found in bone marrow-derived cells (e.g., erythrocytes, white blood cells, mast cells), whereas low levels are found in the liver and brain capillary endothelium (Evers et al., 1996; Robbiani et al., 2000; Wijnholds et al., 1998). Under pathological conditions such as epilepsy, MRP1 can be detected in glial cells of the cortex and hippocampus near to blood vessels within the malformed region and MRP1 can be detected in dysplastic neurons in the cortex (Sisodiya et al., 2002).

To date, the physiological role of only three MRPs has been demonstrated. MRP1 mediates inflammation through the export of leukotriene C_4 from mast cells and macrophages; mice without MRP1 have an altered response to inflammatory stimuli (Robbiani et al., 2000, Schultz et al., 2001, Wijnholds et al., 1997). Furthermore, MRP1 is a protective drug efflux pump in several tissues including epithelia of the colon, urinary collecting duct, oropharynx, and choroid plexus, and the blood-testis barrier due to its presence in the basal plasma membrane of Sertoli cells. MRP2 is a transporter of organic anions from liver into bile (e.g., bilirubin glucuronides). Loss of MRP2 function in humans leads to the mild liver disease called Dubin-Johnson syndrome (Kartenbeck et al., 1996, Paulusma et al., 1997). Loss of MRP6 function leads in human to the skin and eye disease pseudoxanthoma elasticum (Bergen et al., 2000, Le Saux et al., 2000, Ringpfeil et al., 2000), and in mice to ectopic mineralization of connective tissues (Gorgels et al., 2005; Klement et al., 2005). No physiological functions are known yet for the other MRPs, but single knockout

(KO) mice lacking one of the transporters MRP1-6 are healthy and viable (Lorico et al., 1997; Uitto et al., 2003; Wijnholds et al., 1997; Zelcer et al, 2004; Wijnholds, Schinkel and Borst, unpublished data), as are double KO mice that lack MRP4/MRP5 (Wijnholds, Wielinga, and Borst, unpublished data) and triple KO mice that lack MRP1/Mdr1a/Mdr1b (Wijnholds et al., 2000).

Table 1. Tissue distribution, plasma membrane location, and substrate specificity of MRPs

MRP	ABCC or other name	Tissue distribution	Protein in		Plasma membrane location	Preferred substrates
			BBB	BCSFB		
MRP1	ABCC1 MRP	Ubiquitous (low in liver)	-	+	Basolateral	GS-X, Gluc-X MDR drugs, MTX GSH
MRP2	ABCC2 CMOAT cMRP	Liver, kidney, gut	+	-	Apical	GS-X, Gluc-X MDR drugs, MTX GSH
MRP3	ABCC3 MOAT-D CMOAT-2	Liver, kidney, gut, adrenals, pancreas, gallbladder	?	?	Basolateral	Gluc-X, Sulf-X MDR drugs, MTX
MRP4	ABCC4 MOAT-B	Ubiquitous (high in prostate, lung, pancreas, muscle, testis, ovary, bladder, gallbladder)	+	+	Apical and basolateral	NMP analogues, cGMP, cAMP Gluc-X, Sulf-X MTX, GSH
MRP5	ABCC5 MOAT-C PABC11	Ubiquitous (low in liver)	?	+	Basolateral	NMP analogues, cGMP MTX GS-X GSH
MRP6	ABCC6 MOAT-E MLP-1	Liver, kidney	?	?	Basolateral	GS-X peptides?
MRP7	ABCC10	Ubiquitous	?	?	?	?
MRP8	ABCC11	?	?	?	?	NMP analogues, cGMP, cAMP
MRP9	ABCC12	Breast?, testis	?	?		?

Abbreviations: ABC, ATP-binding cassette; ABCC, C group of ABC transporters; GS-X, Gluc-X, Sulf-X: substrate conjugated to glutathione (GSH), glucuronide, or sulfate, respectively; MDR drugs, multidrug resistance drugs; MLP-1, MRP-like protein 1; cMOAT, canalicular multispecific organic anion transporter; MRP, Multidrug resistance protein; MTX, methotrexate; NMP, nucleoside monophosphate; cGMP and cAMP, 3',5'-cyclic GMP and AMP, respectively. MRP1-6 have been reviewed in e.g. in Bodo et al. (2003) and Borst et al. (2000); MRP7 in Chen et al. (2003) and MRP8 in Bera et al. (2001) and Guo et al. (2003), MRP9 in Bera et al. (2002).

Independent gene KO studies in mice have contributed substantially to our present understanding of the physiological function and substrate specificity of human MRP1. MRP1

KO mice are healthy and fertile, but show an altered response to inflammatory stimuli (Robbiani et al., 2000, Schultz et al., 2001, Wijnholds et al., 1997) and a hypersensitivity to toxic drugs such as the anticancer drug etoposide (Lorico et al., 1997; Wijnholds et al., 1997, 1998). In these mice, etoposide causes damage to bone marrow, epithelium of urinary collecting ductules, large intestines, and oropharynx, and Sertoli cells of the testis, (Wijnholds et al., 1998). Furthermore, increased levels of reduced glutathione (GSH) are found in MRP1 KO tissues in accordance with the demonstrated co-transport function of GSH by MRP1 (Rappa et al., 1996).

In MRP1 KO mice etoposide readily passes the choroid plexus due to reduced BCSFB function (Wijnholds et al., 2000). In these experiments, cannulas were implanted into the lateral ventricles of mice lacking MRP1/Mdr1a/Mdr1b or Mdr1a/Mdr1b, CSF samples were taken at regular time intervals and coincidently artificial CSF was introduced in the ventricles to compensate for withdrawal. After intravenous injection of etoposide, levels of etoposide were not significantly increased in total brain tissue suggesting no relevant or a largely redundant role of MRP1 at the BBB of mice lacking Mdr1, but the levels in CSF increased 10-fold suggesting a major role at the BCSFB in preventing MRP1 substrates to pass from the blood into the CSF. These data are supported by Rao et al. (1999) who showed in elegant experiments that the MRP1 substrate sestamibi readily crossed the BCSFB in vivo and in vitro in the absence, but not the presence, of MRP1 inhibitors, strongly suggesting an important role for MRP1 at the BCSFB. Most recently, in situ brain perfusion experiments on wild-type and MRP1 KO mice were used by Cisternino et al. (2003) to demonstrate that MRP1 does not play a significant role in the transport of etoposide and estradiol-17-β-glucuronide (E$_2$17βG) across the luminal membrane of the endothelial cells at the BBB. So, MRP1 localized at the basolateral plasma membrane of the choroid plexus epithelium plays a role in the prevention of drug substrates to enter the CSF via the choroid plexus.

It is likely that other members of the MRP family are active at the BCSFB and BBB. This is exemplified by recent experiments by Lee et al. (2004) who showed that high affinity substrates for MRP1 such as 2,4-dinitrophenyl-S-glutathione (DNP-GS) and E$_2$17βG, were not transported by MRP1 across the BCSFB after intravenous or intracerebroventricular injection (Lee et al., 2004; Nishino et al., 1999). The apparent CSF elimination rate constants for these two substrates did not differ significantly between wild type and MRP1 KO mice. MRP4 and MRP5 are both abundantly expressed in the choroid plexus, DNP-GS is a substrate for MRP5, and E$_2$17βG is a substrate for MRP4, suggesting that MRP4 and MRP5 could also contribute to the BCSFB. It is likely that MRP1 BCSFB function as showed by Wijnholds et al. (2000) could be distinguished from MRP4 and MRP5-mediated efflux because etoposide is poorly transported by MRP4 and MRP5 (Lee et al., 2000; Schuetz et al. 1999, Wijnholds et al., 2000).

The liver canalicular multispecific organic anion transporter, cMOAT or MRP2 or ABCC2, has broad substrate specificity like MRP1 (Kool et al., 1997). It co-transports GSH and neutral drugs, glutathione- and glucuronate-conjugates, and typical MDR drugs (Borst and Oude Elferink, 2002). MRP2 is strongly expressed at the luminal or apical side of epithelium in the liver, kidney, and small intestine. Using confocal laser scanning microscopy and quantitative image analysis, Miller et al. (2000) showed that MRP2, located at the apical plasma membrane of endothelium in isolated rat and pig brain capillaries, transported sulforhodamine 101 and fluorescein methotrexate into the capillary lumen. This transport was inhibited by LTC_4, chlorodinitrobenzene, saquinavir and ritonavir, but not by the P-gp inhibitors PSC833 and verapamil. Recently, Potschka et al. (2003) demonstrated the contribution of MRP2 to efflux at the BBB by showing that the anti-epileptic drug phenytoin accumulated in the brain of MRP2-deficient rats. Furthermore, in wild-type rats, the accumulation of phenytoin increased in the presence of probenecid. Using a model for epilepsy, they could also show that the anticonvulsant activity of phenytoin was markedly higher in MRP2 deficient rats compared to normal rats. In a more recent study using MRP2-deficient rats, Lee et al. (2004) excluded a role for MRP2 in transport of DNP-GS or $E_217\beta G$ across the BCSFB.

In summary, MRP1 and MRP2 are broad specificity plasma membrane organic anion transporters able to transport negatively charged drugs and conjugates of GSH and glucuronate, and to lesser extent sulfate. Some neutrally charged unconjugated drugs are also co-transported with GSH by MRP1 and MRP2. MRP1 and MRP2 are both inhibited by many typical inhibitors of organic anion transport such as sulfinpyrazone and probenecid. No or only little MRP1 is present in human and mouse brain blood capillaries suggesting no major role at the BBB, whereas MRP2 is present in rat brain blood capillaries and recent experiments indicated MRP2-associated pump activity at the BBB. MRP1 is abundantly present in the choroid plexus where it confers BCSFB function by extruding substrates from the CSF towards the blood and restricting the entrance of substrates from the blood to the CSF. Levels of MRP2 at the BCSFB barrier are low, suggesting no major role for MRP2 at the BCSFB.

MRP4 AND MRP5

Lee et al. (1998) was the first to clone human MRP4, also called ABCC4. The MRP4 gene encodes a protein of 1325 amino acids and is amplified in the human T-lymphoid cell line CEM-r1 which is highly resistant to the antiviral agent 9-(2-phosphonyl-methoxyethyl)-adenine (PMEA), an analogue of AMP (Schuetz et al., 1999). These cells efflux PMEA rapidly and subsequent work has shown that transfection of NIH-3T3 cells with MRP4 cDNA confers resistance to PMEA, methotrexate, 6-mercaptopurine (6-MP) and thioguanine (Adachi et al., 2002; Lee et al., 2000). These data indicate that MRP4 is a nucleoside monophosphate transporter.

Several groups cloned and analysed human MRP5, also called ABCC5 (Belinsky et al., 1998; Jedlitschky et al., 2000; McAleer et al., 1999; Suzuki et al., 2000; Wijnholds et al., 2000). MRP5, a protein of 1437 amino acids, effluxes DNP-GS and GSH, and acidic organic dyes such as 5-chloromethylfluorescein diacetate (CMFDA) and 5-fluorescein diacetate (FDA), and this efflux is inhibited by organic anion transport inhibitors such as sulfinpyrazone and benzbromarone (McAleer et al., 1999; Wijnholds et al., 2000).

MRP4 and MRP5 have closely related secondary structures (Belinsky et al., 1998; Lee et al., 1998) and show partial overlap in substrate specificities (Table 1). Both are organic anion pumps with affinity for pyrimidine- and purine-based nucleotide analogues and the cyclic nucleotides cGMP and cAMP. Both MRP4 and MRP5 transport all major thiopurine monophosphates which are important in the efficacy of mercaptopurine, with some differences in the substrate specificity (Wielinga et al., 2002; Wijnholds et al., 2000). For instance, both transport thio-IMP, whereas only MRP5 transports thioxanthosine monophosphate (tXMP). Additionally, during incubation of HEK293 human embryonic kidney cells with thioguanine, the monophosphorylated form of thioguanosine was transported by both MRP4 and MRP5 but the highest transport rate was for MRP4. Recent work has demonstrated that the 3',5'-cyclic nucleotides, cAMP and cGMP are relatively high affinity substrates for MRP4 and MRP5 (Chen et al., 2001, 2002; Jedlitschky et al., 2000; Lai and Tan, 2002; Wielinga et al., 2003). Although, in cells in which cyclic nucleotide synthesis is strongly induced by nitric oxide inducing compounds and phosphodiesterase activity is limited, MRP4 and MRP5 seem to act as low affinity cyclic nucleotide transporters (Wielinga et al., 2003). MRP4 mediates substantial resistance against other acyclic nucleoside phosphonates, whereas MRP5 does not (Reid et al., 2003). MRP4 mediates low-level cladribine resistance, whereas the cytotoxicity of clinically used anticancer nucleosides was not influenced by the overexpression of MRP4 or MRP5. MRP5, but not MRP4, transports the pyrimidine-based antiviral 2',3'-dideoxynucleoside 2',3'-didehydro-2',3'-dideoxythymidine 5'-monophosphate (d4TMP) and its phosphoramidate derivative alaninyl-d4TMP. Further analyses of differences in substrate specificity showed that dipyridamole, dilazep, nitrobenzyl mercaptopurine riboside, sildenafil, trequinsin and MK571 inhibited MRP4 more than MRP5, whereas cyclic nucleotides and monophosphorylated nucleoside analogs were equally poor inhibitors of both pumps. These results strongly suggested that the affinity of MRP4 and MRP5 for nucleotide-based substrates is rather low.

The experiments described above show the need for identifying more relevant substrates for MRP4 and MRP5. Recent experiments demonstrated that MRP4 can release prostaglandins from cells and that prostaglandins (PG) E1 and E2 are good substrates for MRP4 but not for MRP5 or MRP1-3 (Reid et al., 2003). In addition, PGF1α, PGF2α, PGA1 and thromboxane B2 were shown to be high-affinity inhibitors and candidate substrates of MRP4. Membrane vesicles of V79 hamster fibroblasts overproducing MRP4 mediated ATP-dependent cotransport of GSH or S-methyl-glutathione together with cholyltaurine, cholylglycine, or cholate (Rius et al., 2003). The GSH transport could be inhibited by several monoanionic bile salts and MK571. MRP4, but not MRP5, transports glucuronate conjugated substrates such as estradiol $E_217\beta G$. Transport of $E_217\beta G$ by MRP4 in membrane vesicles is inhibited by bile salts, especially by the sulfated derivatives estradiol 3,17-disulphate and taurolithocholate 3-sulphate (Zelcer et al., 2003).

Both proteins are ubiquitously expressed, with relatively high levels of MRP4 in prostate, lung, muscle, bladder, ovary and gallbladder, and with high levels of MRP5 in muscle and brain (Kool et al., 1997; Lee et al., 2000). Both proteins are expressed in the choroid plexus (Choudhuri S et al., 2003; Lee et al., 2004) and brain capillary endothelial cells (Soontornmalai et al., 2006; Zhang et al., 2000, 2004). However the role of these two transporters in the blood-brain and blood-CSF barriers is unknown.

Recently, MRP4 KO mice, that lack the MRP4 protein, were generated (Leggas et al., 2004). These mice showed increased accumulation of the anticancer drug topotecan in brain tissue and CSF. Microdialysis sampling of vesicular CSF of wild type and MRP4 KO mice demonstrated that MRP4 limits substrate penetration into the CSF. In accordance, MRP4 localized to the basolateral membrane of the choroid plexus epithelium. Remarkably, MRP4 localized also to the apical membrane of endothelial cells of the brain capillaries where it limits the entrance of substrates into the brain (Leggas et al., 2004). We have generated MRP5 KO mice that lack the MRP5 transporter protein. These mice do not show an obvious phenotype; the mice are healthy and fertile and do not have a shortened lifespan (Wijnholds and Borst; unpublished results). The physiological role of MRP5 may be hidden by redundancy of MRP transporters, e.g. because of the overlapping substrate specificity and tissue distribution with MRP4. MRP4/MRP5 double KO mice are viable and fertile as well (Wijnholds, Wielinga, and Borst, unpublished results), therefore, elucidation of the role of MRP5 will be analyzed using MRP4/MRP5 double KO mice compared to MRP4 KO mice.

"ORPHAN" ORGANIC ANION EFFLUX ACTIVITIES AT THE BBB AND BCSFB

Entry and efflux of drugs, toxins and xenobiotics to and from the central nervous system occurs largely at the BBB. However, the surface area of the choroid plexus is in the same size range as the luminal area of the capillary endothelial cells of the BBB and is also believed to have an important role in the exchange of substrates (Keep and Jones, 1990; Milhorat, 1976; Spector, 1986, 1990). Knowing the presence or absence of different unidirectional and bidirectional transporters at the BBB and BCSFB may provide insight into the range of drugs, toxins and xenobiotics that can potentially provide a means of detoxification in the brain (reviewed in Hagenbuch et al., 2002, 2003; Schinkel, 2001). Recently Choudhuri and coworkers (2003) demonstrated that, in addition to MRP1, MRP4 and MRP5, various other transporter mRNAs are expressed at moderate to high levels in rat choroid plexus. These transporters include organic anion transporting polypeptides 2 and 3 (Oatp2, Oatp3), organic anion transporters 2 and 3 (Oat2, Oat3), organic cation transporters N1 and N2 (OctN1, OctN2), Menke's metal transporter, divalent metal transporter 1 (DMT1), equilibrative nucleotide transporter 1 (Ent1), constitutive nucleotide transporters 1 and 2 (Cnt1, Cnt2), and peptide transporter 2 (Pept2). Other transporters were expressed at very low levels in the choroid plexus including Oat1, Oct1, Oct2, Oatp1, Oatp4, Oatp5, Oatp12, Oat-K (1/2), bile acid transporters, sodium taurocholate cotransporting polypeptide (Ntcp), bile salt excretory protein (Bsep), ileal bile acid transporter (Ibat), Mdr1a, Mdr1b, Mdr2, AbcG5, AbcG8, Ent2, and Pept1. These mRNA expression studies need to be extended with immunohistochemical studies for precise verification and determination of the subcellular protein localisation.

The very low level of mRNA expression demonstrated for some transporters does not necessarily correlate with the absence of protein and very low levels of efflux pumps may be sufficient for transport (Allen et al., 2000). For example, Rao et al. (1999) showed that mouse, rat and human choroid plexus contain MDR1 P-gp. Vectorial transport studies using the P-gp-specific substrate taxol and P-gp-inhibitors showed that P-gp functionally limits the uptake of substrates from the CSF by conferring an apical to basal drug-permeation barrier at the rat choroid plexus epithelium (Rao et al., 1999). As a second example, Angeletti et al. (1997) showed with an antibody against Oatp1 that Oatp family members are localized at the brush-border membrane of the choroid plexus. In vivo and in vitro studies do suggest that Oatp1 family members in the luminal or apical membrane of the choroid plexus are responsible for the uptake from the CSF of organic anion substrates such as 17β-estradiol and 17β-D-glucuronide. The organic anion transporting polypeptides (Oatps in rodents, OATPs in humans) are a group of membrane polyspecific organic anion transporters classified within the solute carrier family 21A (rodents, *Slc21a*; human, *SLC21A*). They exhibit a wide spectrum of amphipathic transport substrates, including drugs and xenobiotics, bile salts, steroid conjugates, thyroid hormones and neuroactive peptides (Meier et al., 1997). Human OATP-A (*SLC21A3*) and rat Oatp2 (*Slc21a5*) protein have been localized to the BBB using immunolocalization techniques (Gao et al., 1999, 2000). Solute exchange transporters such as the OATPs (e.g. Oatp2) are likely to play a role in the cellular uptake of substrates such as $E_2 17\beta G$ and DHEAS from the brain into the endothelium of brain blood capillaries or from the CSF into the choroid plexus epithelium. These transporters (e.g. Oatp2) are also likely to play a role in the cellular efflux of substrates or their metabolites towards the blood stream (Asaba et al., 2000; Sugiyama et al., 1999, 2001).

Several studies have demonstrated organic anion pump activities across the BBB, from the blood towards the brain, as well as from the brain through the capillary endothelium towards the blood. In addition, several orphan organic anion transport activities have been demonstrated across the BCSFB, from the CSF through the choroid plexus towards the blood. However, the transporters responsible for these transport activities are unknown. MRP1-9 are good candidates for the efflux pumps involved, however elucidation of their role in the activities will require demonstration of orphan transporter activities in wild-type mice compared to MRP1-9 KO mice. Since many of the MRPs show overlap of substrate specificity resulting in possible transporter redundancy, it might be necessary to use mice lacking more than one of the MRPs or to identify more specific substrates and/or inhibitors for each of the MRPs. Here, the efflux of several molecules or molecule classes is described for which the transporter has not been identified and for which MRP-mediated transport is a possibility.

One or a group of orphan efflux pumps transports antiviral drugs such as didanosine (2',3'-dideoxyinosine, ddI) and/or zidovudine (azidothymidine, AZT) across the BCSFB, from the CSF towards the blood, and across the BBB, from the brain towards the blood, via probenecid-sensitive transporter systems (Takasawa et al., 1997). After microinjection of AZT into the cerebral cortex the brain efflux rate of AZT appeared to be significantly inhibited by ddI, probenecid, p-aminohippuric acid, benzylpenicillin and the anion exchange inhibitor 4,4'-diisothiocyanatostilbene-2,2'-disulfonic acid, but not by thymidine (Takasawa et al., 1997). In addition, after microinjection of ddI, the rate of brain efflux of ddI was significantly inhibited by AZT and probenecid, but not by inosine or deoxyinosine (Takasawa et al., 1997). Furthermore, after intracerebroventricular injection of radiolabelled AZT or ddI, transport across the BCSFB of AZT and ddI was significantly inhibited by the coadministration of probenecid (Takasawa et al., 1997). Other investigators obtained similar results (Sawchuk and Hedaya, 1990; Wong et al., 1993). While uptake of zidovudine from the CSF into the choroid plexus epithelium can be inhibited by benzbromarone suggesting a role for members of the solute carrier 22 (SLC22) subfamily of organic anion transporters (OATs) (Koepsell and Endou, 2004; Strazielle et al., 2003) the identity of the major efflux transporters involved is not clear. DdI and ddC transport from blood into the choroid plexus epithelium was recently demonstrated to involve organic anion efflux transporters (Gibbs et al., 2002, 2003). In the ddI experiments, the nucleoside reverse transcriptase inhibitors abacavir, 3'-azido 3'-deoxythymidine and β-L-2',3'-dideoxy-3'-thiacytidine appeared to compete with ddI for transporter binding sites at the choroid plexus. MRP4 and MRP5 do transport some nucleoside analogues and therefore their possible role in the efflux of AZT, ddI, and their metabolites from the choroid plexus epithelium towards the blood stream needs to be examined.

6-MP is used clinically to maintain remission in patients with acute lymphoblastic leukaemia, but 6-MP does not easily enter the brain. Deguchi et al. (2000) performed a quantitative microdialysis technique to measure the efflux transport of 6-MP across the BBB.

Kinetic analyses showed that the 6-MP efflux clearance from brain interstitial fluid to plasma across the BBB was approximately 20-times greater than the influx from plasma to brain. Sulfhydryl-modifying agent N-ethylmaleimide, probenecid and p-aminohippuric acid significantly reduced the efflux clearance, but tetraethylammonium and choline did not, strongly suggesting the participation of organic anion transport proteins in the efflux of 6-MP across the BBB. Both MRP4 and MRP5 are good candidates for this transport function, since both transport thioIMP (Wijnholds et al., 2000; Wielinga et al., 2003).

A probenecid-sensitive efflux pump transports hydroxyurea across the BBB, as demonstrated by the use of a brain perfusion technique in anaesthetized guinea-pigs (Dogruel et al., 2003). Hydroxyurea is used in the treatment of HIV infection in combination with nucleoside analogues, 2'3'-didehydro-3'deoxythymidine (D4T), 2'3'-dideoxyinosine or abacavir. The uptake of radiolabelled hydroxyurea into the brain was increased by D4T, probenecid and digoxin, but not by 2'3'-dideoxyinosine or abacavir. This suggested that hydroxyurea can cross the BBB, but is removed from the brain by a probenecid- and digoxin-sensitive transport mechanism at the BBB, which is affected by D4T. It remains to be tested whether MRPs or OATPs, or both, are involved in this transport.

β-lactam antibiotics such as benzylpenicillin are transported across the BCSFB, from the CSF towards the blood, via a probenecid-sensitive transporter system that has not been identified (Spector and Lorenzo, 1974; Ogawa et al., 1994; Suzuki et al., 1987, 1989). In vivo, after intracerebroventricular administration, radiolabelled benzylpenicillin was eliminated from the CSF much more rapidly than mannitol. Analysis of the elimination clearance from the CSF revealed that approximately two-thirds of the benzylpenicillin elimination was due to active transport across the blood-CSF barrier. Probenecid reduced the transport of benzylpenicillin in a dose-dependent manner. It has been suggested that benzylpenicillin is taken up from the CSF by oat3 in the apical or luminal membrane of the choroid plexus, whereafter it is effluxed by an orphan efflux pump towards the blood (Nagata et al., 2002); the uptake can be inhibited by $E_2 17\beta G$ and cimetidine. The inhibition profile of the efflux needs to be further analyzed and the transporter to be identified.

A probenecid-sensitive orphan efflux pump for anionic herbicides across the BCSFB has been reported for 2,4,5 trichlorophenoxyacetic acid (2,4,5-T) (Kim and Pritchard, 1993). After ventriculocisternal perfusion in the rabbit in vivo, the steady-state clearance of 2,4,5-T from the cerebrospinal fluid exceeded that of inulin and was reduced in a dose-dependent fashion by 2,4-dichlorophenoxyacetic acid and probenecid. The identity of the efflux pump is yet unknown.

An orphan efflux pump transports estrone 3-sulfate by a probenecid-sensitive transport mechanism across the BCSFB thereby regulating the levels of steroid metabolites in the CSF and brain (Abe et al., 1998; Kitazawa et al., 2000; Ohtsuki et al., 2003; Sweet et al., 2002). It has been suggested that estrone-3-sulfate is taken up by oatp3 and oat3 that are localized at the apical plasma membrane of the choroid plexus, whereafter it is effluxed towards the blood by a yet to be identified transporter.

Rat Oatp2 and human OATP-A are strongly expressed at the BBB. Oatp1 and Oatp2 are localized at the apical and/or basolateral domains of the choroid plexus epithelium. It is possible that members of the Oatp/OATP gene family of membrane transporters play a major role in carrier-mediated transport of opioid peptides such as [D-penicillamine(2,5)]enkephalin (DPDPE) and deltorphin II across the BBB and BCSFB of the mammalian brain (Gao et al., 2000). OATP-A-mediated deltorphin II transport was inhibited by the mu-opioid receptor agonist Tyr-D-Ala-Gly-N-methyl-Phe-glycinol, as well as by the endogenous peptide Leu-enkephalin, and the opiate antagonists naloxone and naltrindole. A possible contribution of MRPs in the efflux of opioid peptides from brain endothelium or choroid plexus epithelium towards the blood would be worthwhile to investigate.

Taurocholic acid is effluxed from the brain to blood across the BBB. The transport was shown to be inhibited in the presence of probenecid or an anionic cyclic pentapeptide (BQ-123; an endothelin receptor antagonist) but not by p-aminohippuric acid (Kitazawa et al., 1998). BQ-123 is itself also transported across the BBB and transport is inhibited in the presence of taurocholate. However, kinetic studies indicated that the transport systems are not necessarily the same. Several of the MRPs do transport bile salts or their conjugates with sulfate or glucuronide (Hirohashi et al., 2000; Rius et al., 2003; Sampath et al., 2002; Zelcer et al., 2003) and BQ-123 is a substrate for MRP6 (reviewed in Bodo et al., 2003) suggesting that MRPs may be involved in the efflux of both taurocholic acid and BQ-123.

A further orphan efflux pump may exist for morphine-6-β-D-glucuronide (M6G), an active metabolite of morphine with high analgesic potency but low BBB permeability (Bourassett et al., 2003). Using Mdr1a- and MRP1-deficient mice, it was demonstrated that P-gp and MRP1 are not involved in the transport of M6G at the BBB. The brain uptake of radiolabelled M6G was measured in these mice by in situ brain perfusion technique with and without probenecid, digoxin, or PSC833. Probenecid did not, but digoxin and PSC833 did, increase the brain uptake of M6G, pointing towards a digoxin-sensitive efflux pump (e.g., Oatp2). These experiments do not indicate a significant role for MRPs in M6G transport at the BBB but the involvement of MRPs in the transport across the BBB of other morphine metabolites that are good candidate substrates for MRPs, should be considered.

Prostaglandins are synthesized in the endothelium of the brain capillaries and epithelium of the choroid plexus (DiBenedetto and Bito, 1986; Goehlert et al., 1981), tissues that express MRP4 and OATP. Reid et al. (2003) demonstrated that MRP4 can function as a prostaglandin efflux transporter similar to OATPs and OATs (Hagenbuch and Meier, 2003). However, it has been suggested that prostaglandins are released passively from producing cells by diffusion across the plasma membrane (Schuster, 2002). MRP4-mediated prostaglandin transport is inhibited by several nonsteroidal anti-inflammatory drugs and the leukotriene antagonist MK571 (Chen et al., 2001; Reid et al., 2003; van Aubel et al., 2002). It is certainly possible that MRP4 located in the basolateral membrane of the choroid plexus effluxes high intracellular levels of prostaglandins towards the blood.

CONCLUSION

Several plasma membrane organic anion efflux transporter activities have been demonstrated at the BBB and BCSFB and some of them will turn out to be mediated by MRPs. A detailed study of the subcellular location of MRP family members in brain capillary endothelium and choroid plexus epithelium is needed in order to determine which of these transporters contribute significantly to the brain-periphery barriers. Multiple family-member-specific antibodies against all efflux pumps in human, mouse and rat will have to be generated and the subcellular localisations accurately determined in brain endothelium and choroid plexus epithelium. Given the broad-spectrum substrate recognition properties of these polyspecific organic anion transporters, it might be difficult but not impossible to identify specific substrates and inhibitors. In order to ascribe transport functions to MRPs, we will need gene KO or knockdown or specific inhibitors for each of the individual transporters as well as detailed data about substrate affinities and transport capacity. The knowledge could be used to generate novel transporter-specific inhibitory or stimulatory drugs that alter the properties of the BBB and BCSFB in order to increase the bioavailability of drugs to the brain and/or increase toxic waste product efflux from the brain.

ACKNOWLEDGMENTS

Dutch Cancer Society project number NKI 2001-2473 provided support to J.W. for part of the research described.

REFERENCES

Abe T, Kakyo M, Sakagami H, Tokui T, Nishio T, Tanemoto M, Nomura H, Hebert SC, Matsuno S, Kondo H and Yawo H (1998). Molecular characterization and tissue distribution of a new organic anion transporter subtype (oatp3) that transports thyroid hormones and taurocholate and comparison with oatp2. *J Biol Chem, 273*: 22395-22401.

Adachi M, Sampath J, Lan LB, Sun D, Hargrove P, Flatley R, Tatum A, Edwards MZ, Wezeman M, Matherly L, Drake R and Schuetz J (2002). Expression of MRP4 confers resistance to ganciclovir and compromises bystander cell killing. *J Biol Chem, 277*: 38998-39004.

Allen JD, Brinkhuis RF, Van Deemter L, Wijnholds J and Schinkel AH (2000). Extensive contribution of the multidrug transporters P-glycoprotein and Mrp1 to basal drug resistance. *Cancer Res, 60*: 5761-5766.

Allen JD, Brinkhuis RF, Wijnholds J and Schinkel AH (1999). The mouse Bcrp1/Mxr/Abcp gene: amplification and overexpression in cell lines selected for resistance to topotecan, mitoxantrone, or doxorubicin. *Cancer Res, 59*: 4237-4241.

Angeletti RH, Novikoff PM, Juvvadi SR, Fritschy JM, Meier PJ and Wolkoff AW (1997). The choroid plexus epithelium is the site of the organic anion transport protein in the brain. *Proc Natl Acad Sci USA, 94*: 283-286.

Asaba H, Hosoya K, Takanaga H, Ohtsuki S, Tamura E, Takizawa T and Terasaki T (2000). Blood-brain barrier is involved in the efflux transport of a neuroactive steroid, dehydroepiandrosterone sulfate, via organic anion transporting polypeptide 2. *J Neurochem, 75*: 1907-1916.

Belinsky MG, Bain LJ, Balsara BB, Testa JR and Kruh GD (1998). Characterization of MOAT-C and MOAT-D, new members of the MRP/cMOAT subfamily of transporter proteins. *J Natl Cancer Inst, 90*: 1735-1741.

Bera TK, Iavarone C, Kumar V, Lee S, Lee B and Pastan I (2002). MRP9, an unusual truncated member of the ABC transporter superfamily, is highly expressed in breast cancer. *Proc Natl Acad Sci USA, 99*: 6997-7002.

Bera TK, Lee S, Salvatore G, Lee B and Pastan I (2001). MRP8, a new member of ABC transporter superfamily, identified by EST database mining and gene prediction program, is highly expressed in breast cancer. *Mol Med, 7*: 509-516.

Bergen AA, Plomp AS, Schuurman EJ, Terry S, Breuning M, Dauwerse H, Swart J, Kool M, van Soest S, Baas F, ten Brink JB and de Jong PT (2000). Mutations in ABCC6 cause pseudoxanthoma elasticum. *Nat Genet, 25*: 228-231.

Bodo A, Bakos E, Szeri F, Varadi A and Sarkadi B (2003). The role of multidrug transporters in drug availability, metabolism and toxicity. *Toxicol Lett, 140-141*: 133-143.

Borst P, Evers R, Kool M and Wijnholds J (2000). A family of drug transporters: the multidrug resistance-associated proteins. *J Natl Cancer Inst, 92*: 1295-1302.

Borst P and Elferink RO (2002). Mammalian ABC transporters in health and disease. *Annu Rev Biochem, 71*: 537-92.

Bourasset F, Cisternino S, Temsamani J and Scherrmann JM (2003). Evidence for an active transport of morphine-6-beta-d-glucuronide but not P-glycoprotein-mediated at the blood-brain barrier. *J Neurochem, 86*: 1564-1567.

Chen ZS, Hopper-Borge E, Belinsky MG, Shchaveleva I, Kotova E and Kruh GD (2003a). Characterization of the transport properties of human multidrug resistance protein 7 (MRP7, ABCC10). *Mol Pharmacol, 63*: 351-358.

Chen ZS, Lee K and Kruh GD (2001). Transport of cyclic nucleotides and estradiol 17-beta-D-glucuronide by multidrug resistance protein 4. Resistance to 6-mercaptopurine and 6-thioguanine. *J Biol Chem, 276*: 33747-33754.

Chen ZS, Lee K, Walther S, Raftogianis RB, Kuwano M, Zeng H and Kruh GD (2002). Analysis of methotrexate and folate transport by multidrug resistance protein 4 (ABCC4): MRP4 is a component of the methotrexate efflux system. *Cancer Res, 62*: 3144-3150.

Chen ZS, Robey RW, Belinsky MG, Shchaveleva I, Ren XQ, Sugimoto Y, Ross DD, Bates SE and Kruh GD (2003b). Transport of methotrexate, methotrexate polyglutamates, and 17beta-estradiol 17-(beta-D-glucuronide) by ABCG2: effects of acquired mutations at R482 on methotrexate transport. *Cancer Res, 63*: 4048-4054.

Choudhuri S, Cherrington NJ, Li N and Klaassen CD (2003). Constitutive expression of various xenobiotic and endobiotic transporter mRNAs in the choroid plexus of rats. *Drug Metab Dispos, 31*: 1337-1345.

Cisternino S, Rousselle C, Lorico A, Rappa G and Scherrmann JM (2003). Apparent lack of Mrp1-mediated efflux at the luminal side of mouse blood-brain barrier endothelial cells. *Pharm Res, 20*: 904-909.

Cole SP, Bhardwaj G, Gerlach JH, Mackie JE, Grant CE, Almquist KC, Stewart AJ, Kurz EU, Duncan AM and Deeley RG (1992). Overexpression of a transporter gene in a multidrug-resistant human lung cancer cell line. *Science, 258*: 1650-1654.

Cooray HC, Blackmore CG, Maskell L and Barrand MA (2002). Localisation of breast cancer resistance protein in microvessel endothelium of human brain. *Neuroreport, 13*: 2059-2063.

Deguchi Y, Yokoyama Y, Sakamoto T, Hayashi H, Naito T, Yamada S and Kimura R (2000). Brain distribution of 6-mercaptopurine is regulated by the efflux transport system in the blood-brain barrier. *Life Sci, 66*: 649-662.

DiBenedetto FE and Bito LZ (1986). Transport of prostaglandins and other eicosanoids by the choroid plexus: its characterization and physiological significance. *J Neurochem, 46*: 1725-1731.

Dogruel M, Gibbs JE and Thomas SA (2003). Hydroxyurea transport across the blood-brain and blood-cerebrospinal fluid barriers of the guinea-pig. *J Neurochem, 87*: 76-84.

Doyle LA, Yang W, Abruzzo LV, Krogmann T, Gao Y, Rishi AK and Ross DD (1998). A multidrug resistance transporter from human MCF-7 breast cancer cells. *Proc Natl Acad Sci USA, 95*: 15665-15670.

Evers R, Zaman GJ, Van Deemter L, Jansen H, Calafat J, Oomen LC, Oude Elferink RP, Borst P and Schinkel AH (1996). Basolateral localization and export activity of the human multidrug resistance-associated protein in polarized pig kidney cells. *J Clin Invest, 97*: 1211-1218.

Gao B, Hagenbuch B, Kullak-Ublick GA, Benke D, Aguzzi A and Meier PJ (2000). Organic anion-transporting polypeptides mediate transport of opioid peptides across blood-brain barrier. *J Pharm Exp Ther, 294*: 73-79.

Gao B, Stieger B, Noe B, Fritschy JM and Meier PJ (1999). Localization of the organic anion transporting polypeptide 2 (Oatp2) in capillary endothelium and choroid plexus epithelium of rat brain. *J Histochem Cytochem, 47*: 1255-1264.

Ghersi-Egea JF and Strazielle N (2002). Choroid plexus transporters for drugs and other xenobiotics. *J Drug Target, 10*: 353-357.

Gibbs JE, Jayabalan P and Thomas SA (2003). Mechanisms by which 2',3'-dideoxyinosine (ddI) crosses the guinea-pig CNS barriers; relevance to HIV therapy. *J Neurochem, 84*: 725-734.

Gibbs JE and Thomas SA (2002). The distribution of the anti-HIV drug, 2'3'-dideoxycytidine (ddC), across the blood-brain and blood-cerebrospinal fluid barriers and the influence of organic anion transport inhibitors. *J Neurochem, 80*: 392-404.

Goehlert UG, Ng Ying Kin NM and Wolfe LS (1981). Biosynthesis of prostacyclin in rat cerebral microvessels and the choroid plexus. *J Neurochem, 36*: 1192-1201.

Gorgels TG, Hu X, Scheffer GL, van der Wal AC, Toonstra J, de Jong PT, van Kuppevelt TH, Levelt CN, de Wolf A, Loves WJ, Scheper RJ, Peek R, Bergen AA. (2005) Disruption of Abcc6 in the mouse: novel insight in the pathogenesis of pseudoxanthoma elasticum. *Hum Mol Genet. 14*:1763-73.

Guo Y, Kotova E, Chen ZS, Lee K, Hopper-Borge E, Belinsky MG and Kruh GD (2003). MRP8, ATP-binding cassette C11 (ABCC11), is a cyclic nucleotide efflux pump and a resistance factor for fluoropyrimidines 2',3'-dideoxycytidine and 9'-(2'-phosphonylmethoxyethyl) adenine. *J Biol Chem, 278*: 29509-29514.

Hagenbuch B, Gao B and Meier PJ (2002). Transport of xenobiotics across the blood-brain barrier. *News Physiol Sci, 17*: 231-234.

Hagenbuch B and Meier PJ (2003). The superfamily of organic anion transporting polypeptides. *Biochim Biophys Acta, 1609*: 1-18.

Hipfner DR, Deeley RG and Cole SP (1999). Structural, mechanistic and clinical aspects of MRP1. *Biochim Biophys Acta, 1461*: 359-376.

Hirohashi T, Suzuki H, Takikawa H and Sugiyama Y (2000). ATP-dependent transport of bile salts by rat multidrug resistance-associated protein 3 (Mrp3). *J Biol Chem, 275*: 2905-2910.

Jedlitschky G, Burchell B and Keppler D (2000). The multidrug resistance protein 5 functions as an ATP-dependent export pump for cyclic nucleotides. *J Biol Chem, 275*: 30069-30074.

Jedlitschky G and Keppler D (2002). Transport of leukotriene C4 and structurally related conjugates. *Vitam Horm, 64*: 153-184.

Kartenbeck J, Leuschner U, Mayer R and Keppler D (1996). Absence of the canalicular isoform of the MRP gene-encoded conjugate export pump from the hepatocytes in Dubin-Johnson syndrome. *Hepatology, 23*: 1061-1066.

Keep RF and Jones HC (1990). A morphometric study on the development of the lateral ventricle choroid plexus, choroid plexus capillaries and ventricular ependyma in the rat. *Brain Res Dev Brain Res, 56*: 47-53.

Kim CS and Pritchard JB (1993). Transport of 2,4,5-trichlorophenoxyacetic acid across the blood-cerebrospinal fluid barrier of the rabbit. *J Pharm Exp Ther, 267*: 751-757.

Kitazawa T, Hosoya K, Takahashi T, Sugiyama Y and Terasaki T (2000). In-vivo and in-vitro evidence of a carrier-mediated efflux transport system for oestrone-3-sulphate across the blood-cerebrospinal fluid barrier. *J Pharm Pharmacol, 52*: 281-288.

Kitazawa T, Terasaki T, Suzuki H, Kakee A and Sugiyama Y (1998). Efflux of taurocholic acid across the blood-brain barrier: interaction with cyclic peptides. *J Pharm Exp Ther, 286*: 890-895.

Klement JF, Matsuzaki Y, Jiang QJ, Terlizzi J, Choi HY, Fujimoto N, Li K, Pulkkinen L, Birk DE, Sundberg JP, Uitto J. (2005) Targeted ablation of the abcc6 gene results in ectopic mineralization of connective tissues. *Mol Cell Biol.* 25:8299-310.

Koepsell H and Endou H (2004). The SLC22 drug transporter family. *Pflugers Arch, 447*: 666-676.

Kool M, de Haas M, Scheffer GL, Scheper RJ, van Eijk MJ, Juijn JA, Baas F and Borst P (1997). Analysis of expression of cMOAT (MRP2), MRP3, MRP4, and MRP5, homologues of the multidrug resistance-associated protein gene (MRP1), in human cancer cell lines. *Cancer Res, 57*: 3537-3547.

Kruh GD, Zeng H, Rea PA, Liu G, Chen ZS, Lee K and Belinsky MG (2001). MRP subfamily transporters and resistance to anticancer agents. *J Bioenerg Biomembr, 33*: 493-501.

Lai L and Tan TM (2002). Role of glutathione in the multidrug resistance protein 4 (MRP4/ABCC4)-mediated efflux of cAMP and resistance to purine analogues. *Biochem J, 361*: 497-503.

Leggas M, Adachi M, Scheffer GL, Sun D, Wielinga P, Du G, Mercer KE, Zhuang Y, Panetta JC, Johnston B, Scheper RJ, Stewart CF and Schuetz JD (2004). Mrp4 Confers Resistance to Topotecan and Protects the Brain from Chemotherapy. *Mol Cell Biol, 24*: 7612-7621.

Le Saux O, Urban Z, Tschuch C, Csiszar K, Bacchelli B, Quaglino D, Pasquali-Ronchetti I, Pope FM, Richards A, Terry S, Bercovitch L, de Paepe A and Boyd CD (2000). Mutations in a gene encoding an ABC transporter cause pseudoxanthoma elasticum. *Nat Genet, 25*: 223-227.

Lee K, Belinsky MG, Bell DW, Testa JR and Kruh GD (1998). Isolation of MOAT-B, a widely expressed multidrug resistance-associated protein/canalicular multispecific organic anion transporter-related transporter. *Cancer Res, 58*: 2741-2747.

Lee K, Klein-Szanto AJ and Kruh GD (2000). Analysis of the MRP4 drug resistance profile in transfected NIH3T3 cells. *J Natl Cancer Inst, 92*: 1934-1940.

Lee YJ, Kusuhara H and Sugiyama Y (2004). Do multidrug resistance-associated protein-1 and -2 play any role in the elimination of estradiol-17beta-glucuronide and 2,4-dinitrophenyl-S-glutathione across the blood-cerebrospinal fluid barrier? *J Pharm Sci, 93*: 99-107.

Lorico A, Rappa G, Finch RA, Yang D, Flavell RA and Sartorelli AC (1997). Disruption of the murine MRP (multidrug resistance protein) gene leads to increased sensitivity to etoposide (VP-16) and increased levels of glutathione. *Cancer Res, 57*: 5238-5242.

Maliepaard M, Scheffer GL, Faneyte IF, van Gastelen MA, Pijnenborg AC, Schinkel AH, van De Vijver MJ, Scheper RJ and Schellens JH (2001). Subcellular localization and distribution of the breast cancer resistance protein transporter in normal human tissues. *Cancer Res, 61*: 3458-3464.

McAleer MA, Breen MA, White NL and Matthews N (1999). pABC11 (also known as MOAT-C and MRP5), a member of the ABC family of proteins, has anion transporter activity but does not confer multidrug resistance when overexpressed in human embryonic kidney 293 cells. *J Biol Chem, 274*: 23541-23548.

Meier PJ, Eckhardt U, Schroeder A, Hagenbuch B and Stieger B (1997). Substrate specificity of sinusoidal bile acid and organic anion uptake systems in rat and human liver. *Hepatology, 26*: 1667-1677.

Milhorat TH (1976). Structure and function of the choroid plexus and other sites of cerebrospinal fluid formation. *Int Rev Cytol, 47*: 225-288.

Miller DS, Nobmann SN, Gutmann H, Toeroek M, Drewe J and Fricker G (2000). Xenobiotic transport across isolated brain microvessels studied by confocal microscopy. *Mol Pharmacol, 58*: 1357-1367.

Mitani A, Nakahara T, Sakamoto K and Ishii K (2003). Expression of multidrug resistance protein 4 and 5 in the porcine coronary and pulmonary arteries. *Eur J Pharmacol, 466*: 223-224.

Nagata Y, Kusuhara H, Endou H and Sugiyama Y (2002). Expression and functional characterization of rat organic anion transporter 3 (rOat3) in the choroid plexus. *Mol Pharmacol, 61*: 982-988.

Nies AT, Spring H, Thon WF, Keppler D and Jedlitschky G (2002). Immunolocalization of multidrug resistance protein 5 in the human genitourinary system. *J Urol, 167*: 2271-2275.

Nishino J, Suzuki H, Sugiyama D, Kitazawa T, Ito K, Hanano M and Sugiyama Y (1999). Transepithelial transport of organic anions across the choroid plexus: possible involvement of organic anion transporter and multidrug resistance-associated protein. *J Pharm Exp Ther, 290*, 289-294.

Ogawa M, Suzuki H, Sawada Y, Hanano M and Sugiyama Y (1994). Kinetics of active efflux via choroid plexus of beta-lactam antibiotics from the CSF into the circulation. *Am J Physiol, 266*: R392-R399.

Ohtsuki S, Takizawa T, Takanaga H, Terasaki N, Kitazawa T, Sasaki M, Abe T, Hosoya K and Terasaki T (2003). In vitro study of the functional expression of organic anion transporting polypeptide 3 at rat choroid plexus epithelial cells and its involvement in the cerebrospinal fluid-to-blood transport of estrone-3-sulfate. *Mol Pharmacol, 63*: 532-537.

Paulusma CC, Bosma PJ, Zaman GJ, Bakker CT, Otter M, Scheffer GL, Scheper RJ, Borst P and Oude Elferink RP (1996). Congenital jaundice in rats with a mutation in a multidrug resistance-associated protein gene. *Science, 271*: 1126-1128.

Paulusma CC, Kool M, Bosma PJ, Scheffer GL, ter Borg F, Scheper RJ, Tytgat GN, Borst P, Baas F and Oude Elferink RP (1997). A mutation in the human canalicular multispecific organic anion transporter gene causes the Dubin-Johnson syndrome. *Hepatology, 25*: 1539-1542.

Potschka H, Fedrowitz M and Loscher W (2003). Multidrug resistance protein MRP2 contributes to blood-brain barrier function and restricts antiepileptic drug activity. *J Pharm Exp Ther, 306*: 124-131.

Rao VV, Dahlheimer JL, Bardgett ME, Snyder AZ, Finch RA, Sartorelli AC and Piwnica-Worms D (1999). Choroid plexus epithelial expression of MDR1 P glycoprotein and multidrug resistance-associated protein contribute to the blood-cerebrospinal-fluid drug-permeability barrier. *Proc Natl Acad Sci USA, 96*: 3900-3905.

Rappa G, Lorico A, Flavell RA and Sartorelli AC (1997). Evidence that the multidrug resistance protein (MRP) functions as a co-transporter of glutathione and natural product toxins. *Cancer Res, 57*: 5232-5237.

Reid G, Wielinga P, Zelcer N, de Haas M, Van Deemter L, Wijnholds J, Balzarini J and Borst P (2003a). Characterization of the transport of nucleoside analog drugs by the human multidrug resistance proteins MRP4 and MRP5. *Mol Pharmacol, 63*: 1094-1103.

Reid G, Wielinga P, Zelcer N, van der Heijden I, Kuil A, de Haas M, Wijnholds J and Borst P (2003b). The human multidrug resistance protein MRP4 functions as a prostaglandin efflux transporter and is inhibited by nonsteroidal antiinflammatory drugs. *Proc Natl Acad Sci USA, 100*: 9244-9249.

Ringpfeil F, Lebwohl MG, Christiano AM and Uitto J (2000). Pseudoxanthoma elasticum: mutations in the MRP6 gene encoding a transmembrane ATP-binding cassette (ABC) transporter. *Proc Natl Acad Sci USA, 97*: 6001-6006.

Rius M, Nies AT, Hummel-Eisenbeiss J, Jedlitschky G and Keppler D (2003). Cotransport of reduced glutathione with bile salts by MRP4 (ABCC4) localized to the basolateral hepatocyte membrane. *Hepatology, 38*: 374-384.

Robbiani DF, Finch RA, Jager D, Muller WA, Sartorelli AC and Randolph GJ (2000). The leukotriene C(4) transporter MRP1 regulates CCL19 (MIP-3beta, ELC)-dependent mobilization of dendritic cells to lymph nodes. *Cell, 103*: 757-768.

Sampath J, Adachi M, Hatse S, Naesens L, Balzarini J, Flatley RM, Matherly LH and Schuetz JD (2002). Role of MRP4 and MRP5 in biology and chemotherapy. *AAPS PharmSci, 4*: E14.

Sawchuk RJ and Hedaya MA (1990). Modeling the enhanced uptake of zidovudine (AZT) into cerebrospinal fluid. 1. Effect of probenecid. *Pharm Res, 7*: 332-338.

Schinkel AH (1999). P-Glycoprotein, a gatekeeper in the blood-brain barrier. *Adv Drug Deliv Rev, 36:* 179-194.

Schinkel AH (2001). The roles of P-glycoprotein and MRP1 in the blood-brain and blood-cerebrospinal fluid barriers. *Adv Exp Med Biol, 500:* 365-372.

Schinkel AH and Jonker JW (2003). Mammalian drug efflux transporters of the ATP binding cassette (ABC) family: an overview. *Adv Drug Deliv Rev, 55*: 3-29.

Schinkel AH, Mayer U, Wagenaar E, Mol CA, Van Deemter L, Smit JJ, Van Der Valk MA, Voordouw AC, Spits H, van Tellingen O, Zijlmans JM, Fibbe WE and Borst P (1997).

Normal viability and altered pharmacokinetics in mice lacking mdr1-type (drug-transporting) P-glycoproteins. *Proc Natl Acad Sci USA, 94*: 4028-4033.

Schinkel AH, Smit JJ, van Tellingen O, Beijnen JH, Wagenaar E, Van Deemter L, Mol CA, Van Der Valk MA, Robanus-Maandag EC, te Riele HP, Berns P and Borst P (1994). Disruption of the mouse mdr1a P-glycoprotein gene leads to a deficiency in the blood-brain barrier and to increased sensitivity to drugs. *Cell, 77*: 491-502.

Schinkel AH, Wagenaar E, Mol CA and Van Deemter L (1996). P-glycoprotein in the blood-brain barrier of mice influences the brain penetration and pharmacological activity of many drugs. *J Clin Invest, 97*: 2517-2524.

Schuetz JD, Connelly MC, Sun D, Paibir SG, Flynn PM, Srinivas RV, Kumar A and Fridland A (1999). MRP4: A previously unidentified factor in resistance to nucleoside-based antiviral drugs. *Nat Med, 5*: 1048-1051.

Schultz MJ, Wijnholds J, Peppelenbosch MP, Vervoordeldonk MJ, Speelman P, van Deventer SJ, Borst P and van der PT (2001). Mice lacking the multidrug resistance protein 1 are resistant to Streptococcus pneumoniae-induced pneumonia. *J Immunol, 166*: 4059-4064.

Schuster VL (2002). Prostaglandin transport. *Prost Other Lipid Mediat, 68-69*: 633-647.

Sisodiya SM, Lin WR, Harding BN, Squier MV and Thom M (2002). Drug resistance in epilepsy: expression of drug resistance proteins in common causes of refractory epilepsy. *Brain, 125*: 22-31.

Soontornmalai A, Vlaming ML, Fritschy JM (2006). Differential, strain-specific cellular and subcellular distribution of multidrug transporters in murine choroid plexus and blood-brain barrier. *Neuroscience. 138*:159-69.

Spector R (1990). Drug transport in the central nervous system: role of carriers. *Pharmacol, 40*: 1-7.

Spector R and Goetzl EJ (1986). Leukotriene C4 transport and metabolism in the central nervous system. *J Neurochem, 46*: 1308-1312.

Spector R and Lorenzo AV (1974). The effects of salicylate and probenecid on the cerebrospinal fluid transport of penicillin, aminosalicyclic acid and iodide. *J Pharm Exp Ther, 188*: 55-65.

Strazielle N, Belin MF and Ghersi-Egea JF (2003). Choroid plexus controls brain availability of anti-HIV nucleoside analogs via pharmacologically inhibitable organic anion transporters. *AIDS, 17*: 1473-1485.

Sugiyama D, Kusuhara H, Shitara Y, Abe T, Meier PJ, Sekine T, Endou H, Suzuki H and Sugiyama Y (2001). Characterization of the efflux transport of 17beta-estradiol-D-17beta-glucuronide from the brain across the blood-brain barrier. *J Pharm Exp Ther, 298*: 316-322.

Sugiyama Y, Kusuhara H and Suzuki H (1999). Kinetic and biochemical analysis of carrier-mediated efflux of drugs through the blood-brain and blood-cerebrospinal fluid barriers: importance in the drug delivery to the brain. *J Contr Rel, 62*: 179-186.

Suzuki H, Sawada Y, Sugiyama Y, Iga T and Hanano M (1987). Anion exchanger mediates benzylpenicillin transport in rat choroid plexus. *J Pharm Exp Ther, 243*: 1147-1152.

Suzuki H, Sawada Y, Sugiyama Y, Iga T and Hanano M (1989). Facilitated transport of benzylpenicillin through the blood-brain barrier in rats. *J Pharmacobiodyn, 12*: 182-185.

Suzuki M, Suzuki H, Sugimoto Y and Sugiyama Y (2003). ABCG2 transports sulfated conjugates of steroids and xenobiotics. *J Biol Chem, 278*: 22644-22649.

Suzuki T, Sasaki H, Kuh HJ, Agui M, Tatsumi Y, Tanabe S, Terada M, Saijo N and Nishio K (2000). Detailed structural analysis on both human MRP5 and mouse mrp5 transcripts. *Gene*, *242*: 167-173.

Sweet DH, Miller DS, Pritchard JB, Fujiwara Y, Beier DR and Nigam SK (2002). Impaired organic anion transport in kidney and choroid plexus of organic anion transporter 3 (Oat3 (Slc22a8)) knockout mice. *J Biol Chem*, *277*: 26934-26943.

Takasawa K, Terasaki T, Suzuki H, Ooie T and Sugiyama Y (1997a). Distributed model analysis of 3'-azido-3'-deoxythymidine and 2',3'-dideoxyinosine distribution in brain tissue and cerebrospinal fluid. *J Pharm Exp Ther*, *282*: 1509-1517.

Takasawa K, Terasaki T, Suzuki H and Sugiyama Y (1997b). In vivo evidence for carrier-mediated efflux transport of 3'-azido-3'-deoxythymidine and 2',3'-dideoxyinosine across the blood-brain barrier via a probenecid-sensitive transport system. *J Pharm Exp Ther*, *281*: 369-375.

Uitto J, Matsuzaki Y, Terlizzi J, Li K, Leperi D, Klement J and Pulkkinen L (2003) Pseudoxanthoma elasticumdevelopment of a mouse model by targeted ablation of ABCC6. *Am J Hum Genet*, *73*:1649.

van Aubel RA, Smeets PH, Peters JG, Bindels RJ and Russel FG (2002). The MRP4/ABCC4 gene encodes a novel apical organic anion transporter in human kidney proximal tubules: putative efflux pump for urinary cAMP and cGMP. *J Am Soc Nephrol*, *13*: 595-603.

Wielinga PR, Reid G, Challa EE, van der Heijden I, Van Deemter L, de Haas M, Mol C, Kuil AJ, Groeneveld E, Schuetz JD, Brouwer C, De Abreu RA, Wijnholds J, Beijnen JH and Borst P (2002). Thiopurine metabolism and identification of the thiopurine metabolites transported by MRP4 and MRP5 overexpressed in human embryonic kidney cells. *Mol Pharmacol*, *62*: 1321-1331.

Wielinga PR, van der Heidjen I, Reid G, Beijnen JH, Wijnholds J and Borst P (2003). Characterization of the MRP4- and MRP5-mediated transport of cyclic nucleotides from intact cells. *J Biol Chem*, *278*: 17664-17671.

Wijnholds J (2002). Drug resistance caused by multidrug resistance-associated proteins. *Novartis Found Symp*, *243*: 69-79.

Wijnholds J, deLange EC, Scheffer GL, van den Berg DJ, Mol CA, van der Valk M, Schinkel AH, Scheper RJ, Breimer DD and Borst P (2000a). Multidrug resistance protein 1 protects the choroid plexus epithelium and contributes to the blood-cerebrospinal fluid barrier. *J Clin Invest*, *105*: 279-285.

Wijnholds J, Evers R, van Leusden MR, Mol CA, Zaman GJ, Mayer U, Beijnen JH, van der Valk M, Krimpenfort P and Borst P (1997). Increased sensitivity to anticancer drugs and decreased inflammatory response in mice lacking the multidrug resistance-associated protein. *Nat Med*, *3*: 1275-1279.

Wijnholds J, Mol CA, Van Deemter L, de Haas M, Scheffer GL, Baas F, Beijnen JH, Scheper RJ, Hatse S, De Clercq E, Balzarini J and Borst P (2000b). Multidrug-resistance protein 5 is a multispecific organic anion transporter able to transport nucleotide analogs. *Proc Natl Acad Sci USA*, *97*: 7476-7481.

Wijnholds J, Scheffer GL, van der Valk M, van der Valk P, Beijnen JH, Scheper RJ and Borst P (1998). Multidrug resistance protein 1 protects the oropharyngeal mucosal layer and the testicular tubules against drug-induced damage. *J Exp Med*, *188*: 797-808.

Wong SL, Van Belle K and Sawchuk RJ (1993). Distributional transport kinetics of zidovudine between plasma and brain extracellular fluid/cerebrospinal fluid in the rabbit:

investigation of the inhibitory effect of probenecid utilizing microdialysis. *J Pharm Exp Ther, 264*: 899-909.

Zelcer N, Reid G, Wielinga P, Kuil A, van der Heijden I, Schuetz JD and Borst P (2003). Steroid and bile acid conjugates are substrates of human multidrug-resistance protein (MRP) 4 (ATP-binding cassette C4). *Biochem J, 371*: 361-367.

Zelcer N, Smith A, Scheffer G, Marschall H-U, Wielinga P, Kuil A, van der Valk M, Wijnholds J, Oude Elferink R and Borst P (2003). Generation and characterization of mice lacking the multidrug resistance protein 3 (Abcc3). *PhD Thesis, University of Amsterdam, The Netherlands*.

Zhang Y, Han H, Elmquist WF and Miller DW (2000). Expression of various multidrug resistance-associated protein (MRP) homologues in brain microvessel endothelial cells. *Brain Res, 876:* 148-153.

Zhang Y, Schuetz JD, Elmquist WF and Miller DW (2004). Plasma membrane localization of multidrug resistance-associated protein (MRP) homologues in brain capillary endothelial cells. *J Pharm Exp Ther, 311*:449-55.

In: Multidrug Resistance-Associated Proteins
Editor: Christopher V. Aiello, pp. 179-210

ISBN 1-60021-298-0
© 2007 Nova Science Publishers, Inc.

Chapter 8

ABCC6: FROM PSEUDOXANTHOMA ELASTICUM TO POSSIBLE FUNCTIONS

*Olivier Le Saux[1] and Konstanze Beck[2]**

[1] Department of Cell and Molecular Biology, John A. Burns School of Medicine,
University of Hawaii, Honolulu, HI
[2] Centre for Vascular Research, School of Medical Sciences, University of New South
Wales, Sydney NSW, Australia

ABSTRACT

The 6th member of the sub-family C known as ABCC6 (*alias* MRP6), was first characterized by Kool and co-workers in 1999. ABCC6 is closely related to ABCC1 (*alias* MRP1), the defining member of the sub-family C, which is involved in multidrug-resistance. Predictive analysis indicated that ABCC6 displays a transmembrane structure similar to ABCC1 with three groups of 5, 6 and 6 membrane-spanning domains. In human and rodent, *ABCC6* appears to be constitutively expressed in the liver and kidneys and the encoded 1503 amino acids protein was localized on the basolateral membrane of hepatocytes and renal polarized cells. The substrate specificity of ABCC6 is unknown and only a few molecules were found to be actively transported in vesicular studies. Despite its similarity with ABCC1, there is no indication that ABCC6 is associated with chemotherapy resistance as no correlation between expression and drug resistance was ever observed.

Pseudoxanthoma elasticum (PXE) is an autosomal recessive disorder characterized by a generalized accumulation of calcified elastic fibers that results in dermal abnormalities. The skin manifestations are the prevailing characteristics of PXE and are associated with ocular and vascular symptoms. The PXE phenotype is highly heterogeneous and no correlation between the multiple gene alterations and the variable symptoms could be established. The genetic linkage analysis that permitted the

---

* Addresses for correspondence: Konstanze Beck, PhD, Centre for Vascular Research, School of Medical Sciences, University of New South Wales, Sydney NSW 2052, Australia, E-mail: *k.beck@unsw.edu.au* or Olivier Le Saux, Ph.D. University of Hawaii, John A. Burns School of Medicine, Honolulu, HI 9813. E-mail: *lesaux@hawaii.edu.*

identification of the first few mutations failed to reveal any locus heterogeneity suggesting that ABCC6 is solely responsible for PXE. Up to now, more than 140 mutations have been identified. The vast majority of these disease-causing changes are single nucleotide substitutions resulting in missense, nonsense and splice variants while a few others are large and small deletions or insertions. Most of the nucleotide variants seemed to cluster in specific domains of the protein such as the ATP-binding folds or a large cytoplasmic loop suggesting that PXE arises from the lack of transport activity. In prototypic elastic fiber diseases or in disorders caused by mutations in other ABCC genes, the development of the phenotype is usually consistent with the apparent function of the encoded protein. In contrast, there is no obvious connection between ABCC6 and elastic fiber synthesis or deposition. Therefore, it was suggested that PXE is a metabolic disease with ABCC6 involved in a detoxification process. At the present time, a handful of divergent approaches based on mouse models and *in vitro* studies aim specifically at gathering clues about these obscure and most likely indirect processes resulting from the absence of ABCC6 function in unspecified tissues and ultimately affecting elastic fibers.

INTRODUCTION

The ATP-binding cassette (ABC) represents the largest family of transmembrane proteins. These proteins bind ATP and use the energy to drive the transport of various molecules across cell membranes. ABC transporters are classified based on the sequence and organization of their ATP-binding domains. The human ATP-binding cassette (ABC) gene family consists of 48 members divided into seven subgroups; A through G. Genetic lesions in at least 14 of these genes cause heritable diseases [Klein et al. 1999; Stefkova et al. 2004]. About a third of all these ABC transporter-related diseases are linked to genes from the single sub-group C. The widely known cystic fibrosis is among these disorders and one of the latest additions to this group is pseudoxanthoma elasticum that stems from mutation in the *ABCC6* gene.

PSEUDOXANTHOMA ELASTICUM (PXE)

Clinical Symptoms of Pseudoxanthoma Elasticum

Pseudoxanthoma elasticum (PXE) is a rare heritable disorder characterized by ocular, vascular and skin abnormalities that result from the accumulation of morphologically abnormal, calcified elastic fibres in the affected tissues [Uitto and Shamban 1987]. The skin manifestations are the most prevailing characteristic of PXE, but the ocular and cardiovascular symptoms are responsible for the morbidity of the disease.

The first description of the clinical signs of PXE appeared in the literature more than a century ago. During the years 1881, 1884 and 1889, cases reports by the physician Rigal, Baltzer and Chauffard respectively reported similar dermal histological finding that were then attributed to xanthomas [Rigal 1881; Balzer 1884; Chauffard 1889]. These cases and others were reviewed by Darier in 1896 and he concluded that these dermal occurrences actually represented a unique and independent disease entity, distinct from the xanthomas and involving elastic tissues. To mark this distinction, Darier proposed the term "pseudoxanthome élastique" which remains largely used to this day [Darier 1896]. The fundamental histopathological features of PXE, i.e. the calcification of elastic fibres, were first described in 1901 by von Tannenhain [von Tannenhain 1901] and Werther seemed to have been the first to suggest PXE as a congenital trait [Werther 1904].

Dermal Manifestations

The skin lesions are generally the first signs of PXE to be observed during childhood or adolescence and often progress slowly and unpredictably. Therefore, a dermatologist makes frequently the initial diagnosis. The accumulation of abnormal calcified elastic fibres in the mid-dermis produces these skin lesions, which consist of yellowish papules and plaques and laxity with loss of elasticity. These lesions can be seen on the face, neck, axilla, antecubital fossa, popliteal fossa, groin, and periumbilical area [Uitto and Shamban 1987; Neldner 1988; Truter et al. 1996; Uitto et al. 1998]. The diagnosis must be confirmed by skin biopsy of an affected area that will show calcification of fragmented elastic fibers in the mid- and lower dermis (Figure 1).

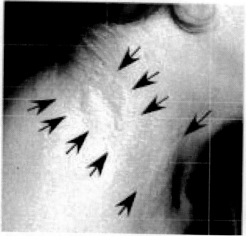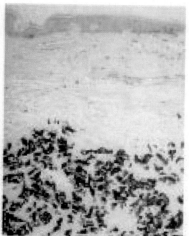

Figure 1: Dermal manifestation of PXE. Left panel: picture of skin lesion on the neck of a PXE patient (arrows). Reproduced with permission. Right panel: calcium stain of a section of a skin biopsy showing calcified elastic fibers (black) in the lower dermis.

Ocular Manifestations

Another typical characteristic of PXE are ocular lesions due to the accumulation of abnormal elastic fibers in the Bruch's membrane, resulting in angioid streaks [Weenink et al. 1996]. Doyne was the first to describe these ocular streaks in 1889 [Doyne 1889], and Knapp introduced the term "Angioid streaks" for their resemblance to blood vessels [Knapp 1892]. The combination of PXE and ocular manifestations was initially referred to as the Gronblad-Strandberg syndrome, after the names of two ophthalmologists who independently related the occurrence of angioid streaks to *Pseudoxanthoma elasticum* in 1929 [Groenblad 1929]. Angioid streaks are completely asymptomatic and can remain undetected late in life until retinal haemorrhages occur unless a retinal examination is performed earlier. The majority of PXE patients will develop ocular manifestations during their second decade of life. Bilateral angioid streaks are normally seen as linear gray or dark red lines with irregular serrated edges lying beneath normal retinal blood vessels (Figure 2) and represent breaks in the Bruch's membrane. The Bruch's membrane is not in a true sense a "membrane" but rather a heterogeneous elastin-rich layer separating the chorioid from the retina. The elastic laminae of the Bruch's membrane is comprised between two layers of collagen (type I, III and IV) which lie in direct contact with the basement membranes of the retinal pigmented epithelium (RPE) and the capillaries in the choriocapillary layer of the choriod.

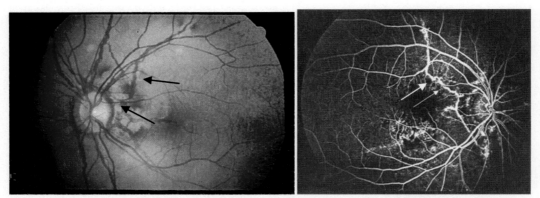

Figure 2: Left panel: Retinal fundus photography of angiod streaks (Arrows. Right panel: A Retinal fluorescein angiography. Pictures from *www.pxe.org* or reproduced with permission.

As a consequence of angioid streaks, a PXE patient will progressively develop chorioidal neovascularisation with a subsequent hemorrhagic detachment of the fovea and later scarring. Optic nerve drusen may also be associated with angioid streaks and results in visual field deficits and even advanced visual impairment. The cause of angioid streaks formation is uncertain but the consequences are clearly vascular.

Cardiovascular Manifestations

The common cardiovascular complications of PXE are due to the presence of abnormal calcified elastic fibres in the internal elastic lamina of medium-sized arteries (Figure 3). The broad spectrum of phenotypes includes premature atherosclerotic changes, intimal fibroplasia causing angina or intermittent claudication or both, early myocardial infarction and hypertension [Nishida et al. 1990; Lebwohl et al. 1993].

The fibrous thickening of the endocardium and atrioventricular valves can also result in restrictive cardiomyopathy and/or mitral valve prolapse. Approximately 10% of PXE patients also develop gastrointestinal bleeding and central nervous system complications (such as stroke and dementia) as a consequence of systemic arterial wall mineralization [Eddy and Farber 1962; Neldner 1988]. Renovascular hypertension and atrial septal aneurysm can be seen in PXE patients as well [Bertulezzi et al. 1998].

Strikingly, lung abnormalities are not a significant phenotypic feature of PXE, even though pulmonary tissues appear to also present elastic fiber mineralization [Lebwohl et al. 1993; Gheduzzi et al. 2003].

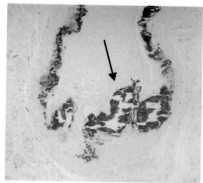

Figure 3: Calcium stain of a duodenum artery from a diseased PXE patient. As indicated by the arrow, the elastic laminae show a considerable amount of mineral deposits.

Diagnostic

The initial diagnosis of PXE is usually based on the presence of typical yellowish, cobblestone-like papular skin lesions in bilaterally symmetrical flexural sites (neck, antecubital focea, axilla, groins and popliteal spaces). The lateral neck is often the first site to be diagnosed and a trained dematologist can make an early diagnosis. A small punch biopsy from lesional area gives a positive histological confirmation of calcified elastic fibers in the deep dermis. The retina is the other main tissue to look for PXE-specific manifestations generally by funduscopic examination. However, the characteristic angioid streaks may not be visible in the early stages of the disease and usually appear a few years after the onset of the skin lesions. The initial clinical determination of cardiovascular involvement in PXE should include an history of intermittent claudication, gastrointestinal bleeding, angina pectoris, hypertension, and exercise-related fatigue of the upper and lower extremities and an evaluation of the pulse status at various peripheral locations. It is important to note that at the time of the first examination, the three disease manifestations (skin, ocular and cardiovascular symptoms) may not necessarily be found all at once. With progressing age, however, all sites will manifest clinical signs and symptoms of PXE but with considerable clinical heterogeneity. F.M. Pope indeed described a wide spectrum of clinical manifestations of PXE and categorized them into different diagnostic subclasses in the 1970s [Pope 1974; Pope 1975]. Pope's classification has been often referred to but became gradually obsolete when the general understanding of the disease evolved over time and also because some of his observations which have not been made in earlier investigations [Eddy and Farber 1962], could not be confirmed in subsequent reports [Neldner 1988]. An additional shortcoming of this classification was the frequent need to reclassify patients as their disease progressed. A consensus conference in 1992 [Lebwohl et al. 1994] concluded that all patients eventually fell into a single phenotype of the disease involving the skin, the eyes, and the cardiovascular system, although with considerable clinical heterogeneity. This conference defined PXE as a pleiotropic disease to explain the many different facets of the clinical manifestations. Three major diagnostic criteria and two minor diagnostic criteria were established [Lebwohl et al. 1994]. Although these criteria are certainly helpful for the diagnostic PXE and counseling families, this classification will probably have to be amended notably by taking into account molecular information as well as the latest development in research.

CLINICAL GENETICS

Inheritance and Prevalence

Even though the first formal description of PXE was performed over a century ago [Darier 1896], a large number of cases of PXE have been reported in the past three decades. PXE appears to be inherited as an autosomal recessive (AR) or sporadic phenotype but kindreds with autosomal dominant (AD) inheritance have also been described. The recent abundance of literature dealing with inheritance is bringing to a close a long-standing debate of the transmission of PXE.

The first attempt at defining the mode of transmission of PXE was performed by Berlyne and co-workers [Berlyne et al. 1961]. They suggested that PXE could be inherited as a partial X-linked recessive disorder, which implied that patients would tend to be of the same gender. However, this hypothesis was rapidly refuted, as it was evident that PXE affects males and females. A dual mode of inheritance was later suggested by Pope [Pope 1974], generalizing the notion of different types of PXE. Two dominant and two recessive forms of PXE were thus described based on different inherited phenotypes and similar proportions of dominant and recessive forms of the disease were proposed. For example, the AR PXE type II, the most infrequent type of PXE, is characterized by generalized skin changes with no vascular or ocular manifestations. In 1988, Neldner proposed a revised classification arguing that the various symptoms observed by Pope, which defined the four subtypes of PXE, were more likely to correspond to different stages of an age-dependent phenotype. In contrast to Pope, he concluded that a higher proportion (97%) of AR inheritance existed [Neldner 1988]. However, the ensuing literature continued to describe patients with considerable phenotypic variability and severity, further sustaining the notion of PXE subtypes with the underlying suggestion that genetic heterogeneity may be responsible for the different phenotypes [Viljoen et al. 1987]. Indeed, Viljoen suggested the existence of a fifth subtype inherited as an AR PXE in South Africa [Viljoen 1988]. DePaepe and co-workers reiterated, in 1991, the possibility of distinct forms of PXE in Belgium and Afrikaner populations [De Paepe et al. 1991]. In later discussions, however, researchers agreed that only 2 forms of PXE existed, a primarily recessively inherited disorder and a minor dominant form with incomplete penetrance [Uitto et al. 1998].

The general prevalence of PXE is not precisely known although it's frequently reported at 1/100,000 despite the lack of supporting data. Today, many scientists styding PXE and notably a patient support group called PXE International Inc. suggest that the actual prevalence of PXE might be higher, perhaps close to 1/25,000. This estimate proposed by PXE International Inc was based on a census study in the population of East coast of the United State. Such a prevalance would translate in a heterozygote carriers frequency of about 1/80.

In Europe, Trip and co-workers. reported that the prevalence of the most frequent mutation (R1141X) was particularly elevated in individuals with coronary artery disease and also in the general Dutch population [Trip et al, 2002]. Because this mutation represents roughly one third of the mutations found in this population, the prevalence of heterozygote carriers in this population could be estimated at 1/45. This rate of heterozygote carriers of ABCC6 mutations is surprisingly elevated for a disease considered as rare. However, given the heterogenous manifestations of PXE, the variable severity and the difficulties to unambiguously diagnose this disorder, one could suggest that PXE is grossly underdiagnosed and that the true overall carrier frequency might be comprised between 1/45 and 1/80.

Partial Manifestations in Heterozygous Carriers

In the decades leading to identification of the gene, there were numerous examples of dermal "elastic fibers changes" or cardiovascular abnormalities ranging from hypertension to myocardial infarction, in family members of severely affected individuals. Some of these cases of partial expression were often assumed as dominant inheritance with 10 to 20 % penetrance [Altman et al. 1974; Langness et al. 1974; Ross et al. 1978; Stutz et al. 1985]. In 1988, Neldner could not reach a definitive conclusion as to what phenotype could be accounted as dominant PXE or partial manifestations, short of a molecular diagnosis. He recognized the "complexities and possible consequences of the carriers status" in the genetic counseling of PXE patients [Neldner 1988]. The conclusion of an example of genetic counseling in an apparent dominant case of PXE based only on ultrastructural examination of skin biopsies provides us with an illustration of a possible inadequate diagnosis based on partial phenotype in obligate carriers in an AR pedigree [Hausser and Anton-Lamprecht 1991]. Indeed, we now know that the PXE phenotype, as observed in several heterozygous carriers, ranges from sub-clinical manifestations to visible lesions [van Soest et al. 1997; Bacchelli et al. 1999; Rubegni et al. 2000; Ringpfeil et al. 2006]. The spectrum of these partial phenotypes somewhat overlaps with that of the less severely affected PXE patients. There is, therefore, a certain continuum in the PXE phenotype between heterozygous carriers and PXE patients, which make the clinical diagnosis of the less severe forms of PXE equivocal.

The identification of PXE gene in 2000 had a positive influence on the debate on inheritance patterns of PXE, which is intrinsically linked to the issue of adequate diagnosis and the presence of subtle clinical symptoms in heterozygous carriers. However, while adding some fuel to the fire, the advent of a molecular diagnosis for PXE has also helped extinguish it. Various groups investigated those families with apparent AD transmission after the identification of the PXE gene. All displayed pseudo-dominant inheritance with the mutated alleles being transmitted in an AR fashion [Cai et al. 2000; Chassaing et al. 2004; Miksch et al. 2005]. In fact, there is no hard evidence to support autosomal dominant inheritance while a large body of data points to simple autosomal recessive inheritance for PXE [Plomp et al. 2004; Chassaing et al. 2005; Ringpfeil et al. 2006]. Indeed, there is no report describing PXE in three generation families. Moreover, both dominant and recessive forms of PXE have been linked to the same chromosomal region at 16p13.1 and only ABCC6 mutations were found in families described with AR or AD inheritance. Finally, the same mutations have been identified in recessive and dominant families [Bergen et al. 2000; Cai et al. 2000; Le Saux et al. 2000], which represents an unlikely scenario given the apparent lack of locus heterogeneity [Bacchelli et al. 1999; Cai et al. 2000]. In fact, the various subtypes of a disorder or a dual mode of inheritance for a disease are often due to mutations in different genes or different mutations in the same gene. Epidermilysis bullosa (EB) is an excellent illustration of this principle. The recent generation of PXE knockout mouse models further supports the notion of exclusive AR inheritance [Gorgels et al. 2005; Klement et al. 2005]. Therefore, the current consensus is that PXE is exclusively an autosomal recessive disease even though there are still many aspects of this disease that remain unexplained such as the heterogeneity of the PXE phenotype and its possible relationship with diet or other environmental factors. In a recent article, Dr. Bergen adequately summarized the current perspective on this issue as "(these) findings mark the end of the autosomal dominant PXE segregation myth" [Bergen 2006].

MOLECULAR GENETICS

The PXE Gene: Identification of an Unlikely Culprit

As abnormal elastic fiber morphology is such a characteristic feature of the PXE phenotype, several groups had used a candidate gene approach in an attempt to identify gene mutations responsible for the PXE phenotype. Polymorphic markers in genes encoding known elastic fiber proteins (tropoelastin, lysyl oxidase, fibrillin 1 and 2) were used in a linkage and sib pair analysis, performed with families apparently presenting autosomal recessive and autosomal dominant forms of PXE. No obvious linkage between these markers and the PXE phenotype was found [Christiano et al. 1992; Christiano and Uitto 1994; Raybould et al. 1994]. This unsuccessful candidate gene approach prompted several laboratories to consider a systematic genome search. Struk and co-workers noticed a significant linkage of the PXE phenotype to a 5 cM region at 16p13 [Struk et al. 1997]. van Soest and colleagues reported the same locus at 16p13.1 in a large consanguineous Dutch family [van Soest et al. 1997]. The PXE gene was later confined to a 800kb locus containing several candidate genes [Bacchelli et al. 1999] and subsequently resized to about 500kb [Cai et al. 2000]. These candidate genes encoded an isoform of myosin heavy chain (MYH11), the multidrugresistance–associated proteins ABCC1 and ABCC6 (also known as MRP1 and MRP6, respectively), an unknown protein called pM5 (later denominated Nodal Modulator 1 or NOMO1) and two identical unknown proteins initially referred to as UNK and subsequently termed Nuclear Pore Interacting Protein or NPIP. The centromeric region containing NOMO1 and the NPIP genes turned out to be a duplicated region, which has been re-positioned on the telomeric side of the PXE locus on the current published sequence of the human chromosome 16 (www. www.ncbi.nlm.nih.gov). It is noteworthy that the published sequence centromeric to the PXE gene (ABCC6) harbours a gene homolog to NOMO1 called NOMO3.

The various groups involved in the final search for PXE mutations screened the exons of the several candidate genes for mutations using single-strand conformation polymorphism (SSCP), heteroduplex analysis (HA) or direct sequencing. All groups identified similar mutations in a single gene called *ABCC6* [Bergen et al. 2000; Cai et al. 2000; Le Saux et al. 2000].

The PXE Gene Encodes an ABC Transporter

As opposed to other elastic fiber diseases such as Supravalvular Aortic Stenosis (SVAS), Marfan syndrome and *Cutis laxa*, mutations responsible for the development of the PXE phenotype were found in a gene encoding an ABC transporter, which has no obvious relation with elastic fibers. *ABCC6* belongs to the subfamily C of the ATP binding cassette (ABC) gene super-family. The sub-family includes 13 members (*ABCC1* to *ABCC13*) notably those genes involved in drug-resistance such as *MRP1 to 6* (*ABCC1-6*) but also the cystic fibrosis transmembrane conductance regulator gene (*ABCC7* or *CFTR*) and the sulfonylurea receptor genes (*ABCC8* and *9* or *SUR*). The *ABCC6* gene consists of 31 exons spanning about 73 kb on chromosome 16. The *ABCC6* mRNA, sizing about 6 kb, has an open reading frame of 4.5 kb encoding a 1503 amino acid protein. Two ABCC6 pseudogenes homologous to the 5' of ABCC6 (exon 1-9, and 1-4) were recently identified and are located closely to ABCC6 [Germain 2001; Pulkkinen et al. 2001]. The *ABCC6* gene is transcribed primarily in liver and kidneys (See below).

ABCC6 Mutations

After the identification of *ABCC6* as the gene responsible for the development of the PXE phenotype, several groups conducted systematic mutational screening with cohorts of PXE patients of various sizes. To date, these studies identified 141 disease-causing nucleotide variants affecting 26 out of the 31 *ABCC6* exons (Figure 4, Table 1). Among these mutations, 75 are missense mutations (53% of the total), 17 are nonsense mutations, 15 are mutations potentially affecting splicing, 4 represent small insertions leading to frameshift and 30 are small and large deletions.

Remarkably, *ABCC6* mutations are distributed in clusters notably in the C-terminal end of the protein while variants considered as neutral appeared to be evenly distributed [Le Saux et al. 2001; Chassaing et al. 2005]. This unequal distribution is more pronounced if one considers only missenses variants. Among the 75 different missense mutations known in ABCC6, the vast majority involve amino acids in intracellular domains while only a few are located in transmembrane regions and extracellular regions. More than half of those missenses mutations are located in 7 exons; exon 24 that encodes a large cytoplasmic loop of 70 amino acids and the exons encoding both nucleotide-binding folds (NBFs, exons 16-18 and 28-30). The presence of 13 variants in the 70 amino acids domain, 7 affecting arginyl residues, underscores its importance, yet the function of this region is unknown. The NBFs contain 43% of all missense mutations, which clearly illustrates the importance of ATP-mediated transport activity for the overall ABCC6 function and the development of the PXE phenotype. Moreover, the relative distribution of variants between the two NBFs is unequal with 8 missense variants being located in the N-terminal NBF while 24 are found in the C-terminal NBF (Figure 4). This supports the notion that the NBFs of ABCC6 are functionally non-equivalent [Le Saux et al. 2001]. Functional studies have been initiated in Dr. Varadi's laboratory with selected missense variants affecting the 70 amino acids loop and the C-terminal NBF. Thus far, the results indicate that the mutant proteins either have no ATP-dependent transport activity and are properly targeted to the basolateral membrane (V1298F, G1303R, G1312S) or the protein is fully functional but is retained intracellularly in polarized cells [Ilias et al. 2002; Fülöp et al. 2006].

Deletions Mediated by Alu Repeats

Three large intragenic deletions have been characterized thus far; ABCC6del23–29, ABCC6del23–25 and ABCC6del15. These deletions seem to have been mediated by *Alu* repeats (*Alu*SX and *Alu*Jo/Jb) [Le Saux et al. 2001; Pulkkinen et al. 2001; Katona et al. 2005]. The analysis of the non-coding regions of *ABCC6* has indeed revealed a high proportion of repetitive elements [Pulkkinen et al. 2001], suggesting that this gene might be susceptible to significant amount of genomic rearrangements. For example, *ABCC6* intronic sequences contained 38 *Alu*SX repeats. The presence of these numerous repetitive sequences suggested that a significant fraction of undetected mutations might derive from DNA rearrangements that are difficult to detect using a conventional PCR-based approach [Le Saux et al. 2001]. However, the limited number of such deletions found thus far indicate that this type of large deletion will not be as prevalent as initially thought.

Allelic Heterogeneity

Most of the 141 pathogenic mutations appear to be unique or may be restricted to a few kindred, which further illustrates the high degree of allelic heterogeneity in PXE. However, two variants (Ex23-29del and R1141X) are recurrent mutations. The frequency of these two recurrent mutations differs in the various population groups studied. The deletion Ex23-29 represents 28% of the detected mutations in the US population and 4% in a European cohort, whereas mutation R1141X represents about 4% of the detected mutations in the US population and 28% in the European population [Le Saux et al. 2001]. Furthermore, the frequency of the R1141X mutation varies between European PXE populations, 44.7% in Germans [Hendig et al. 2005], 30% in the Dutch population [Hu et al. 2003], 26% in Italian patients [Gheduzzi et al. 2004], and 13% in the French population [Chassaing et al. 2004]. The frequent occurrence of R1141X in certain European PXE groups is most likely due to founder effects as evidenced in the Dutch, French and Italian cohorts [Hu et al. 2003; Chassaing et al. 2004; Gheduzzi et al. 2004]. A few other allelic variants with elevated local frequency may also be identical-by-descent. For instance, the residue R518 is recurrently mutated in French and Italian patients with PXE [Chassaing et al. 2004; Gheduzzi et al. 2004]. In the Afrikaners of South Africa, a European-derived population that settled at the Cape of Good Hope in the 17th century, 3 missense variants were found to co-segregate with 3 specific haplotypes also indicated a founder origin of PXE in this largely consanguineous population [Le Saux et al. 2002). The most common variant (R1339C) accounted for 53% of the PXE alleles, whereas other mutant alleles appeared at lower frequencies ranging from 3% to 12%. These mutations were also identified in American or European populations but at lower frequency [Le Saux et al. 2001; Gheduzzi et al. 2004]. A similar analysis involving Afrikaners and individuals of Mexican ancestries detected the same R1339C variant segregating in a common haplotype environment, which confirmed the founder origin of this allele [Miksch et al. 2005]. Interestingly, R1339C was also found in an individual of European ancestries within a distinct haplotype, which prompted the authors to conclude that this mutant allele can independently occur in various region of the world [Miksch et al. 2005]. Away from Europe and European-derived populations, the Japanese PXE population is of particular interest. Indeed, this PXE cohort of Asian ancestry presented mutations distinct from those found in Western nations probably indicating that PXE arose separately in Japan and Europe. Two of the Japanese mutant alleles, 2542delG and Q378X accounted for 53% and 25% of the identified mutated alleles [Noji et al. 2004]. Regrettably, the authors did not perform haplotype analysis with these samples, which might have provided molecular support to the founder origin of PXE in these Islands. Nevertheless, one may tentatively suggest that similar to the presence of founder mutations in the Afrikaners of South Africa with PXE, mutant alleles might have arrived in the Japanese archipelago either with the first settlers in the centuries B.C. or arose independently in Japan.

The mutation detection rate reported so far ranged from 55% in the initial studies [Le Saux et al. 2001; Hu et al. 2003] to 97% in a more recent analysis [Miksch et al. 2005]. The lack of mutation detection in certain cases was frequently attributed to technical and physical restrictions such as the widely used PCR-based methods to examine the coding regions and adjacent sequences. Based on the recent literature [Chassaing et al. 2005; Miksch et al. 2005] and our own experience, it appears that applying direct sequencing of all 31 exons of ABCC6 combined with PCR detection of known deletions will give the best results with a mutation detection rate close to 100%.

Table 1.

nucleotide	amino acid	exon	status	origin	no. of alleles	reference
nonsense mutations (n=17)						
373G->T	E125X	4	ch	India	1	[Miksch et al. 2005]
595C->T	Q199X	5	hm	Japan	2	[Yoshida et al. 2005]
681C->G	Y227X	7	ch	Italy		[Meloni et al. 2001]
1132C->T	Q378X	9	ht, hm, ch	nd	6	[Cai et al. 2001]
			hm, ch	Italy	5	[Gheduzzi et al. 2004]
			hm, ch	US, Germany	6	[Miksch et al. 2005]
1552C->T	R518X	12	ch	Italy	1	[Meloni et al. 2001]
			ch, hm	Italy	9	[Gheduzzi et al. 2004]
			hm, ht	France	3	[Chassaing et al. 2004]
			ch	Germany	1	[Miksch et al. 2005]
2161G->A	W721X	17	ch	US	1	[Miksch et al. 2005]
2247C->T	Q749X	17	ht, ch	Holland	2	[Hu et al. 2003]
2304C->A	Y768X	18	ch	SA	4	[Le Saux et al. 2002]
			ch	SA	1	[Miksch et al. 2005]
2524C->T	Q842X	19	ch	CH	1	[Miksch et al. 2005]
3088C->T	R1030X	23	ht	SA	1	[Le Saux et al. 2002]
			ht, ch	Italy	3	[Gheduzzi et al. 2004]
3421C->T	R1141X	24	hm, ch	Italy, UK, Belgium	10	[Le Saux et al. 2000]
			ht	Holland	2	[Bergen et al. 2000]
			hm, ht	CH, US	3	[Struk et al. 2000]
			ch, ht	UK, US	4	[Ringpfeil et al. 2000]
			ch, ht, hm	Germany, US, UK, Belgium	38	[Le Saux et al. 2001]
			ch	nd	2	[Cai et al. 2001]
			ch, ht	SA	4	[Le Saux et al. 2002]

Table 1. (Continued)

nucleotide	amino acid	exon	status	origin	no. of alleles	reference
			hm, ch, ht	Holland	22	[Hu et al. 2003]
			hm, ch, ht	Italy	24	[Gheduzzi et al. 2004]
			ch, hm	France	4	[Chassaing et al. 2004]
			ch, hm	CH, SA, Germany, US, UK	45	[Miksch et al. 2005]
3427C>T	R1143X	24	ht	US	1	[Le Saux et al. Unpublished]
3490C->T	R1164X	24	hm	US	1	[Struk et al. 2000]
			ch	Germany, UK	2	[Ringpfeil et al. 2001]
			ch	nd	1	[Cai et al. 2001]
			ch	Italy	1	[Meloni et al. 2001]
			ht	France	1	[Chassaing et al. 2004]
			ch, hm	UK, US	9	[Miksch et al. 2005]
3668G->A	W1223X	26	ch	France	1	[Chassaing et al. 2004]
3709C->T	Q1237X	26	ch	Belgium	1	[Le Saux et al. 2001]
3823C->T	R1275X	27	ch	Italy	1	[Gheduzzi et al. 2004]
4192C->T	R1398X	29	ch	Belgium	1	[Le Saux et al. 2001]
missense mutations (n=75)						
386G->A	G129E	4	ch	US	1	[Miksch et al. 2005]
676G->A	G226R	7	nd	nd	nd	[Chassaing et al. 2005]
743C->T	L248F	7	ch	US	1	[Miksch et al. 2005]
951C->A	S317R	8	ch	SA	1	[Miksch et al. 2005]
1064T->G	L355R	9	ch	US	1	[Miksch et al. 2005]
1091C->G	T364R	9	ch	nd	1	[Pulkkinen et al. 2001]
			ch	Italy	1	[Gheduzzi et al. 2004]
			ch	US	1	[Miksch et al. 2005]
1108A->G	N370D	9	ch	US	2	[Miksch et al. 2005]
1171A->G	R391G	9	ch	France	1	[Chassaing et al. 2004]
			ch	US	2	[Miksch et al. 2005]
1192A->G	S398G	10	ch	UK	1	[Miksch et al. 2005]
1233T->G	N411K	10	ht	US	1	[Le Saux et al. 2001]
			ch	Italy	1	[Gheduzzi et al. 2004]
1318T->G	C440G	10	ch	Italy	1	[Gheduzzi et al. 2004]
1363G->C	A455P	11	nd	nd	?	[Uitto et al. 2001]
1484T->A	L495H	12	ch	Germany	1	[Miksch et al. 2005]

Table 1. (Continued)

nucleotide	amino acid	exon	status	origin	no. of alleles	reference
1505A->T	K502M	12	nd	nd	nd	[Chassaing et al. 2005]
1553G->A	R518Q	12	ch, ht	US, Belgium	2	[Le Saux et al. 2001]
			ht	SA	1	[Le Saux et al. 2002]
			ch	Italy	3	[Gheduzzi et al. 2004]
			hm, ch	Morocco, France	3	[Chassaing et al. 2004]
			hm, ch	CH, US	4	[Miksch et al. 2005]
1652T->C	F551S	13	ch	US	1	[Miksch et al. 2005]
1703T->C	F568S	13	ch	US	1	[Le Saux et al. 2001]
1781C->T	A594V	14	ch	US	2	[Miksch et al. 2005]
1798C->T	R600G	14	ch	Italy	1	[Gheduzzi et al. 2004]
2018T->C	L673P	16	ch	SA	1	[Le Saux et al. 2002]
2030T->C	L677P	16	ch	US	1	[Miksch et al. 2005]
2252T->A	M751K	18	ht	Germany	5	[Hendig et al. 2005]
2263G>A	G755R	18	ht	US	1	[Le Saux et al. Unpublished]
2278C->T	R760W	18	ht	Germany	2	[Hendig et al. 2005]
			ch	US	1	[Miksch et al. 2005]
2294G->A	R765Q	18	ht	Germany	1	[Le Saux et al. 2001]
			ch	Holland	1	[Hu et al. 2003]
			ht	Germany	3	[Hendig et al. 2005]
			ch	US	1	[Miksch et al. 2005]
2297C->A	A766D	18	hm	Turkey	2	[Chassaing et al. 2004]
2342C->T	A781V	18	nd	nd	nd	[Chassaing et al. 2005]
2419C->T	R807W	19	ch	US	1	[Miksch et al. 2005]
2420G->A	R807Q	19	nd	nd	nd	[Chassaing et al. 2005]
			ch	Germany	1	[Miksch et al. 2005]
2428G->A	V810M	19	ch	Italy	1	[Gheduzzi et al. 2004]
2458G->C	A820P	19	ch	Italy	1	[Gheduzzi et al. 2004]
2552T->C	L851P	19	ht	Germany	1	[Hendig et al. 2005]
2855T->G	F952C	22	ht	Germany	1	[Hendig et al. 2005]
2965G->C	G992R	22	nd	nd	nd	[Chassaing et al. 2005]
3168C->A	D1056E	23	ch	India	1	[Miksch et al. 2005]
3340C->T	R1114C	24	ch	Italy	1	[Gheduzzi et al. 2004]
			ch	US	1	[Miksch et al. 2005]
3341G->A	R1114H	24	ht	Holland	1	[Hu et al. 2003]

Table 1. (Continued)

nucleotide	amino acid	exon	status	origin	no. of alleles	reference
3341G->C	R1114P	24	ht	UK	1	[Le Saux et al. 2001]
			hm	US	2	[Le Saux et al. 2000]
3362C->G	S1121W	24	ch	Germany	1	[Le Saux et al. 2001]
3362C->T	S1121L	24	hm, ch	CH	3	[Miksch et al. 2005]
3380C->T	M1127T	24	ch	Italy	1	[Gheduzzi et al. 2004]
3389C->T	T1130M	24	hm	Holland	2	[Hu et al. 2003]
			ch	Italy	1	[Gheduzzi et al. 2004]
			ch, ht	France, Algeria	2	[Chassaing et al. 2004]
3398G>C	G1133A	24	ht	US	1	[Le Saux et al. Unpublished]
3412C->T	R1138W	24	hm	US	1	[Ringpfeil et al. 2000]
			ch	US	1	[Miksch et al. 2005]
3413G->C	R1138P	24	ch	Germany	1	[Le Saux et al. 2001]
3413G->A	R1138Q	24	ch	UK, US	2	[Le Saux et al. 2001]
			ch	nd	1	[Le Saux et al. 2000]
			ht	UK	1	[Ringpfeil et al. 2000]
			ch	SA	3	[Le Saux et al. 2002]
			ch	Italy	1	[Gheduzzi et al. 2004]
			hm	France	2	[Chassaing et al. 2004]
			ch	SA, US	3	[Miksch et al. 2005]
3415G>A	A1139T	24	ht	US	1	[Le Saux et al. Unpublished]
3491G->A	R1164Q	24	ch	US	1	[Miksch et al. 2005]
3608G->A	G1203D	25	ch	Germany	1	[Le Saux et al. 2001]
3661C->T	R1221C	26	ch	Holland	1	[Hu et al. 2003]
			ch	Japan	1	[Noji et al. 2004]
			ch	US	2	[Miksch et al. 2005]
3703C->T	R1235W	26	hm	CH	2	[Miksch et al. 2005]
3712G->C	D1238H	26	ch	Algeria	1	[Chassaing et al. 2004]
3892G->T	V1298F	28	ht	US	2	[Le Saux et al. 2001]
3895G->A	G1299S	28	nd	nd	nd	[Chassaing et al. 2005]
3902C->T	T1301I	28	ch	Belgium	1	[Le Saux et al. 2001]
3904G->A	G1302R	28	hm	US	4	[Le Saux et al. 2001]
			ht	Holland	1	[Hu et al. 2003]
			ch	US	1	[Miksch et al. 2005]
3907G->C	A1303P	28	ch	Belgium, US	4	[Le Saux et al. 2001]
			ch	Holland	1	[Hu et al. 2003]

Table 1. (Continued)

nucleotide	amino acid	exon	status	origin	no. of alleles	reference
			ch	US	1	[Miksch et al. 2005]
3919T->C	S1307P	28	nd	nd	nd	[Chassaing et al. 2005]
3940C->T	R1314W	28	hm, ht	US	3	[Le Saux et al. 2001]
			hm	US	2	[Le Saux et al. 2000]
3941G->A	R1314Q	28	ch	Germany	1	[Le Saux et al. 2001]
			ch	US	1	[Miksch et al. 2005]
3961G->A	G1321S	28	ht	US	1	[Le Saux et al. 2001]
4004T->G	L1335P	28	ht	France	1	[Chassaing et al. 2004]
4015C->T	R1339C	28	hm	Mexico, SA	4	[Struk et al. 2000]
				US	2	[Le Saux et al. 2001]
			ht, hm, ch	SA	18	[Le Saux et al. 2002]
			ht, hm	Italy	3	[Gheduzzi et al. 2004]
			hm, ch	SA, Germany, Mexico	11	[Miksch et al. 2005]
4016G->T	R1339L	28	ch	US	1	[Miksch et al. 2005]
4016G->A	R1339Q	28	hm, ch	CH, US	5	[Miksch et al. 2005]
4036C->T	P1346S	28	ch	Italy	1	[Gheduzzi et al. 2004]
4041G->C	Q1347H	28	hm	US	2	[Le Saux et al. 2001]
4060G->C	G1354R	29	ch	nd	1	[Pulkkinen et al. 2001]
4069C->T	R1357W	29	ch	Japan	1	[Noji et al. 2004]
			ch	US	1	[Miksch et al. 2005]
4081G->A	D1361N	29	ch	Germany	1	[Le Saux et al. 2001]
4182G->T	K1394N	29	ch	Holland	1	[Hu et al. 2003]
4198G->A	E1400K	29	ch	Italy	2	[Gheduzzi et al. 2004]
			hm, ch	Morocco	3	[Chassaing et al. 2004]
4209C->A	S1403R	30	ht	Germany	1	[Hendig et al. 2005]
4271T->C	I1424T	30	ht	US	1	[Le Saux et al. 2001]
4377C->T	R1459C	30	ht	Holland	1	[Hu et al. 2003]
deletions (n=30)						
ABCC6del	no protein	all	ht	Holland	1	[Bergen et al. 2000]
ABCC6del	no protein	all	ht	nd	1	[Miksch et al. 2005]
ABCC6,ABCC1,M YH11	no protein	all	ch	Italian	1	[Meloni et al. 2001]
ABCC6,ABCC1,M YH11	no protein	all	ch	Holland	1	[Hu et al. 2003]
ABCC6,ABCC1,M YH11 +5genes del	no protein	all	ht	nd	1	[Miksch et al. 2005]
ABCC6,ABCC1,M YH11 +7genes del	no protein	all	ht	nd	1	[Miksch et al. 2005]
ABCC6del1-21	no protein	1-21	ht	CH	1	[Miksch et al. 2005]
105delA	fs	2	ch	US	1	[Miksch et al. 2005]

Table 1. (Continued)

nucleotide	amino acid	exon	status	origin	no. of alleles	reference
179-187del	R60-Y62del	2	ch	nd	1	[Pulkkinen et al. 2001]
			ch	US	1	[Miksch et al. 2005]
179-195del	fs	2	ht	Belgium	1	[Le Saux et al. 2001]
220-222del	V74del	3	hm	France	2	[Chassaing et al. 2004]
960delC	fs	8	ch	Italy	1	[Meloni et al. 2001]
1088-1120del	Q363-R373del	9	ch	Algeria	1	[Chassaing et al. 2004]
ABCC6del15	fs	15	hm	SA	2	[Le Saux et al. 2002]
1944del22	fs	16	ht	Holland	1	[Bergen et al. 2000]
			ch, ht	Holland	2	[Hu et al. 2003]
1995delG	fs	16	ht	Germany	1	[Le Saux et al. 2001]
			ht	Germany	3	[Hendig et al. 2005]
2322delC	fs	18	ht	US	1	[Le Saux et al. 2001]
2542delG	fs	19	nd	nd	?	[Uitto et al. 2001]
			hm	Japan	2	[Noji et al. 2004]
2835-2850del16	fs	22	ht	Germany	1	[Hendig et al. 2005]
ABCC6del23-29	fs	23-29	ch	Germany, UK, Greece	4	[Ringpfeil et al. 2001]
			ch	US, Europe	26	[Le Saux et al. 2001]
			hm, ch, ht	Holland	13	[Hu et al. 2003]
			ch	France	2	[Chassaing et al. 2004]
			ch	CH, US	19	[Miksch et al. 2005]
3106delTTT	F1036del	23	ch	US	1	[Miksch et al. 2005]
3141delCTT	F1048del	23	ch	US	1	[Miksch et al. 2005]
3343-3345del	F1048del	23	nd	nd	nd	[Chassaing et al. 2005]
ABCC6del24-25	fs	24-25	ch	Hungary	1	[Katona et al. 2005]
3775delT	fs	27	ht	US	1	[Le Saux et al. 2000]
			hm	Holland	2	[Bergen et al. 2000]
			hm	Europe	2	[Le Saux et al. 2001]
			ht	SA	1	[Le Saux et al. 2002]
			hm, ch, ht	Holland	5	[Hu et al. 2003]
			ch	US	2	[Miksch et al. 2005]
3912delG	fs	28	ch	US	1	[Miksch et al. 2005]
4104delC	fs	29	ch	Belgium	1	[Le Saux et al. 2001]
			ch	SA	1	[Le Saux et al. 2002]
4182delG	fs	29	hm, ch, ht	Holland	6	[Hu et al. 2003]
4318delA	fs	30	hm	Italy	2	[Gheduzzi et al. 2004]
4434delA	fs	31	hm	Germany	2	[Hendig et al. 2005]

Table 1. (Continued)

nucleotide	amino acid	exon	status	origin	no. of alleles	reference
insertions [n=4]						
938-939insT	fs	8	ht	UK	1	[Le Saux et al. 2001]
			ch, ht	SA	2	[Le Saux et al. 2002]
3544insC	fs	25	ch	Italy	1	[Gheduzzi et al. 2004]
3769insC	fs	27	ch	US	2	[Miksch et al. 2005]
4220insAGAA	fs	30	ht	Holland	2	[Bergen et al. 2000]
			ht	Holland	1	[Hu et al. 2003]
splice site mutations (n=15)						
IVS8+2delTG	splicing	i-8	nd	nd	nd	[Chassaing et al. 2005]
IVS13-29T->A	splicing	i-13	nd	nd	nd	[Chassaing et al. 2005]
IVS14-5T->G	splicing	i-14	nd	nd	nd	[Chassaing et al. 2005]
IVS15-1G->C	splicing	i-15	ht	US	1	[Le Saux et al. unpublished]
2248-2_2248-1del	splicing: del ex 18	i-17	ch	Italy	1	[Gheduzzi et al. 2004]
IVS17-12delTT	splicing	i-17	ch	Holland	1	[Hu et al. 2003]
IVS21+1G->T	splicing	i-21	ch	US, Germany	7	[Le Saux et al. 2001]
			nd	nd	?	[Uitto et al. 2001]
			ch	nd	2	[Le Saux et al. 2000]
			ht	Germany	7	[Hendig et al. 2005]
			ch	US	5	[Miksch et al. 2005]
IVS23-3_-38del-3.-5insAGA	splicing	i-23	ch	US	1	[Miksch et al. 2005]
IVS24+1G->A	splicing	i-24	ht	US	1	[Le Saux et al. Unpublished]
IVS24-1G->A	splicing	i-24	hm	US	2	[Miksch et al. 2005]
IVS25-3C->A	splicing	i-25	ch	France	1	[Chassaing et al. 2004]
3735G->T	splicing E1245D	26	ch	US	1	[Miksch et al. 2005]
3735G->A	splicing E1245E	26	ch	US	1	[Miksch et al. 2005]
IVS26-1G->A	splicing	i-26	ch	Belgium	1	[Le Saux et al. 2001]
			ch	Greece	2	[Ringpfeil et al. 2000]
			ch	Italy	2	[Gheduzzi et al. 2004]
			ch	US	1	[Miksch et al. 2005]
IVS27-6G->A	splicing	i-27	ch	US	1	[Miksch et al. 2005]

A total of 141 PXE-causing mutations in ABCC6 have been identified so far. Abbreviations: ch= compound heterozygous, hm= homozygous, ht= heterozygous, fs= frameshift, i= intron, CH= Switzerland, SA= South Africa, UK= United Kingdom, US= USA, nd= not determined. Note: IVS13-29T>A is listed as a mutation in Chassaing et al. 2005 but the authors feel that this sequence variant is unlikely to be causative given its intronic position.

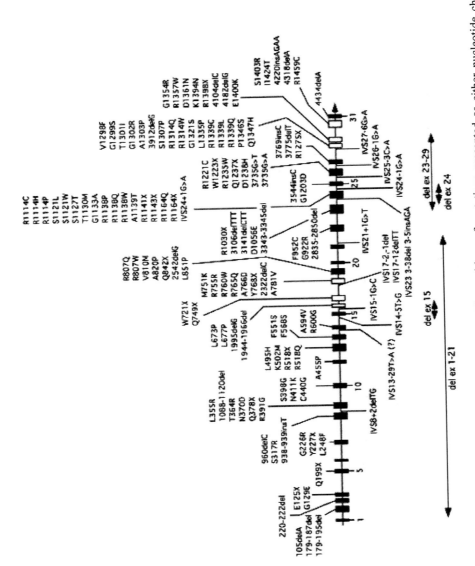

Figure 4: Localization of mutations causing PXE in the ABCC6 gene. The positions of mutations presented as either nucleotide changes or amino acid substitutions are indicated with respect to the exon/intron structure of ABCC6. Boxes represent exons drawn approximately to scale. The number of every fifth exon is indicated. Horizontal lines with arrows indicate 4 of the large deletions involving some ABCC6 exons. Larger deletions with breakpoints both upstream and downstream of ABCC6 and removing all exons are listed in Table 1.

Genotype-Phenotype Correlation

After the identification of *ABCC6* mutations, it was expected to rapidly see emerge a correlation between the phenotype and the various types and positions of mutations that would notably explain the high phenotypic heterogeneity. All studies involving large cohorts of patients have thus far failed to identify any element of correlation [Le Saux et al. 2001; Chassaing et al. 2004; Gheduzzi et al. 2004]. Remarkably, one study did report a correlation between mutation type and the age of onset but since the authors did not extend their analysis to all 31 exons of *ABCC6*, their results are questionable [Hendig et al. 2005]. The high degree of allelic heterogeneity encountered in these studies certainly made such an approach difficult. In fact, some authors even noted significant intra-familial phenotypic variation, which is suggestive of the contribution of factors other than the strict *ABCC6* allelic background. The development and severity of the PXE phenotype seem to be determined by a number of other unknown factors. One may speculate that these factors could be environmental such as nutrition, hormones, lifestyle, environmental factors, or even medical history. PXE-like symptoms have been associated with several other clinical disorders such as certain cases of chronic renal failure, long-term use of penicilamine or even dermal contact with dry saltpeter [Nielsen et al. 1978; Bolognia and Braverman 1992; Coatesworth et al. 1998]. Although, in these cases the lesions described were reminiscent of PXE, they appeared circumstantial as no sign of systemic PXE was reported. In contrast, the complete clinical spectrum of PXE (dermal, ocular and vascular) that has been associated with hemoglobinopathies such as beta-thalassemia appears to occur independently of *ABCC6* mutations [Hamlin et al. 2003]. This fact clearly supports the notion that the pathomechanism that leads to elastic fiber calcification is open to epigenetic influences. Although, no other obvious loci have been implicated in the development of the PXE phenotype [Struk et al. 1997; van Soest et al. 1997], various genetic determinants could alter the severity or the progression of the disease. For example, PXE seems to affect more female than male but the exact reason is unknown. Also, the metabolic pathway that stems from the loss of ABCC6 function and leads to elastic fiber calcification is certainly complex involving multiple intervening steps. Some of the steps could be genetically determined, such as the synthesis and availability of ABCC6 substrates and the transport capacity for these metabolites by similar transporters. Since ABC transporters are ubiquitous in the body, several may display overlapping functions. The loss of ABCC6 function may in part be partially compensated for by other transporters. Therefore, based on current data, the likelihood that any direct correlation would emerge between the type and position of a mutation in *ABCC6* and the clinical symptoms and/or the severity of the phenotype is low.

PXE AND BETA-GLOBIN DISEASES

The striking increase in beta-thalassemia patient survival over the past decade has focused attention on metabolic abnormalities deriving from consequences of this hemoglobinopathy. In recent years, the development of clinical and histopathologic manifestations of elastic tissue defects resembling inherited PXE has been reported in patients with beta-thalassemia, sickle cell disease, and sickle thalassemia [Aessopos et al. 1989;

Aessopos et al. 1992; Aessopos et al. 1997; Aessopos et al. 1998]. In a recent study involving beta-thalassemia patients of age 30 and older, Aessopos and co-workers (2002) showed that 20% of the affected subjects displayed skin lesions and 85% revealed one or more of the three typical dermal, cardiovascular or ocular PXE manifestations [Aessopos et al. 2002]. The clinical manifestations of PXE are particularly frequent in cases with thalassemia intermedia, due to the higher survival rate of these patients [Aessopos et al. 2002]. The similarities between the PXE-like syndrome associated with beta-thalassemia and inherited PXE are striking. Indeed, the clinical phenotype consists of all skin, ocular, and vascular manifestations with variable severity. The symptoms are age-dependent but with a later onset, generally after the second decade of life. Moreover, a recent study demonstrated that the skin lesions were structurally indistinguishable from inherited PXE as demonstrated by light and electron microscopy. Furthermore, these lesions were accompanied by identical extracellular matrix changes [Baccarani-Contri et al. 2001]. These results suggest that a common pathomechanism for elastic fiber defects between inherited PXE and beta-thalassemia exists and is most likely to be linked to ABCC6 activity. The PXE-like syndrome is, however, believed to be acquired rather than inherited [Aessopos et al. 2002; Hamlin et al. 2003] and may be related to the consequences of the primary disease i.e. the hemoglobinopathies. The high prevalence of acquired PXE symptoms in association with beta-thalassemia implicates elastic tissue injury as one of the main abnormalities associated with these diseases and the co-existence of the two phenotypes introduces a novel pathogenetic aspect of PXE and a new and an important research challenge.

ABCC6, A MRP FAMILY MEMBER

ABCC6/Abcc6 Transcriptional Regulation

Because *ABCC6* is constitutively expressed in a limited range of tissues [Beck et al. 2003; Kool et al. 1999], the transcriptional regulation of this gene appears tightly controlled. To date, there are only a handful of studies that have focused on the *ABCC6* promoter as a potential site for PXE mutations and to delineate its transcriptional regulation. The first report showed that the proximal promoter of the human *ABCC6* gene contains an activator sequence that is transcriptionally dependent on DNA-methylation, which may play a role in the tissue specificity [Aranyi et al. 2005]. More recently, Jiang et al. cloned about 2.6kb of the human *ABCC6* promoter but mostly focused their work on the proximal promoter region [Jiang et al. 2005]. The authors notably showed that the human *ABCC6* proximal promoter can be modulated by pro-inflammatory cytokines such as TGF-beta and that stimulating-protein 1 (Sp1) is a likely activator of *ABCC6* transcription. However, inflammation processes are not a major characteristic of PXE and the transcription factors that determine the tissue-specificity of ABCC6 were only partially defined. One of us (OLS) also explored the transcriptional regulation of the murine *Abcc6* gene. The choice of the mouse gene is explained by the small size and the well defined promoter region [Douet et al, 2006]. In this work, about 3.0 kb of the *Abcc6* gene promoter was cloned. The 5'-flanking region of the mouse *Abcc6* gene was found to contain a proximal TATA-less promoter requiring an intact CCAAT-box and Sp1 binding for its basal expression. We found a liver-specific *cis*-acting enhancer region located between -1.6kb and -2.9kb. Further analysis showed for the first time that the HNF4α and NF-E2 transcription factors are key regulators of *mAbcc6* gene expression both *in vitro* and *in vivo*, while HNF1α is not. These results are consistent with the tissue distribution of Abcc6 primarily found in liver and in kidneys as HNF4α is known to provide transcriptional signals essentially in liver and kidney while HNF1α promotes gene expression primarily in kidney, spleen and to a lower extent in liver. The identification of NF-E2 was quite surprising since this transcription factor is an essential regulatory element controlling the pathways of heme and globin synthesis. Based on these results, one could speculate that ABCC6/Abcc6 functional might be related to a detoxification function with respect to the hemoglobin metabolism or heme recycling in liver. This is particularly intriguing since there is a high incidence of PXE manifestations in Mediterranean patients with beta-thalassemia, sickle cell and sickle thalassemia. These diseases all derive from genetic lesions leading to an abnormal or reduced production of beta-globin while the PXE manifestations associated with the beta-thalassemias don't seem to derive from ABCC6 mutations [Hamlin et al. 2003]. Could the *ABCC6* expression be critically influenced by altered NF-E2 in beta-thalassemia patients? Ongoing studies should provide an answer to this question.

Tissue Distribution of ABCC6

The tissue distribution of rat and mouse Abcc6 and human ABCC6 has been studied by several investigators analyzing tissues for Abcc6/ABCC6 mRNA and protein content in rodents and humans. By northern blots analysis, rat Abcc6 mRNA was found to be predominantly expressed in the liver and to a lesser extent in kidney, small intestine, and colon. This study found Abcc6 protein predominantly localized to the basolateral membrane of hepatocytes in rat liver and the authors suggested that Abcc6 might fulfill a housekeeping transport function involved in the regulation of paracellular and/or transcellular solute movement from blood into bile [Madon et al. 2000].

Similarly, in mice, Abcc6 mRNA is most abundant in liver, with lesser amounts detected in kidney, small intestine and colon by RNase protection assay. Using sensitive *in situ* hybridization, we also detected murine Abcc6 mRNA in brain, retina, skin, trachea, myocardium, aorta, tongue and stomach in this study. Using a polyclonal antibody this broad tissue distribution was confirmed for the Abcc6 protein. The presence of Abcc6 in epithelial cell in a variety of murine tissues, in neurons, muscle cells and leukocytes suggested a complex multifunctional role for Abcc6 [Beck et al. 2003]. In contrast, the study by Gorgels et al. only detected Abcc6 protein in basolateral membranes of hepatocytes and proximal tubules epithelial cells, but not in eye, skin or blood vessels of the kidney in mice [Gorgels et al. 2005]. A recent study employed a nested RT-PCR strategy to address the significance of low level of *Abcc6* expression in murine tissues other than liver and kidney [Matsuzaki et al. 2005]. As previously shown [Beck et al. 2003], Abcc6 mRNA was found to be most abundant in liver and lower amounts were found in kidney and small intestine, whereas Abcc6 cDNA derived from total RNA of brain, stomach, tongue and eye was only detected after two rounds of 30 amplification cycles. In these tissues, the authors identified additional RT-PCR products representing aberrantly spliced Abcc6 mRNA species containing premature termination codons. Similar results were obtained from cultured human keratinocytes and skin fibroblasts.

The authors suggest that the low levels of expression found in these tissues may represent illegitimate transcription potentially leading to the synthesis of a non functional protein [Matsuzaki et al. 2005].

Human ABCC6 mRNA was found to be highly expressed in liver and kidney and to a low or very low extent in a few other tissues such as lung, duodenum, pancreas, and colon by RNase protection assay [Kool et al. 1999] and by RT-PCR in skin, retina, vessel wall, placenta and leukocytes [Bergen et al. 2000; Le Saux et al. 2000; Hu et al. 2003]. Using *in situ* hybridization we confirmed this ubiquitous distribution of ABCC6 mRNA in humans. We detected the ABCC6 protein in numerous human tissues such as liver, kidney, colon, pancreas, lung, brain, and stomach, where we found a strikingly strong immunostaining for ABCC6 in enteroendocrine G cells [Beck et al. 2005b]. Another study however, reported considerable immunostaining for human ABCC6 only in the liver and kidney, and could not detect any ABCC6 protein in other tissues examined [Scheffer et al. 2002].

To assess a possible role for ABCC6 in multidrug resistance, the (over)expression of ABCC6 was analyzed in a panel of resistant human cell lines. ABCC6 overexpression in these cell lines was found to be invariably associated with amplification of the adjacent ABCC1 gene suggesting that ABCC6 does not contribute to the multidrug resistance of the cell lines analyzed [Kool et al. 1999].

Taken together, these studies demonstrate high expression levels for ABCC6/Abcc6 in liver in humans and rodents followed by lower expression levels in kidney and intestines [Kool et al. 1999; Madon et al. 2000; Beck et al. 2003; Matsuzaki et al. 2005]. Whereas some reports found very low level of expression in other tissues such as skin, eye, blood vessels, lung and stomach [Kool et al. 1999; Bergen et al. 2000; Le Saux et al. 2000; Beck et al. 2003; Beck et al. 2005b], others failed to detect ABCC6/Abcc6 protein in tissues other than liver and kidney [Scheffer et al. 2002; Gorgels et al. 2005]. Low expression levels of ABCC6/Abcc6 in tissues other than liver and kidney could represent illegitimate transcription as suggested by Matsuzaki et al. [Matsuzaki et al. 2005]. Alternatively, transport active ABCC6/Abcc6 could indeed be present in low amounts in various cell types and tissues fulfilling a complex multifunctional role [Beck et al. 2003].

The ABCC6 Protein

Human ABCC6 mRNA endcodes a 1503 amino acid polypeptide. Within the MRP family, ABCC6 has the highest similarity to ABCC1 with 45% amino acid identity. Based on this similarity, ABCC6 is predicted to have a similar structure as ABCC1 characterized by the presence of the extra N-terminal extension with five transmembrane spanning segments (TMD0) connected by a cytoplasmic linker (L0) to a Pgp-like core consisting of two transmembrane domains (TMD1, TMD2) with 6 transmembrane segments each and two nucleotide binding folds (NBF1, NBF2) located in the cytoplasm. The extracellular sequences have two putative glycosylation sites [Borst et al. 1999].

Rat Abcc6 was found to be localized at the lateral and, to a lesser extent, at the canalicular plasma membrane of hepatocytes in the liver [Madon et al. 2000], whereas human ABCC6 appears to be located exclusively at the basolateral cell membrane in hepatocytes and proximal tubule epithelial cells in the kidney [Scheffer et al. 2002]. When expressed by retroviral transduction in polarized mammalian (MDCKII) cells, human ABCC6 was also found to be exclusively localized to the basolateral membrane and was glycosylated at Asn15, which is located in the extracellular N-terminal region [Sinko et al. 2003].

ATP Dependant Trans-membrane Transport of Model Substrates by ABCC6 in vitro

The physiological substrate of ABCC6 is unknown to date, but a few molecules were found to be actively transported in vesicular studies. Transport studies in vesicles isolated from Sf9 cells expressing rat Abcc6 identified the anionic cyclopentapeptide and endothelin receptor antagonist BQ-123 as an Abcc6 substrate [Madon et al. 2000]. ATP binding and hydrolysis by rat Abcc6 has been demonstrated in a yeast expression system [Cai et al. 2002].

Using isolated membranes from Sf9 cells expressing human ABCC6 Ilias et al. demonstrated ATP binding and ATP-dependent active transport of the glutathione conjugates leukotriene C_4 and N-ethylmaleimide S-glutathione and of the cyclopentapeptide BQ-123. Probenecid, benzbromarone and indomethacin specifically inhibited transport of N-ethylmaleimide S-glutathione. Three missense mutant forms of ABCC6 previously identified in PXE patients showed abolished transport activity for the tested model substrates suggesting a direct link between the loss of ABCC6 transport activity and the development of the PXE phenotype [Ilias et al. 2002]. Another study confirmed ATP-dependent transport of BQ123 and leukotriene C_4 by human ABCC6 and identified S-(2, 4-dinitrophenyl)glutathione as *in vitro* substrate suggesting a possible function as glutathione conjugate pump for ABCC6. Analysis of the drug sensitivity of ABCC6-transfected cells revealed low levels of resistance to several natural product agents, including etoposide, teniposide, doxorubicin, and daunorubicin indicating that ABCC6 is able to confer low levels of resistance to certain anticancer agents [Belinsky et al. 2002].

In vitro cultured human dermal fibroblasts from normal and PXE subjects have been analyzed for their ability to accumulate and release fluorescent clacein. The authors claim that calcein accumulation was significantly higher and calcein release was significantly slower in fibroblasts from PXE patients compared to control fibroblasts suggesting ABCC6 dependent calcein export. Verapamil, benzbromarone and indomethacin interfered with the extrusion of calcein from *in vitro* cultured human skin fibroblasts [Boraldi et al. 2003].

Active transporters of the ABCC subfamily preferentially transport anionic compounds such as glutathione and other organic anion conjugates and have therefore been suggested to help protect their host against toxic compounds. However, active MRP transporters, such as ABCC6, that are located at the basolateral side of renal and hepatic epithelial cells would pump drugs into the body, rather than into bile or urine for disposal [Borst et al. 1999]. The elucidation of genuine physiological transport substrate(s) of ABCC6 and its biological function will be an important step in determining how the loss of ABCC6 function leads to the development of the phenotype observed in PXE patients.

HOW DOES LOSS OF ABCC6 FUNCTION LEAD TO THE PXE PHENOTYPE?

Since the discovery of the PXE gene, the most intriguing question has been how ABCC6 deficiency leads to the phenotype observed in PXE patients. Is the connective tissue in PXE patients directly affected by a loss of ABCC6 transport function in extracellular matrix (ECM) producing cells? If this were the case, compounds locally extruded by ABCC6 into the ECM could directly or indirectly ensure the correct assembly of elastic fibers and/or be necessary for the maintenance of elastic fiber integrity over time. In an initial attempt to address this question, we analyzed Abcc6 expression levels and tissue distribution in embryonic murine development. However, Abcc6 was not found in all tissues synthesizing tropoelastin, nor could we detect any increase of Abcc6 expression levels associated with increased elastin production at these early developmental stages suggesting that the presence of Abcc6 in elastin depositing tissues may not be necessary to ensure proper elastic fiber deposition [Beck et al. 2005a].

The predominant expression of ABCC6 in liver and kidney is the basis of an alternative hypothesis proposing that PXE is a primary metabolic rather than a primary connective tissues disease. It was suggested that in the absence of functional ABCC6 certain metabolic compounds may accumulate resulting in the progressive calcification of elastic fibers, which would also explain the delayed onset of the clinical manifestations and the progressive nature of the calcification process [Uitto et al. 2001].

A handful of divergent approaches based on mouse models and *in vitro* studies aim specifically at gathering clues about the obscure and most likely indirect processes resulting from the absence of ABCC6 function in unspecified tissues and ultimately affecting elastic fibers.

In vitro Cellular Studies towards Understanding ABCC6 Function

To address the question, if ABCC6 deficiency in PXE patients could induce a persistent imbalance in circulating metabolite(s), which may impair the synthetic abilities of normal elastoblasts or specifically alter elastic fiber assembly, we have compared the deposition of elastic fiber proteins in cultures of fibroblasts derived from PXE and unaffected individuals. We found that PXE fibroblasts cultured with normal human serum deposited structurally normal elastic fibers. When maintained in the presence of serum from PXE patients however, normal and PXE fibroblasts as well as normal smooth muscle cells deposited abnormal aggregates of elastic fibers indicating that certain metabolites present in PXE sera interfered with the normal assembly of elastic fibers *in vitro*. Our study supports the hypothesis that PXE is a primary metabolic disorder with secondary connective tissue manifestations [Le Saux et al. 2006]. Serum fetuin-A, an inhibitor of calcification, has recently been shown to be present at lower concentrations in the serum of PXE patients compared to unaffected family members and control subjects [Hendig et al. 2006]. Could fetuin-A be one of the metabolites altered in PXE serum leading to progressive mineralization of elastic fibers in PXE?

Since certain hemolytic disorders result in similar clinical and histopathological damage as seen in PXE patients, Pasquali-Ronchetti and coworkers hypothesized that PXE lesions may result from chronic oxidative stress in PXE cells as a consequence of ABCC6 deficiency. Such mild oxidative stress due to the imbalance between production and degradation of oxidant species was suggested to result from the loss of mitochondrial membrane potential with overproduction of H_2O_2 in PXE dermal fibroblasts compared to fibroblasts from patients undergoing surgical treatment for breast cancer [Pasquali-Ronchetti et al. 2006]. In another study, iron accumulation resulting from hemolysis, increased iron absorption and multiple blood transfusions was suspected to lead to acquire elastic tissue defects in patients with hemolytic disorders. Normal human skin fibroblasts cultured in the presence of low iron concentrations induced a significant increase in the synthesis of tropoelastin and deposition of insoluble elastin, whereas higher iron concentrations inducing intracellular reactive oxygen species production no longer stimulated elastogenesis. These results suggest that extreme fluctuations in intracellular iron levels may result in impaired elastic fiber production [Bunda et al. 2005].

The Abcc6 -/- Mouse Develops a PXE like Phenotype

Using conventional gene targeting two laboratories have generated Abcc6 deficient mice (Abcc6-/-) that develop a phenotype that shares calcification of elastic fibers and other features with human PXE pathology making this animal model a useful tool to further investigate the etiology of PXE [Klement et al. 2005; Gorgels et al. 2005].

The Abcc6-/- mice created by the group of Dr. Uitto present with aberrant mineralization of soft tissues in organs affected by PXE in humans. Complete necropsies revealed profound mineralization of the skin, arterial blood vessels, and retina. Electron microscopy revealed mineralization affecting both elastic structures and collagen fibers. Mineralization of vibrissae was noted as early as 5 weeks of age and was progressive with age in Abcc6-/- mice [Klement et al. 2005].

Abcc6-/- mice created in Dr. Bergen's laboratory also spontaneously developed calcification of elastic fibers in blood vessel walls and in the Bruch's membrane in the eye, whereas, no clear abnormalities were seen in the dermal extracellular matrix. Calcification of blood vessels was most prominent in small arteries in the cortex of the kidney, but in old mice, it occurred also in other organs and in the aorta and vena cava. Abcc6-/- mice developed a 25% reduction in plasma HDL cholesterol. No changes in serum mineral balance were found [Gorgels et al. 2005].

CONCLUSION

ABCC6 as several other ABC transporters of the same family are thought to actively export metabolites from the basolateral or apical sides of polarized cells [Madon et al. 2000; Beck et al. 2003]. ABCC6 is particularly abundant in renal proximal tubules and hepatocytes and is also present in numerous epithelial cell types [Beck et al. 2005b]. Remarkably, non-polarized cells such as arterial SMC, dermal fibroblasts, and other connective tissue cells capable of elastic fiber synthesis, present moderate or low levels of ABCC6 expression [Beck et al. 2005b]. The basic functions of these cells seem to be affected by ABCC6 deficiency and could be responsible for the major phenotypic changes observed in PXE. However, the endogenous substrates of ABCC6 are presently not known and the exact pathomechanism underlying the PXE phenotype is only a matter of speculation. And this is where most research groups now tend to focus their attention. What caused the extensive phenotypical heterogeneity? What is the tissue basis for PXE and what is the exact relationship between ABCC6 and elastic fibers? These are (arguably) the principal questions needing answer.

Hopefully, the study of the connection between PXE and the beta-thalassemias and the availability of two mouse models of PXE will provide vital clues that will help us understand the function of ABCC6 and ultimately will define the complex pathophysiology of this disease.

REFERENCES

Aessopos, A., Farmakis, D. & Loukopoulos, D. (2002). Elastic tissue abnormalities resembling pseudoxanthoma elasticum in beta thalassemia and the sickling syndromes. *Blood*, 99, 30-35.

Aessopos, A., Samarkos, M., Voskaridou, E., Papaioannou, D., Tsironi, M., Kavouklis, E., Vaiopoulos, G., Stamatelos, G. & Loukopoulos, D. (1998). Arterial calcifications in beta-thalassemia. *Angiology*, 49, 137-143.

Aessopos A, Farmakis D, Karagiorga M, Rombos I, Loucopoulos D (1997) Pseudoxanthoma elasticum lesions and cardiac complications as contributing factors for strokes in beta-thalassemia patients. *Stroke* 28:2421-2424.

Aessopos, A., Savvides, P., Stamatelos, G., Rombos, I., Tassiopoulos, T., Karagiorga, M., Kaklamanis, P. & Fessas, P. (1992). Pseudoxanthoma elasticum-like skin lesions and angioid streaks in beta- thalassemia. *Am J Hematol*, 41, 159-164.

Aessopos, A., Stamatelos, G., Savvides, P., Rombos, I., Tassiopoulos, T. & Kaklamanis, P. (1989). Pseudoxanthoma elasticum and angioid streaks in two cases of beta-thalassaemia. *Clin Rheumatol*, 8, 522-527.

Altman, L.K., Fialkow, P.J., Parker, F. & Sagebiel, R.W. (1974). Pseudoxanthoma elasticum. An underdiagnosed genetically heterogeneous disorder with protean manifestations. *Arch Intern Med*, 134, 1048-1054.

Aranyi, T., Ratajewski, M., Bardoczy, V., Pulaski, L., Bors, A., Tordai, A. & Varadi, A, (2005). Identification of a DNA methylation-dependent activator sequence in the pseudoxanthoma elasticum gene, ABCC6. *J Biol Chem*, 280, 18643-18650.

Baccarani-Contri, M,, Bacchelli, B., Boraldi, F., Quaglino, D., Taparelli, F., Carnevali, E., Francomano, M.A., Seidenari, S., Bettoli, V., De Sanctis, V. & Pasquali-Ronchetti, I. (2001). Characterization of pseudoxanthoma elasticum-like lesions in the skin of patients with beta-thalassemia. *J Am Acad Dermatol*, 44, 33-39.

Bacchelli, B., Quaglino, D., Gheduzzi, D., Taparelli, F., Boraldi, F., Trolli, B., Le Saux, O., Boyd, C.D. & Ronchetti IP (1999). Identification of heterozygote carriers in families with a recessive form of pseudoxanthoma elasticum (PXE). *Mod Pathol*, 12, 1112-1123.

Balzer, F. (1884). Recherches sur les caractères anatomiques du xanthelasma. *Arch Physiol* (Serie 3), 4, 65-80.

Beck, K., Dang, K. & Boyd, C.D. (2005a). The tissue distribution of murine Abcc6 (Mrp6) during embryogenesis indicates that the presence of Abcc6 in elastic tissues is not required for elastic fiber assembly. *J Mol Histol,* 36, 167-170.

Beck, K., Hayashi, K., Dang, K., Hayashi, M. & Boyd, C.D. (2005b). Analysis of ABCC6 (MRP6) in normal human tissues. *Histochem Cell Biol,* 123, 517-528.

Beck, K., Hayashi, K., Nishiguchi, B., Le Saux, O., Hayashi, M. & Boyd, C.D. (2003). The Distribution of Abcc6 in Normal Mouse Tissues Suggests Multiple Functions for this ABC Transporter. *J Histochem Cytochem,* 51, 887-902.

Belinsky, M.G., Chen, Z.S., Shchaveleva, I., Zeng, H. & Kruh, G.D. (2002). Characterization of the drug resistance and transport properties of multidrug resistance protein 6 (MRP6, ABCC6). *Cancer Res,* 62, 6172-6177.

Bergen, A.A. (2006). Pseudoxanthoma elasticum: the end of the autosomal dominant segregation myth. *J Invest Dermatol,* 126, 704-705.

Bergen, A.A., Plomp, A.S., Schuurman, E.J., Terry, S., Breuning, M., Dauwerse, H., Swart, J., Kool, M., van Soest, S., Baas, F., ten Brink, J.B. & de Jong, P.T. (2000). Mutations in ABCC6 cause pseudoxanthoma elasticum. *Nat Genet,* 25, 228-231.

Berlyne, G.M., Bulmer, M.G. & Platt, R.L. (1961). The genetics of pseudoxanthoma elasticum. *Quart J Med,* 30, 201-212.

Bertulezzi, G., Paris, R., Moroni, M., Porta, C., Nastasi, G. & Amadeo, A. (1998). Atrial septal aneurysm in a patient with pseudoxanthoma elasticum. Acta Cardiol, 53, 223-225.

Bolognia, J.L. & Braverman, I. (1992). Pseudoxanthoma-elasticum-like skin changes induced by penicillamine. *Dermatology,* 184, 12-18.

Boraldi, F., Quaglino, D., Croce, M.A., Garcia Fernandez, M.I., Tiozzo, R., Gheduzzi, D., Bacchelli, B. & Pasquali Ronchetti, I. (2003). Multidrug resistance protein-6 (MRP6) in human dermal fibroblasts. Comparison between cells from normal subjects and from Pseudoxanthoma elasticum patients. *Matrix Biol,* 22, 491-500.

Borst, P., Evers, R., Kool, M. & Wijnholds, J. (1999). The multidrug resistance protein family. *Biochim Biophys Acta,* 1461, 347-357.

Bunda, S., Kaviani, N. & Hinek, A. (2005). Fluctuations of intracellular iron modulate elastin production. *J Biol Chem,* 280, 2341-2351.

Cai, J., Daoud, R., Alqawi, O., Georges, E., Pelletier, J. & Gros, P. (2002). Nucleotide binding and nucleotide hydrolysis properties of the ABC transporter MRP6 (ABCC6). *Biochemistry,* 41, 8058-8067.

Cai, L., Lumsden, A., Guenther, U.P., Neldner, S.A., Zach, S., Knoblauch, H., Ramesar, R., Hohl, D., Callen, D.F., Neldner, K.H., Lindpaintner, K., Richards, R.I. & Struk, B. (2001). A novel Q378X mutation exists in the transmembrane transporter protein ABCC6 and its pseudogene: implications for mutation analysis in pseudoxanthoma elasticum. *J Mol Med,* 79, 536-546.

Cai, L., Struk, B., Adams, M.D., Ji, W., Haaf, T., Kang, H.L., Dho, S.H., Xu, X., Ringpfeil, F., Nancarrow, J., Zach, S., Schaen, L., Stumm, M., Niu, T., Chung, J., Lunze, K., Verrecchia, B., Goldsmith, L.A., Viljoen, D., Figuera, L. E., Fuchs, W., Lebwohl, M., Uitto, J., Richards, R., Hohl, D. & Ramesar, R. (2000). A 500-kb region on chromosome 16p13.1 contains the pseudoxanthoma elasticum locus: high-resolution mapping and genomic structure. *J Mol Med,* 78, 36-46.

Chassaing, N., Martin, L., Calvas, P., Le Bert, M. & Hovnanian, A. (2005). Pseudoxanthoma elasticum: a clinical, pathophysiological and genetic update including 11 novel ABCC6 mutations. *J Med Genet,* 42, 881-892.

Chassaing, N., Martin, L., Mazereeuw, J., Barrie, L., Nizard, S., Bonafe, J.L., Calvas, P, & Hovnanian, A. (2004). Novel ABCC6 mutations in pseudoxanthoma elasticum. *J Invest Dermatol,* 122, 608-613.

Chauffard, M.A. (1889). Xanthélasma disséminé et symétrique et sans insuffisance hépatique. *Bull Soc Med Paris (*Ser 3), 6, 412-419.

Christiano, A.M., Lebwohl, M.G., Boyd, C.D. & Uitto, J. (1992). Workshop on pseudoxanthoma elasticum: molecular biology and pathology of the elastic fibers. Jefferson Medical College, Philadelphia, Pennsylvania, June 10, 1992. *J Invest Dermatol,* 99, 660-663.

Christiano, A.M. & Uitto, J. (1994). Molecular pathology of the elastic fibers. J Invest Dermatol, 103, 53S-57S.

Coatesworth, A.P., Darnton, S.J., Green, R.M., Cayton, R.M. & Antonakopoulos, G.N. (1998). A case of systemic pseudo-pseudoxanthoma elasticum with diverse symptomatology caused by long-term penicillamine use. *J Clin Pathol,* 51, 169-171.

Darier, J. (1896). Pseudo-xanthome élastique. III ème congrès Intern de Dermat de Londres, 289-295.

De Paepe, A., Viljoen, D., Matton, M., Beighton, P., Lenaerts, V., Vossaert, K., De Bie, S., Voet, D., De Laey, J.J. & Kint, A. (1991). Pseudoxanthoma elasticum: similar autosomal recessive subtype in Belgian and Afrikaner families. *Am J Med Genet,* 38, 16-20.

Douet V., VanWart C.M., Heller M.B., Reinhard S. and Le Saux O. (2006). HNF4α and NF-E2 are key transcriptional regulators of the murine *Abcc6* gene expression. *Biochimica et Biophysica Acta,* 1759: 426-436.

Doyne (1889). Chorioidal and retinal changes the result of blows on the eye. *Trans. Ophthalmol. Soc.* UK, 9, 128.

Eddy, D.D. & Farber, E.M. (1962). Pseudoxathoam elasticum. Internal manifestatons: a report of cases and a review of the literature. Arch Dermatol, 86, 729-740.

Fülöp, K., Ilias, A., Sinkó, E., Homolya, L., Sarkadi, B. & Váradi, A. (2006). Analysis of missense PXE-mutants of ABCC6/MRP6. ATP-binding cassette (ABC) proteins: from multidrug resistance to genetic diseases FEBS special meeting, Innsbruck, Austria.

Germain, D.P. (2001). Pseudoxanthoma elasticum: evidence for the existence of a pseudogene highly homologous to the ABCC6 gene. *J Med Genet,* 38, 457-461.

Gheduzzi, D., Guidetti, R., Anzivino, C., Tarugi, P., Di Leo, E., Quaglino, D. & Ronchetti, I.P. (2004). ABCC6 mutations in Italian families affected by pseudoxanthoma elasticum (PXE). *Hum Mutat,* 24, 438-439.

Gheduzzi, D., Sammarco, R., Quaglino, D., Bercovitch, L., Terry, S., Taylor, W. & Ronchetti, I.P. (2003). Extracutaneous ultrastructural alterations in pseudoxanthoma elasticum. *Ultrastruct Pathol,* 27, 375-384.

Gorgels, T.G., Hu, X., Scheffer, G.L., van der Wal, A.C., Toonstra, J., de Jong, P.T., van Kuppevelt, T.H., Levelt, C.N., de Wolf, A., Loves, W.J., Scheper, R.J., Peek, R. & Bergen, A.A. (2005). Disruption of Abcc6 in the mouse: novel insight in the pathogenesis of pseudoxanthoma elasticum. *Hum Mol Genet,* 14, 1763-1773.

Groenblad, E. (1929). Angioid streaks: pseudoxanthoma elasticum: vorloeufige mitteilung. *Acta Ophthalmol* (Copenh), 7, 329.

Hamlin, N., Beck, K., Bacchelli, B., Cianciulli, P., Pasquali-Ronchetti, I. & Le Saux, O. (2003). Acquired Pseudoxanthoma elasticum-like syndrome in beta-thalassaemia patients. *Br J Haematol,* 122, 852-854.

Hausser, I. & Anton-Lamprecht, I. (1991). Early preclinical diagnosis of dominant pseudoxanthoma elasticum by specific ultrastructural changes of dermal elastic and collagen tissue in a family at risk. *Hum Genet,* 87, 693-700.

Hendig, D., Schulz, V., Arndt, M., Szliska, C., Kleesiek, K. & Gotting, C. (2006). Role of Serum Fetuin-A, a Major Inhibitor of Systemic Calcification, in Pseudoxanthoma Elasticum. *Clin Chem,* 52(2), 227-234.

Hendig, D., Schulz, V., Eichgrun, J., Szliska, C., Gotting, C. & Kleesiek, K. (2005). New ABCC6 gene mutations in German pseudoxanthoma elasticum patients. *J Mol Med,* 83, 140-147.

Hu, X., Plomp, A., Wijnholds, J., Ten Brink, J., van Soest, S., van den Born, L.I., Leys, A., Peek, R., de Jong, P.T. & Bergen, A.A. (2003). ABCC6/MRP6 mutations: further insight into the molecular pathology of pseudoxanthoma elasticum. *Eur J Hum Genet,* 11, 215-224.

Ilias, A., Urban, Z., Seidl, T.L., Le Saux, O., Sinko, E., Boyd, C.D., Sarkadi, B. & Varadi, A. (2002). Loss of ATP-dependent transport activity in pseudoxanthoma elasticum-associated mutants of human ABCC6 (MRP6*). J Biol Chem,* 277, 16860-16867.

Jiang, Q., Matsuzaki, Y., Li, K. & Uitto, J. (2005). Transcriptional Regulation and Characterization of the Promoter Region of the Human ABCC6 Gene. *J Invest Dermatol,* 126(2), 325-335.

Katona, E., Aslanidis, C., Remenyik, E., Csikos, M., Karpati, S., Paragh, G. & Schmitz, G. (2005). Identification of a novel deletion in the ABCC6 gene leading to Pseudoxanthoma elasticum. *J Dermatol Sci,* 40, 115-121.

Klein, I., Sarkadi, B. & Varadi, A. (1999). An inventory of the human ABC proteins. *Biochim Biophys Acta,* 1461, 237-262.

Klement, J.F., Matsuzaki, Y., Jiang, Q.J., Terlizzi, J., Choi, H.Y., Fujimoto, N., Li, K., Pulkkinen, L., Birk, D.E., Sundberg, J.P. Uitto, J. (2005). Targeted ablation of the abcc6 gene results in ectopic mineralization of connective tissues. *Mol Cell Biol,* 25, 8299-8310.

Kool, M., van der Linden, M., de Haas, M., Baas, F. & Borst, P. (1999). Expression of human MRP6, a homologue of the multidrug resistance protein gene MRP1, in tissues and cancer cells. *Cancer Res,* 59, 175-182.

Knapp, H. (1892). On the formation of dark angioid streaksas an unusual metamorphosis of retinal hemorrhage. *Arch Ophthalmol,* 21, 289-292.

Langness, U., Kreysel, H.W., Thiel, H.J., Paetzold, O.H. & Lerche, W. (1974). [Clinical and genetic aspects of the Darier-Gronblad-Strandberg syndrome (author's transl)]. *Med Klin,* 69, 1229-1234.

Le Saux, O., Bunda, S., Vanwart, C.M., Douet, V., Got, L., Martin, L. & Hinek, A. (2006). Serum Factors from Pseudoxanthoma Elasticum Patients Alter Elastic Fiber Formation In Vitro. *J Invest Dermatol,* 126(7), 1497-1505.

Le Saux, O., Beck, K., Sachsinger, C., Treiber, C., Goring, H.H.H., Curry, K., Johnson, E.W., Bercovitch, L., Marais, A.S., Terry, S.F., Viljoen, D.L. & Boyd, C.D. (2002). Evidence for a founder effect for pseudoxanthoma elasticum in the Afrikaner population of South Africa. *Hum Genet,* 111, 331-338.

Le Saux, O., Beck, K., Sachsinger, C., Silvestri, C., Treiber, C., Goring, H.H.H., Johnson, E.W., De Paepe, A., Pope, F.M., Pasquali-Ronchetti, I., Bercovitch, L., Marais, A.S., Viljoen, D.L., Terry, S.F. & Boyd, C.D. (2001). A spectrum of ABCC6 mutations is responsible for pseudoxanthoma elasticum. *Am J Hum Genet*, 69, 749-764.

Le Saux, O., Urban, Z., Tschuch, C., Csiszar, K., Bacchelli, B., Quaglino, D., Pasquali-Ronchetti, I., Pope, F.M., Richards, A., Terry, S., Bercovitch, L., de Paepe, A. & Boyd, C.D. (2000). Mutations in a gene encoding an ABC transporter cause pseudoxanthoma elasticum. *Nat Genet*, 25, 223-227.

Lebwohl, M., Neldner, K., Pope, F.M., De Paepe, A., Christiano, A.M., Boyd, C.D., Uitto, J. & McKusick, V.A. (1994). Classification of pseudoxanthoma elasticum: report of a consensus conference. *J Am Acad Dermatol*, 30, 103-107.

Lebwohl, M., Halperin, J. & Phelps, R.G. (1993). Brief report: occult pseudoxanthoma elasticum in patients with premature cardiovascular disease. *N Engl J Med*, 329, 1237-1239.

Madon, J., Hagenbuch, B., Landmann, L., Meier, P.J. & Stieger, B. (2000). Transport function and hepatocellular localization of mrp6 in rat liver. Mol Pharmacol, 57, 634-641.

Matsuzaki, Y., Nakano, A., Jiang, Q.J., Pulkkinen, L. & Uitto, J. (2005). Tissue-specific expression of the ABCC6 gene. *J Invest Dermatol*, 125, 900-905.

Meloni, I., Rubegni, P., De Aloe, G., Bruttini, M., Pianigiani, E., Cusano, R., Seri, M., Mondillo, S., Federico, A., Bardelli, A.M., Andreassi, L., Fimiani, M. & Renieri, A. (2001). Pseudoxanthoma elasticum: Point mutations in the ABCC6 gene and a large deletion including also ABCC1 and MYH11. *Hum Mutat*, 18, 85.

Miksch, S., Lumsden, A., Guenther, U.P., Foernzler, D., Christen-Zach, S., Daugherty, C., Ramesar, R.K., Lebwohl, M., Hohl, D., Neldner, K.H., Lindpaintner, K., Richards, R.I. & Struk, B. (2005). Molecular genetics of pseudoxanthoma elasticum: type and frequency of mutations in ABCC6. *Hum Mutat*, 26, 235-248.

Neldner, K.H. (1988). Pseudoxanthoma elasticum. *Int J Dermatol*, 27, 98-100.

Nielsen, A.O., Christensen, O.B., Hentzer, B., Johnson, E. & Kobayasi, T. (1978). Salpeter-induced dermal changes electron-microscopically indistinguishable from pseudoxanthoma elasticum. *Acta Derm Venereol*, 58, 323-327.

Nishida, H., Endo, M., Koyanagi, H., Ichihara, T., Takao, A. & Maruyama, M. (1990). Coronary artery bypass in a 15-year-old girl with pseudoxanthoma elasticum. *Ann Thorac Surg*, 49, 483-485.

Noji, Y., Inazu, A., Higashikata, T., Nohara, A., Kawashiri, M.A., Yu, W., Todo, Y., Nozue, T., Uno, Y., Hifumi, S. & Mabuchi, H. (2004). Identification of two novel missense mutations (p.R1221C and p.R1357W) in the ABCC6 (MRP6) gene in a Japanese patient with pseudoxanthoma elasticum (PXE). *Intern Med*, 43, 1171-1176.

Pasquali-Ronchetti, I., Garcia-Fernandez, M.I., Boraldi, F., Quaglino, D., Gheduzzi, D., De Vincenzi Paolinelli, C., Tiozzo, R., Bergamini, S., Ceccarelli, D. & Muscatello, U. (2006). Oxidative stress in fibroblasts from patients with pseudoxanthoma elasticum: possible role in the pathogenesis of clinical manifestations. *J Pathol*, 208, 54-61.

Plomp, A.S., Hu, X., de Jong, P.T. & Bergen, A.A. (2004). Does autosomal dominant pseudoxanthoma elasticum exist? *Am J Med Genet A*, 126, 403-412.

Pope, F.M. (1974). Two types of autosomal recessive pseudoxanthoma elasticum. *Arch Dermatol*, 110, 209-212.

Pope, F.M. (1975). Historical evidence for the genetic heterogeneity of pseudoxanthoma elasticum. *Br J Dermatol,* 92, 493-509.

Pulkkinen, L., Nakano, A., Ringpfeil, F, & Uitto, J. (2001). Identification of ABCC6 pseudogenes on human chromosome 16p: implications for mutation detection in pseudoxanthoma elasticum. *Hum Genet,* 109, 356-65.

Raybould, M.C., Birley, A.J., Moss, C., Hulten, M. & McKeown, C.M. (1994). Exclusion of an elastin gene (ELN) mutation as the cause of pseudoxanthoma elasticum (PXE) in one family. *Clin Genet,* 45, 48-51.

Rigal, D. (1881). Observation pour servir à l'histoire de la chéloide diffuse xanthélasmique. *Ann Dermatol Syphilol,* 2, 491-501.

Ringpfeil, F., McGuigan, K., Fuchsel, L., Kozic, H., Larralde, M., Lebwohl, M. & Uitto, J. (2006). Pseudoxanthoma elasticum is a recessive disease characterized by compound heterozygosity. *J Invest Dermatol,* 126, 782-786.

Ringpfeil, F., Nakano, A., Uitto, J. & Pulkkinen, L. (2001). Compound heterozygosity for a recurrent 16.5-kb Alu-mediated deletion mutation and single-base-pair substitutions in the ABCC6 gene results in pseudoxanthoma elasticum. *Am J Hum Genet,* 68, 642-52.

Ringpfeil, F., Lebwohl, M.G., Christiano, A.M. & Uitto, J. (2000). Pseudoxanthoma elasticum: mutations in the MRP6 gene encoding a transmembrane ATP-binding cassette (ABC) transporter. *Proc Natl Acad Sci* U S A, 97, 6001-6006.

Ross, R., Fialkow, P.J. & Altman, L.K. (1978). Fine structure alterations of elastic fibers in pseudoxanthoma elasticum. *Clin Genet,* 13, 213-223.

Rubegni, P., Mondillo, S., De Aloe, G., Agricola, E., Bardelli, A.M. & Fimiani, M. (2000). Mitral valve prolapse in healthy relatives of patients with familial Pseudoxanthoma elasticum. *Am J Cardiol,* 85, 1268-1271.

Scheffer, G,L., Hu, X., Pijnenborg, A.C., Wijnholds, J., Bergen, A.A. & Scheper, R.J. (2002). MRP6 (ABCC6) detection in normal human tissues and tumors. *Lab Invest,* 82, 515-518.

Sinko, E., Ilias, A., Ujhelly, O., Homolya, L., Scheffer, G.L., Bergen, A.A., Sarkadi, B. & Varadi, A. (2003). Subcellular localization and N-glycosylation of human ABCC6, expressed in MDCKII cells. *Biochem Biophys Res Commun,* 308, 263-269.

Stefkova, J., Poledne, R. & Hubacek, J.A. (2004). ATP-binding cassette (ABC) transporters in human metabolism and diseases. *Physiol Res,* 53, 235-243.

Struk, B., Cai, L., Zach, S., Ji, W., Chung, J., Lumsden, A., Stumm, M., Huber, M., Schaen, L., Kim, C.A., Goldsmith, L.A., Viljoen, D., Figuera, L.E., Fuchs, W., Munier, F., Ramesar, R., Hohl, D., Richards, R., Neldner, K.H. & Lindpaintner, K. (2000). Mutations of the gene encoding the transmembrane transporter protein ABC-C6 cause pseudoxanthoma elasticum. *J Mol Med,* 78, 282-286.

Struk, B., Neldner, K.H., Rao, V.S., St Jean, P. & Lindpaintner, K. (1997). Mapping of both autosomal recessive and dominant variants of pseudoxanthoma elasticum to chromosome 16p13.1. *Hum Mol Genet,* 6, 1823-1828.

Stutz, S.B., Schnyder, U.W. & Vogel, A. (1985). [Clinical aspects and genetics of pseudoxanthoma elasticum]. *Hautarzt,* 36, 265-268.

Trip M.D., Smulders Y.M., Wegman J.J., Hu X., Boer J.M., ten Brink J.B., Zwinderman A.H., Kastelein J.J., Feskens E.J., Bergen A.A. (2002). Frequent mutation in the ABCC6 gene (R1141X) is associated with a strong increase in the prevalence of coronary artery disease. *Circulation,* 106(7):773-775.

Truter, S., Rosenbaum-Fiedler, J., Sapadin, A. & Lebwohl, M. (1996). Calcification of elastic fibers in pseudoxanthoma elasticum. *Mt Sinai J Med,* 63, 210-215.

Uitto, J., Pulkkinen, L. & Ringpfeil, F. (2001). Molecular genetics of pseudoxanthoma elasticum: a metabolic disorder at the environment-genome interface? *Trends Mol Med,* 7, 13-17.

Uitto, J., Boyd, C.D., Lebwohl, M.G., Moshell, A.N., Rosenbloom, J. & Terry, S. (1998). International Centennial Meeting on Pseudoxanthoma Elasticum: progress in PXE research. *J Invest Dermatol,* 110, 840-842.

Uitto, J. & Shamban, A. (1987). Heritable skin diseases with molecular defects in collagen or elastin. *Dermatol Clin,* 5, 63-84.

van Soest, S., Swart, J., Tijmes, N., Sandkuijl, L.A., Rommers, J. & Bergen, A.A. (1997). A locus for autosomal recessive pseudoxanthoma elasticum, with penetrance of vascular symptoms in carriers, maps to chromosome 16p13.1. *Genome Res,* 7, 830-834.

von Tannehain, E.G. (1901). Zur Kenntnis des Pseudoxanthoma elasticum (Darier). *Wien Klin Wochenschr,* 14, 1038-1041.

Viljoen, D. (1988). Pseudoxanthoma elasticum (Gronblad-Strandberg syndrome). *J Med Genet,* 25, 488-490.

Viljoen, D.L., Beatty, S. & Beighton, P. (1987). The obstetric and gynaecological implications of pseudoxanthoma elasticum. *Br J Obstet Gynaecol,* 94, 884-888.

Weenink, A.C., Dijkman, G. & de Meijer, P.H. (1996). Pseudoxanthoma elasticum and its complications: two case reports. *Neth J Med,* 49, 24-29.

Werther, (1904). über pseudoxanthoma elasticum. *Arch Dermatol Syph,* 69, 23-36.

Yoshida, S., Honda, M., Yoshida, A., Nakao, S., Goto, Y., Nakamura, T., Fujisawa, K. & Ishibashi, T. (2005). Novel mutation in ABCC6 gene in a Japanese pedigree with pseudoxanthoma elasticum and retinitis pigmentosa. *Eye,* 19, 215-217.

In: Multidrug Resistance-Associated Proteins
Editor: Christopher V. Aiello, pp. 211-236

ISBN 1-60021-298-0
© 2007 Nova Science Publishers, Inc.

Chapter 9

An Herbal Medicine, Inchinkoto, Enhances Multidrug Resistance-Associated Protein 2-Mediated Choleresis Development of New Pharmacotherapeutic Strategies for Cholestatic Liver Diseases

Junichi Shoda,[1] Masahiro Yamamoto,[2] Hirotoshi Utsunomiya,[3] Koji Oda[4] and Hiroshi Suzuki[5]

[1]Department of Gastroenterology, Institute of Clinical Medicine, The University of Tsukuba Graduate School of Comprehensive Human Sciences, Ibaraki, Japan
[2]Kampo and Pharmacognosy Laboratory, Central Research Laboratories, Tsumura & Co., Ibaraki, Japan
[3]Department of Pathology, Wakayama Medical College, Wakayama, Japan
[4]Division of Surgical Oncology, Department of Surgery, Nagoya University Graduate School of Medicine, Aichi, Japan
[5]Department of Pharmacy, The University of Tokyo Hospital, Faculty of Medicine, The University of Tokyo, Tokyo, Japan.

ABSTRACT

Plants contain abundant bioactive materials. A Kampo (Chinese/Japanese herbal) medicine, Inchinkoto (ICKT), and its ingredients exert potent choleretic effects by a "bile acid-independent" mechanism. However, details underlying the choleresis have not been fully clarified. The ATP-dependent, apical conjugate export pump, termed multidrug resistance-associated protein 2 (Mrp2; Abcc2), is the major driving force for bile acid-independent bile flow. Therefore, the experiments were designed to determine whether ICKT or its ingredients potentiate Mrp2-mediated choleresis *in vivo*. Biliary secretion of Mrp2 substrates and protein mass, subcellular localization, and the steady-state messenger RNA (mRNA) level of Mrp2 were assessed in rat liver after an infusion of genipin, an intestinal bacterial metabolite of geniposide that is a major ingredient of ICKT. The function of Mrp2 was also assessed by the ATP-dependent uptake of Mrp2-specific substrates using canalicular membrane vesicles (CMVs) from the liver. Infusion of genipin rapidly increased bile flow and biliary secretion of bilirubin conjugates and reduced glutathione, but did not increase bile acid secretion. The ATP-dependent uptake of Mrp2 substrates was significantly stimulated in the CMVs from the liver. These effects were not observed in Eisai hyperbilirubinemic rats (Mrp2-deficient rats). Under these conditions, genipin treatment increased the protein mass of Mrp2 in the CMVs but not the mRNA level. In immunoelectron-microscopic studies, a significant increase in Mrp2 density in the canalicular membrane was observed in the genipin-treated liver when compared to the vehicle-treated liver. Genipin, a major active ingredient in ICKT, may enhance the bile acid-independent secretory capacity of hepatocytes, mainly by an Mrp2-mediated mechanism through stimulation of exocytosis and insertion of the transporter protein into canalicular membranes. Therefore, ICKT may be a potent therapeutic agent for a number of cholestatic liver diseases.

INTRODUCTION

Kampo medicine is a Japanese traditional medicine that was developed from traditional herbal medicine originating in ancient China [1]. In Japan, a number of Kampo medicines are now manufactured on a modern industrial scale, whereby the quality and quantity of ingredients are standardized under strict, scientific quality controls.

One such medicine, Inchinkoto (ICKT), has been recognized as a "magic bullet" for the treatment of jaundice and has long been used in Japan and China as a choleretic and hepatoprotective agent for various types of liver diseases. ICKT consists of a mixture of three medicinal herbs: *Artemisia capillaris* Spica, Gardenia Fructus and Rei Rhizoma. Several major ingredients responsible for the beneficial effect of orally administered ICKT and its mechanisms of action have been identified. Genupin, which is an intestinal metabolite of geniposide (a major ingredient of Gardenia Fructus), has been demonstrated to have potent choleretic [2] and hepatoprotective effects [3]. The choleretic effect results in increased bilirubin and reduced glutathione (GSH) secretion into the bile, which in turn exerts subsequent bile acid-independent bile formation. The hepatoprotective effect is related to the potent antiapoptotic action of genipin, mediated via interference with apoptotic signaling pathways in mitochondria [4]. 6,7-Dimethylesculetin, a major ingredient of *Artemisia capillaris* Spica, increases the expression of various components (sinusoidal and canalicular organic anion transporters, carrier proteins and a conjugating enzyme) involved in bilirubin metabolic pathways through activation of constitutive androstane receptor (CAR) signaling [5].

Although no well-controlled clinical studies have been conducted, experimental investigations [3,4,6,7] and several case reports demonstrating possible beneficial effects of ICKT in severe liver disorders, many of which are currently untreatable, encourage future research to establish its effectiveness in the treatment of cholestatic liver diseases.

CHOLESTASIS AND MULTIDRUG RESISTANCE-ASSOCIATED PROTEINS

Cholestasis is defined as failure of normal amount of bile to reach the duodenum. This leads to hepatic and systemic accumulation of potentially toxic biliary constituents such as bilirubin and bile acids, resulting in liver damage and jaundice [8]. Cholestasis results from diverse etiologies, including genetic and acquired forms of cholestatic diseases. Acquired cholestasis can be divided into hepatocellular or obstructive in origin. The former type includes disorders such as primary biliary cirrhosis, cholestasis secondary to sepsis (endotoxic shock), drug-induced cholestasis, pregnancy- or total parenteral nutrition-induced cholestasis. The latter type includes cholestasis because of pancreatobiliary disorders such as stones or carcinomas. These cholestatic disorders are commonly associated with defective function of transport systems involved in the biliary excretion of those solutes that are identified to be primary driving forces for bile formation.

Hepatic uptake and secretion of bile acids and non-bile acid organic anions are mediated by specific transporter proteins at the basolateral and canalicular membranes of hepatocytes and cholangiocytes (Figure 1) [9,10]. Multidrug resistance-associated protein 2 (Mrp2; Abcc2) functions as a multispecific organic anion transporter of the hepatocellular canalicular membrane [11-15] and mediates the efflux of a wide variety of organic anions, including bilirubin glucuronides, glutathione (GSH), glutathione conjugates, and sulfated and glucuronidated bile acids [13,14,16]. Mrp2-dependent secretion of these solutes largely contributes to the bile acid-independent fraction of bile flow [17,18], which accounts for about half of the bile flow in rats [19,20]. Experimental cholestasis has been associated with impaired Mrp2-mediated transport [21,22] as well as down-regulation and altered localization of Mrp2 [8]. An impairment of Mrp2 function may lead to a reduction in bile acid-independent canalicular bile flow, since the biliary excretion of reduced GSH, an important determinant of bile acid-independent bile flow [23]. These findings provide the molecular basis for impairment of biliary secretion of a broad range of anionic conjugates and the development of jaundice in human subjects with cholestasis [18].

Obstructive cholestasis is one of the most important issues in the field of hepatobiliary surgery, since long-standing cholestasis causes hepatic fibrosis [24], which is associated with a deterioration of liver functions, and since hepatobiliary surgery is associated with high rates of postoperative mortality and morbidity [25,26]. It is postulated that hyperbilirubinemia may be due to, in part, to latent damage to the hepatic transport system of bile as a result of persistent bile duct obstruction. However, the underlying mechanisms by which bile duct obstruction impairs bile secretion, particularly in humans, are not fully understood, and methods to evaluate the function of bile secretion for cholestatic liver have not yet been established.

Moreover, it is likely that hepatic impairments associated with obstructive cholestasis is improved by a relief of biliary obstruction in animal experiments [24,27] and clinical studies [24,28,29]. Percutaneous transhepatic biliary drainage (PTBD) has been thought to be an effective method of reducing jaundice and also of lessening liver injury through toxic bile acid retention. Interest should be focused on the expression levels of canalicular membrane transporter proteins in the cholestatic liver of patients undergoing PTBD, since the transport of biliary constituents across the canalicular membrane is the rate-limiting step in bile formation and the impairment of canalicular transport systems should play a major role in the pathogenesis of cholestasis. The efficacy of PTBD, the decreasing rate of hyperbilirubinemia after drainage, may depend on the capability of the cholestatic liver to produce and secrete bile, which in turn depends on the expressions and functional activities of canalicular membrane transporters in the liver.

Hepatocytes

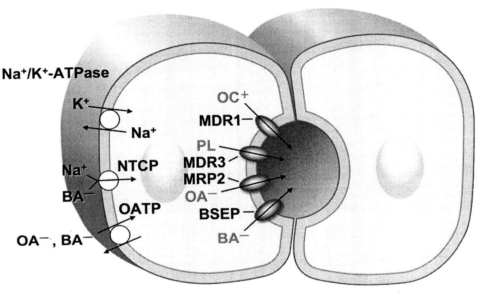

Figure 1. Sinusoidal and canalicular membrane transporters in rat hepatocytes. Na^+-dependent bile acid (BA) uptake at a sinusoidal membrane is mediated by NTCP and is driven by the electrochemical Na^+ gradient generated and maintained by the Na^+/K^+-ATPase. The Na^+-independent hepatic uptake of organic anions (OA^-) and BA is mediated by members of the OATP family. Transport across the canalicular membrane represents the rate-limiting step in the overall blood-to-bile transfer of most endogenous bile constituents and xenobiotics. It is driven mainly by ATP-dependent export pumps, which belong to the superfamily of the ATP-binding cassette (ABC) transporters. Several multidrug-resistance proteins (MDR) were identified in canalicular membranes. MDR1 mediates canalicular excretion of amphiphilic organic cations and other hydrophobic compounds, while MDR3 functions as a flippase, translocating phosphatidylcholine (PC) from the inner to the outer leaflet of this membrane domain, thus facilitating canalicular excretion of phospholipids. Canalicular excretion of BA is mediated by another ABC transporter, BSEP. Excretion of non-BA OA^-, such as bilirubin diglucuronides, as well as sulfated and glucuronidated BA, is mediated by MRP2.

In our previous paper of clinical study [30], the expression levels of the canalicular membrane transporters MRP2 and bile salt exporting pump (BSEP) for bilirubin conjugate and bile acid in the liver of patients with obstructive cholestasis who had undergone preoperative PTBD, and the results were correlated with the impairment of bile formation and secretion.

A total of 24 patients who had experienced obstructive cholestasis and had undergone preoperative PTBD were included in the study. These 24 patients were classified into two groups, a well-drained group (group I) and a poorly drained (group II) group, according to the efficacy of PTBD based on the degree of daily secretion of bilirubin and total bile acid in the drained bile. The "well-drained" patients were defined as those with bilirubin secretion of more than 200 mg/day and bile acid secretion increasing to over 5 mmoles/day during the drainage period, and the "poorly drained" patients as those with bilirubin secretion of less than 200 mg/day and bile acid secretion of less than 5 mmoles/day during the whole drainage period.

The steady-state mRNA levels of MRP2 and BSEP in the liver were determined by RT-PCR. Figure 2 shows the PCR-assisted amplifications of their mRNAs in the liver specimens from representative cases of control subjects, group I patients and group II patients. The mRNA levels of MRP2 and BSEP in the liver were preserved in 14 patients in group I but slightly decreased in 10 patients in group II compared to the levels in 18 control subjects. The protein levels of MRP2 in the cholestatic liver of patients undergoing PTBD were evaluated by immunoblot analysis using specific pAbs (Figure 3). The protein level of MRP2 was preserved in the liver specimens from the patients in group I but decreased in the specimens from the patients in group II.

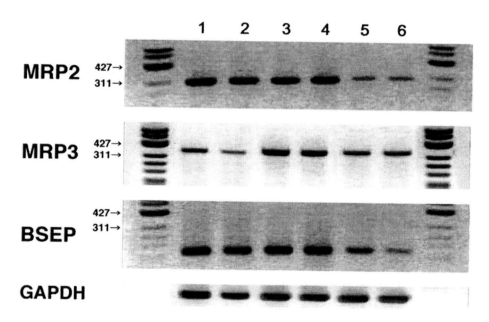

Figure 2. RT-PCR-assisted amplifications of MRP2, MRP3 and BSEP mRNAs in liver tissue specimens from control subjects, cholestatic patients well-drained by PTBD (patients in group I), and patients poorly drained by PTBD (patients in group II). *Lanes* 1 & 2, control subjects; *Lanes* 3 & 4, patients in group I; *Lanes* 5 & 6, patients in group II. The abundance of GAPDH mRNA was determined as an internal standard. The PCR products were 300 bp for MRP2, 357 bp for MRP3, 167 bp for BSEP, and 311 bp for GAPDH.

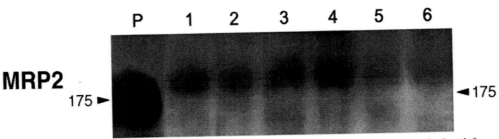

Figure 3. Immunoblot analysis of MRP2 in the crude plasma membrane fractions isolated from liver tissue specimens of control subjects, cholestatic patients well-drained by PTBD (patients in group I), and patients poorly drained by PTBD (patients in group II). *Lane* P, positive control; *Lanes* 1 & 2, control subjects; *Lanes* 3 & 4, patients in group I; *Lanes* 5 & 6, patients in group II.

The immunohistochemical expressions of MRP2 and BSEP were studied in the liver sections from control subjects and cholestatic patients undergoing PTBD, and the results are shown in Figure 4. In the immunofluorescence stainings of MRP2 and BSEP, their stainings outlined the canalicular membrane domain of the liver sections from both the control subjects and the patients in group I. The linear and intense staining pattern may correlate with the preserved mRNA and protein levels of MRP2 and also the preserved mRNA level of BSEP in their liver. However, in the liver sections from patients in group II, the stainings of MRP2 and BSEP disrupted a linear and intense localization in the canalicular membrane domain and appeared fuzzy, compared to the staining pattern in the liver sections from control subjects. These results may correlate with the decreased mRNA and protein levels of MRP2 and also the decreased mRNA level of BSEP in their liver. The diminished canalicular membrane localization of MRP2 and BSEP suggest their impaired function in the liver. The magnitude of these alterations was greater for the patients in group II than for those in group I.

The biological function [32,33] and histological localization of MRP3 [32,34] in the liver have been recently reported. Consistent with the findings in a recent study,18 the immunostaining of MRP3 was mostly observed in the epithelia of both intrahepatic bile ducts and proliferated bile ductules in the cholestatic liver sections. A proliferation of bile ductules due to obstructive cholestasis may explain the increased mRNA level of MRP3 in the liver. Since cholangiocytes, accounting for only 3-5% of the hepatocyte population, play an important role in determining the bile flow and pH of hepatic bile through absorption and/or secretory processes [35], the biological function of MRP3 in the biliary epithelia is of particular interest. Recently, Hirohashi et al. [36] reported that MRP3 mediates the uptake of mono- and divalent bile acids in an ATP-dependent manner, suggesting that MRP3 functions as an organic anion transporter for bile acid as well as bilirubin conjugates [33].

Based on the results, the mRNA levels of MRP2 and BSEP were preserved in the cholestatic liver of patients well-drained by PTBD but reduced in the liver of patients poorly drained. The immunostaining of MRP2 and BSEP represented a fuzzy canalicular membrane localization in the liver of patients poorly drained, in contrast to the linear and intense localization in the liver of control subjects and the diminished canalicular membrane localization of MRP2 and BSEP was associated with the impairment of biliary bilirubin and bile acid secretion.

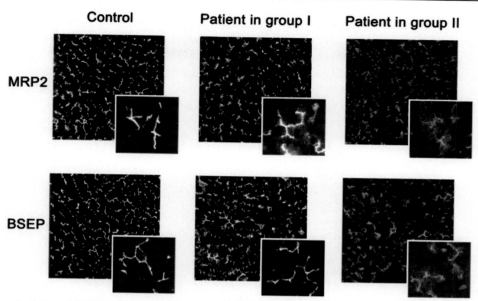

Figure 4. Immunofluorescence localization of MRP2 and BSEP in liver tissue sections. Liver specimens were obtained from a control subject, a cholestatic patient well-drained by PTBD (a patient in group I), and a patient poorly drained by PTBD (a patient in group II). The immunofluorescence stainings of MRP2 and BSEP outlined the canalicular membrane domain of the liver sections from the control subject and the well-drained patient. However, in the section from the poorly drained patient, the stainings disrupted a linear and intense localization in the canalicular membrane domain and appeared fuzzy. The magnitude of the alterations was greater in the patients in group II than in those in group I.

Other important findings in the study are that the mRNA levels of MRP3, an inducible transporter for organic anions such as bilirubin conjugate and bile acid, was increased in the liver of cholestatic patients (Figure 2), and the immunostaining was observed mostly in the epithelia of both intrahepatic bile ducts and proliferated bile ductules and, to a lesser extent, in the hepatocytes surrounding the portal tracts (Figure 5). MRP3 is initially referred to as MRP-like protein 2 and has been cloned from the liver of cMOAT/MRP2-deficient rats (EHBR) [31], since MRP3 acts as an inducible transporter to compensate for the reduced function of MRP2 and/or BSEP in the cholestatic liver and extrudes accumulated bile acids from the liver into blood. In addition, MRP3 may be involved in bilirubin conjugate and bile acid transport in cholangiocytes since MRP3 is extensively expressed on the lateral membrane of intrahepatic bile duct epithelia in the human liver [32].

It has been noticed that long-standing biliary obstruction and complication of cholangitis associated with biliary infection have a large influence on the hepatic secretory function of cholestatic patients through inflammation-related oxidative stress on the liver. In animals with LPS/cytokine-induced cholestasis, a rapid redistribution of canalicular membrane transporters, from the canalicular membrane to an intracellular subapical compartment, is observed in their liver [37,38]. This is quite similar to the immunohistochemical expressions of MRP2 and BSEP in the cholestatic liver poorly drained by PTBD. The greater impairment in the expression of canalicular transporters in the cholestatic liver of patients poorly drained may be causatively related to inflammatory processes in the hepatobiliary system (i.e., local cholangitis) rather than attributable to a secondary response to the long-standing injury by biliary obstruction. Not only a variation in the protein amount but also its subcellular translocation can lead to altered canalicular transport. It seems that in obstructive cholestasis, the expression levels of MRP2 and BSEP in the liver may be altered at both the gene transcription and the post-transcriptional levels, i.e., impaired intracellular sorting or targeting of the transporter proteins, impaired protein activation, and increased protein degradation [39].

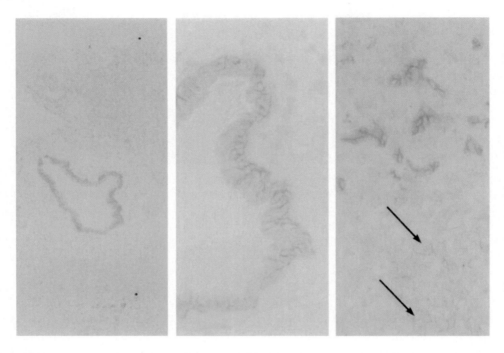

Figure 5. Immunohistochemical localization of MRP3 in liver tissue sections. Liver specimens were obtained from a control subject (left & middle) and a cholestatic patient well-drained by PTBD (right; a patient in group I). The immunostaining of MRP3 was found mostly in the epithelia of intrahepatic bile ducts (left: original magnification x 25), predominantly at the basolateral domain (middle: original magnification x 100), in the epithelia of the proliferated bile ductules (right: original magnification x 62), and, to a lesser extent, in the hepatocytes surrounding the portal tracts (right: original magnification x 62).

Moreover, in our recent paper [40], the association of impaired expression levels of hepatic MRP2 with posthepatectomy hyperbilirubinemia was investigated in patients with biliary tract carcinoma. Liver failure with severe hyperbilirubinemia develops in 8.7 to 32% of patients who have undergone extensive liver resection for biliary tract carcinoma [41-48]. The mortality rates of the patients who developed hyperbilirubinemia after major hepatectomy for such diseases are very high [49]. In fact, severe hyperbilirubinemia has been demonstrated to play a role in the development of postoperative septic complications leading to liver failure, by suppressing bacteriocidal activity of neutrophils [49] or by evoking bacterial translocation from the gut [50]. In the study, expression levels of MRP2 were determined in liver tissue specimens before hepatectomy from patients with biliary tract carcinoma in order to clarify whether chronic bile duct obstruction causes the down-regulation of hepatic MRP2 expression in humans and whether the MRP2 expression level before hepatectomy in the anticipated remnant liver is associated with the subsequent development of posthepatectomy hyperbilirubinemia.

To directly determine the effect of chronic bile duct obstruction on the hepatic MRP2 expression, the expression levels were compared between the cholestatic and noncholestatic lobes in 7 patients. The protein levels in the cholestatic lobes were 45% of those in the noncholestatic lobes, and the immunostaining of MRP2 in the cholestatic lobes was weak and not restricted to the bile canaliculi (Figure 6). For another 39 patients, the MRP2 expression was graded with the immunohistochemical staining as follows: grade I, strong and delineating the canalicular membrane; grade III, weak and fuzzy and frequent absent from the hepatocytes; and grade II, between grades I and III (Figure 7). Of six patients with grade-III MRP2 expression, three died of liver failure and three survived with (n=1) or without (n=3) liver failure. Of seven patients with grade-II MRP expression, one had developed severe hyperbilirubinemia. None of the patients with grade-I MRP2 expression developed severe hyperbilirubinemia or died. The correlation of the MRP2 expression in the anticipated remnant liver with the posthepatectomy severe hyperbilirubinemia was evaluated in these patients. The results have shown that postoperative maximum bilirubin levels were significantly correlated with the immunohistochemical expression levels of MRP2 in the anticipated remnant liver (Figure 8).

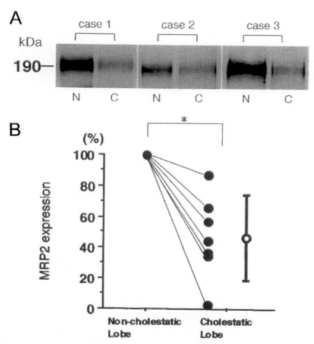

Figure 6. Immunoblot analysis of MRP2 in the noncholestatic and cholestatic lobes of patients with biliary tract carcinoma. a, The MRP2 protein levels are reduced in the cholestatic lobes (C), compared with the levels in the noncholestatic lobes (N). b, Densitometric analysis revealed that the MRP2 protein levels in the cholestatic lobes were 45% of that in the noncholestatic lobes (*$P<0.005$ by the Wilcoxon signed-ranks test). The MRP2 expression in the cholestatic lobe is presented as the percentage of that in the noncholestatic lobe set to 100%.

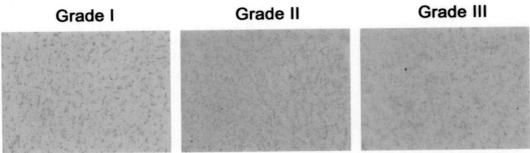

Figure 7. Grading and quantification of hepatic MRP2 expression. Immunohistochemical localization of canalicular MRP2 protein was graded. Grade I, strong labeling is restricted to the hepatocyte apical membrane delineating the bile canaliculi; grade II, intermediate between grades I and III; and grade III, the staining is weak, fuzzy and frequently absent among the hepatocytes.

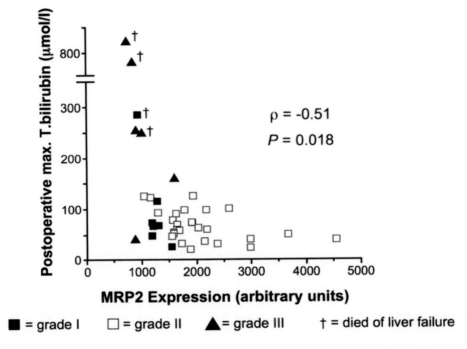

Figure 8. Clinical outcome of the study patients and correlation between canalicular MRP2 expression and postoperative maximum serum bilirubin. Each of the study patients (n = 39) was blotted by the quantified MRP2 expression and the postoperative maximum bilirubin level. *dagger*, died of liver failure; *open square*, MRP2 grade I; *closed square*, MRP2 grade II; *closed triangle*, MRP2 grade III. Postoperative maximum bilirubin levels were significantly correlated with MRP2 expression in the liver tissues taken before hepatectomy ($\rho = -0.51$, $P = 0.018$ by Spearman's rank correlation).

These findings of the study were in agreement with those of animal models with cholestasis [18,37,38,51-58]. The decreased canalicular localization of the protein was accompanied by the intracellular localization of the protein in pericanalicular vesicular structures, the findings suggesting endocytosis and translocation of the MRP2 protein [51]. The alteration in the MRP2 expression in patients with chronic biliary obstruction might be affected by the structural changes of the liver, such as hepatocyte swelling and tissue fibrosis, due to long-standing bile duct obstruction. In terms of clinical perspective, it is of clinical importance that patients with impaired MRP2 expression in the anticipated remnant liver have an increased risk for posthepatectomy severe hyperbilirubinemia. Considering that the presence of preoperative cholangitis is a risk factor for the development of posthepatectomy liver failure [42,55], it is plausible that the preoperative cholangitis may be causatively associated with the decrease in MRP2 expression in such patients in as much as endotoxin and inflammatory cytokines are known to diminish the levels of plasma membrane transporters [18,37,38,52,54].

Thus, cholestasis has been associated with impaired Mrp2-mediated transport [21,22] as well as down-regulation and altered localization of Mrp2 [18]. These findings provide the molecular basis for impairment of biliary secretion of a broad range of anionic conjugates and the development of jaundice in human subjects with cholestasis [18]. In cholestatic patients, a reduced expression of MRP2 can occur at the mRNA level to a lesser extent [30,56]. Importantly, intact MRP2 messenger RNA (mRNA) levels, despite reduced canalicular MRP2 immunostaining in severely cholestatic and jaundiced patients [30], suggest that the potential mechanisms for the regulation of MRP2 expression in cholestatic liver diseases in humans include not only changes in the rate of transcription but also posttranscriptional/posttranslational changes [30,37,51]. Decreased hepatic MRP2 expression, caused by biliary obstruction due to carcinoma, is a possible risk factor for posthepatectomy severe hyperbilirubinemia. Therefore, stimulation and restoration of defective expression and function of MRP2 in cholestasis may be an important target for specific pharmacotherapeutic interventions [57].

CHOLERETIC ACTIONS OF INCHINKOTO

In the medical treatment book "Shang han za bing lun: medical text by Zhang Zhong jing comprised of the Shang han lun and the Jin kui yao lue" written in China in the beginning of the 3rd century A.D., Inchinkoto (Yin-Chen-Hao-Tang in Chinese) had already been described as the effective drug for the treatment for jaundice. Modern phytochemistry has identified various choleretic compounds from Inchinkoto and its constituent herbs since the third decade of 20th century. Major ingredients, capirallisin and 6,7-dimethylescuretin from *Artemisia Capirallis* Spica and geniposide from Gardenia Fructus are among them. The choleretic effect of ICKT and its ingredients has been examined in the experimental animals since mid-1970s by several investigators in Japan. These studies have suggested that the choleretic effect of ICKT is largely bile-salt independent, and is contributed by multiple ingredients including capillarisin, 6,7-dimethylescuretin, and geniposide via distinct mechanisms. However, the detailed mechanisms by which ICKT and the ingredients exert the choleretic effect had not been clarified until recently. The advances in research of bile formation and hepatocellular transporters have opened a road to the understanding the mechanisms of action of the agents as described in the following paragraphs.

GENIPOSIDE/GENIPIN

Geniposide, a major ingredient of Gradenia Fructus, is an iridoid compound whose content is several [58] to 15 (unpublished observation) % of ICKT, and in the case of oral administration, geniposide is converted to its aglycone, genipin by intestinal bacteria (Figure 9). Takeda and colleagues have investigated the choleretic effect of genipin [59] and related iridoid compounds and their relationships between structures and choleretic actions [60] and demonstrated that the effect is mediated by bile-salt independent canalicular bile formation and that the hemiacetal moiety of iridoid compounds play an important role. Recently, Shoda and Yamamoto et al [61] have reported that the enhancement of the bile acid-independent bile formation by genipin is mediated by the rapid stimulation of exocytosis and insertion of multispecific organic anion transporter MRP2 (multidrug resistance-associated protein 2, Abcc2) into the bile canaliculi (Figure 10). Infusion of genipin rapidly increased bile flow by 230% and biliary secretion of bilirubin conjugates by 513% and reduced glutathione (GSH) by 336% which are transported mainly by Mrp2 (Figure 11). Excretion of bile acid did not change by genipin infusion (Figure 11). The kinetic analysis of canalicular membrane vesicles prepared from genipin-treated rat liver has elucidated the enhanced ATP-dependent transport of various Mrp2-specific substrates by about 200% (Figure 12) is due to the increased amount of Mrp2 in canalicular membrane (Figure 13). These effects of genipin were completely abrogated in Mrp2-defficient Eisai hyperbilirubinemic rats (Figure 12). The effect of genipin is rapid (within 30 min) and is not accompanied with the increase in Mrp2 mRNA and total amount of Mrp2 protein in whole cells (Figure 13); therefore, genipin is supposed to enhance the redistribution of Mrp2 into canalicular membrane. This assumption was supported by the immunohistochemical studies of Mrp2 on light and electron microscopy (Figures 14 and 15). Furthermore, in an *in vitro* experiment, to determine the effect of genipin on redistribution of Mrp2 to remaining apical domain, hepatocyte couplets were cultured for 1 hour in the presence or absence of 100 □M genipin. In the absence of genipin, Mrp2 was found to be localized throughout the cytosol with a preference for the region close to the plasma membrane and the remaining apical region (Figure 16). However, in the presence of genipin, a large concentration of probably vesicular Mrp2 was found to be localized at the cell-to-cell contact site, representing the apical pole, which in turn suggests that more Mrp2-containing vesicles are recruited to the apical domain and that a small apical vacuole is forming (Figure 16). The results indicate that genipin treatment stimulates a sorting and targeting of Mrp2 protein on the canalicular membrane in hepatocyte couplets.

However, many questions remains to be answered: a) what are the mechanisms underlying these changes in expression/localization? (e.g., alterations of the signaling balance, activation/inhibition of transcriptional factors, impairment of motor protein function, etc); b) can changes in expression/localization of canalicular membrane transporters be not only prevented but also reversed by factors counteracting these dysfunction? Satisfactory answers to these questions could allow the design of new therapeutic strategies in liver pathobiology involving secretory impairment.

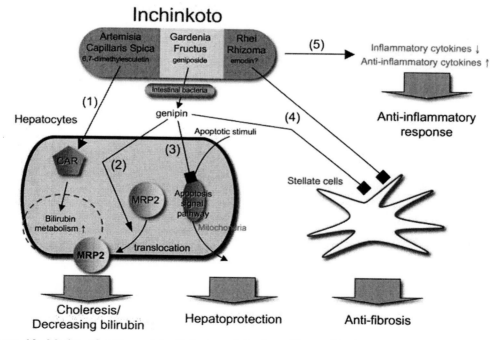

Figure 9. Structures of geniposide (left), genipin (middle), and genipin 1-*O*-β-*D*-glucuronide (right). A major ingredient of Inchinkoto (ICKT), geniposide, is converted to an active metabolite, genipin, by intestinal bacteria. Genipin is then transported to the liver via portal circulation and subject to conjugation (mainly with glucuronide). By thin-layer chromatographic (TLC) and/or high-performance liquid chromatographic (HPLC) analyses, about 20% of infused genipin was secreted into the bile as the main metabolite 1-*O*-β-*D*-glucuronide (unpublished observation). Unconjugated genipin was detected, but the amount was ca. 1/50 of that of genipin-1-*O*-β-*D*-glucuronide. The other unidentified metabolites detected in the bile were also in small amounts.

Figure 10. Modes of action of Inchinkoto and its ingredients. (1) 6,7-Dimethylescuretin activates bilirubin metabolism *via* a constitutive androstane receptor (CAR). (2) Genipin enhances translocation of multidrug transporter-associated protein 2 (MRP2) into the canalicular membrane. (3) Genipin interferes with mitochondrial apoptotic signal pathways. (4) Anthraquinones inhibit the activation of hepatic stellate cells. (5) Inchinkoto modulates cytokine responses *in vivo*.

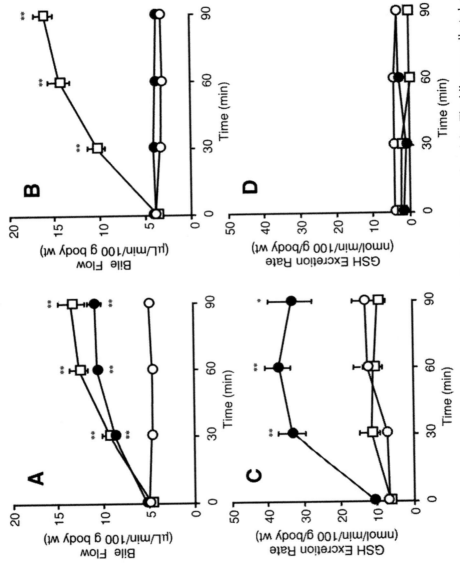

Figure 11. Bile flow (A & B) and rate of biliary secretion of GSH (C & D) after bolus infusion of genipin. The bile was collected over a 30-minute period before infusion in SDRs (A & C) and Mrp2-defective EHBRs (B & D), and the initial values of bile flow and rate of GSH secretion were calculated. The rats were continuously infused with a vehicle (O), genipin (●) or UDC (□). The choleretic activity and rate of GSH secretion were measured at 30 minute-intervals over a 90 minute-period. Data are given as means ± SEM (n = 6). **P<0.01, significantly different from the vehicle-treated group.

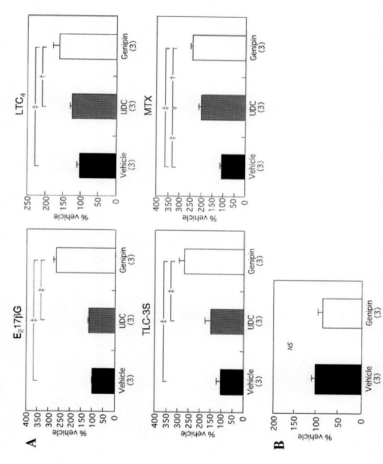

Figure 12. A: ATP-dependent uptake of Mrp2 substrates into canalicular membrane vesicles in SDRs. Livers were harvested 30 minutes after intravenous administration of vehicle, genipin or UDC. Canalicular membrane vesicles from vehicle-, UDC-, or genipin-treated SDR livers were incubated at 37°C for 2 minutes in a medium containing 100 nM [³H]E217βG, 100 nM [³H]LTC4, 100 nM [³H] TLC-3S, or 100 nM [³H] MTX in the presence and absence of ATP. ATP-dependent uptake of the ligands was calculated by subtracting the ligand uptake in the absence of ATP from that in the presence of ATP. Data are expressed as percentages of the values obtained in the vehicle- treated rats. Each column and vertical bar represents the mean ± SEM of triplicate determinations. †$P<0.05$, ‡$P<0.01$, significantly different from the two groups. B: ATP-dependent uptake of [³H]E217βG into canalicular membrane vesicles in EHBRs. Livers were harvested 30 minutes after intravenous administration of vehicle or genipin. Canalicular membrane vesicles from vehicle- or genipin-treated EHBR liver tissues were incubated at 37°C for 2 minutes in a medium containing 100 nM [³H]E217βG in the presence and absence of ATP.

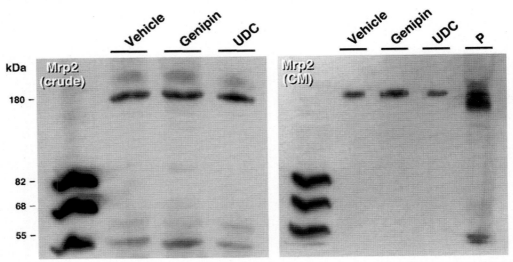

Figure 13. Immunoblot analysis of Mrp2 in crude plasma membrane (crude) fractions and canalicular membrane (CM) fractions isolated from livers of vehicle-, genipin-, and UDC-treated SDRs. Membrane-enriched fractions were prepared from rat livers 30 minutes after intravenous administration of vehicle, UDC or genipin. Immunoblotting was performed with 100 μg of crude plasma membrane fractions or with 2 μg of CM fractions, and the blots were probed with the pAb raised against Mrp2. P, positive control. The membrane vesicles from LLC-PK1 cells transfected with rat Mrp2 cDNA were used as a positive control for Mrp2.

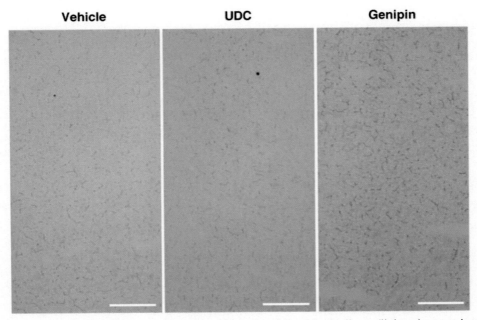

Figure 14. Immunohistochemical localizations of Mrp2 and Bsep in the livers (light-microscopic view). Liver sections were prepared from SDR livers 30 minutes after intravenous administration of vehicle, UDC or genipin. Mrp2 immunostaining shows a diffuse and linear pattern outlining the canalicular membrane domain of each liver section from vehicle-, UDC-, and genipin-treated rats. Bars, 100 μm. The immunostaining of Mrp2 was more intense and more diffuse in the bile canaliculi in genipin-treated livers compared to that in vehicle- and UDC-treated livers.